STRESS AND HEALTH:
NEW RESEARCH

STRESS AND HEALTH: NEW RESEARCH

KIMBERLY V. OXINGTON
EDITOR

Nova Biomedical Books
New York

Copyright © 2005 by Nova Science Publishers, Inc.

All rights reserved. No part of this book may be reproduced, stored in a retrieval system or transmitted in any form or by any means: electronic, electrostatic, magnetic, tape, mechanical photocopying, recording or otherwise without the written permission of the Publisher.

For permission to use material from this book please contact us:
Telephone 631-231-7269; Fax 631-231-8175
Web Site: http://www.novapublishers.com

NOTICE TO THE READER
The Publisher has taken reasonable care in the preparation of this book, but makes no expressed or implied warranty of any kind and assumes no responsibility for any errors or omissions. No liability is assumed for incidental or consequential damages in connection with or arising out of information contained in this book. The Publisher shall not be liable for any special, consequential, or exemplary damages resulting, in whole or in part, from the readers' use of, or reliance upon, this material.

This publication is designed to provide accurate and authoritative information with regard to the subject matter covered herein. It is sold with the clear understanding that the Publisher is not engaged in rendering legal or any other professional services. If legal or any other expert assistance is required, the services of a competent person should be sought. FROM A DECLARATION OF PARTICIPANTS JOINTLY ADOPTED BY A COMMITTEE OF THE AMERICAN BAR ASSOCIATION AND A COMMITTEE OF PUBLISHERS.

Library of Congress Cataloging-in-Publication Data

Stress and health : new research / Kimberly V. Oxington (editor).
    p. ; cm.
Includes bibliographical references and index.
ISBN 1-59454-244-9 (hardcover)
1. Stress (Physiology)
[DNLM: 1. Stress, Psychological--complications. 2. Stress, Psychological--physiopathology. 3. Behavioral Research. 4. Psychophysiologic Disorders--etiology. WM 172 S913204 2004] I. Oxington, Kimberly V.
QP82.2.S8S855   2004
616.9'8--dc22
    2004030809

Published by Nova Science Publishers, Inc. ✢ *New York*

CONTENTS

Preface		vii
Chapter I	Parental Stress and Child Behavioral Adjustment in Children with Congenital Heart Disease *Karen J. Visconti*	1
Chapter II	Stress, Cardiovascular Disease and Hypertension *Pedro Armario, Raquel Hernández del Rey, Pere Castellanos, Mari Cruz Almendros and Montserrat Martín-Baranera*	43
Chapter III	Of Stress, Mice and Men: A Radical Approach to Old Problems *Rubina Mian, Graeme McLaren and David W. Macdonald*	61
Chapter IV	Growth in Early Life is Associated with Stress Symptoms In Adults *Yin Bun Cheung*	81
Chapter V	Evaluating Parental Stress Experiences Following Preterm Birth *Rosalind Lau and Carol Morse*	103
Chapter VI	Cortisol Responses to Experimental Stress in Patients with Whiplash Associated Disorder *Mariëtte Blokhorst, Pinel Schrijver, Stefan Meeldijk, Rob Hermans, Richel Lousberg, Gerrit Zilvold*	125
Chapter VII	Cytokines in Behavioral Medicine Research: Importance for Psychological States of Stress, Depression and Fatigue and Health Outcomes *Shamini Jain and Paul J. Mills*	143
Chapter VIII	Effect of Stress on Male and Female Fertility: Literature Review *Naomi Schneid-Kofman and Eyal Sheiner*	173

Chapter IX	Brief Cognitive-Behavioral Couples Support Groups Developed to Manage the Stress of IVF Treatment *Mary Ellen McNaughton-Cassill, John Michael Bostwick, Nancy J. Arthur, Randal D. Robinson and Gregory S. Neal*	**187**
Chapter X	Psychological Adjustment of Short Interval Follow–Up Mammography- A French Study About 129 Patients *B. Barreau, S. Tastet, A. Hubert*	**203**
Index		**221**

PREFACE

Stress is a physical response to an undesirable situation. Mild stress can result from missing the bus, standing in a long line at the store or getting a parking ticket. Stress can also be severe. Divorce, family problems, an assault, or the death of a loved one, for example, can be devastating. One of the most common sources of both mild and severe stress is work. Stress can be short-term (acute) or long-term (chronic). Acute stress is a reaction to an immediate threat — either real or perceived. Chronic stress involves situations that aren't short-lived, such as relationship problems, workplace pressures, and financial or health worries. Stress is an unavoidable consequence of life. As Hans Selye (who coined the term as it is currently used) noted, "Without stress, there would be no life". However, just as distress can cause disease, it seems plausible that there are good stresses that promote wellness. Stress is not always necessarily harmful. Winning a race or an election can be just as stressful as losing, or more so, but may trigger very different biological responses. Increased stress results in increased productivity up to a point. This new book deals with the dazzling complexity of this good-bad phenomenon and presents up-to-date research from throughout the world.

The birth of a child can be stressful enough for many parents, but when the child is born with a medical complication, the experience can take on a whole new level of fear and anxiety. Congenital heart disease is the most common birth defect affecting children. Chapter I will provide a review of research on the behavioral and emotional adjustment of children with cardiac disorders as well as factors that may affect child adjustment, such as parental stress, family social support, child intelligence, and child language development.

As presented in Chapter II, psychosocial factors could be important determinants of cardiovascular disease. Anger, hostility, depression, anxiety and other personality factors and character traits have been related to an increased risk of cardiovascular disease. A high level of anger in response to stress is associated in young men with an increased risk of subsequent premature cardiovascular disease, especially myocardial infarction. The mechanisms by which stress causes vascular injury are not very well known, but some studies have demonstrated that mental stress induces endothelial dysfunction.

The tremendous destructive capabilities of reactive oxygen species in stress related disorders has become apparent only recently, although in early historical times the ancients may have been aware of the devastating power of stress on well-being. Chapter III explores ancient myths and modern techniques surrounding stress-induced immunosupression in species as diverse as mice and humans, investigating techniques and mechanisms, and speculating on possible therapeutic interventions.

In humans, concentrations of stress hormones in adults are related to birth weight. Furthermore, growth stunted children had higher levels of salivary cortisol concentrations and higher heart rates than non-stunted children. Studies have demonstrated that fetal and postnatal growth retardation has a negative impact on some aspects of psychological health in children and adolescents, but it is not known whether the impact is transient or not. In chapter IV, the author reports the findings from a cohort study of over 11,000 persons followed from birth to age 42. Chapter V presents a controlled prospective longitudinal study that was carried out to evaluate stress experiences of parents whose preterm infants were admitted to a special care nursery in a tertiary level maternity hospital. Findings revealed that parents of preterm infants reported higher subjective stress levels than parents of term infants within the first week of their infant's birth but returned lower objective markers of stress. Mothers of preterm infants were more anxious and stressed when compared to fathers of preterm infants.

As reported in Chapter VI, an experiment was carried out to explore cortisol levels and cortisol response as a result from a mental stress task, in patients with a Whiplash Associated Disorder (WAD) compared to healthy subjects and subjects in a relax-control condition. In addition, it was investigated whether the amount and appraisal of severity of daily hassles predicted cortisol response. As was expected, results revealed that WAD patients had significant higher cortisol levels in time. Although the differences were not significant, there seems to be a trend towards an increase in cortisol concentrations after performing a mental stress task in the experimental WAD group, compared to the healthy control group and relax control groups.

Cytokines are important immune transmitters that mediate effects of psychological states on disease processes and health outcomes. Cytokines have diverse effects not only on immune system function but also on the central nervous system and hypothalamic-pituitary axis activity, providing multiple routes for their actions. Alterations in cytokine levels have been identified in a number of disorders that are particularly important to stress and behavioral medicine research. The purpose of Chapter VII is to familiarize the behavioral medicine researcher with cytokines, providing descriptions of their classifications, functions, techniques of measurement and interactions with physiological systems relevant to stress and negative psychological states.

The review in Chapter VIII was aimed to determine the connection between psychological stress and both male and female infertility. Many cultures consider reproduction to be of great importance, an obligatory achievement expected of any established couple. Infertility therefore may result in stress to a couple trying to conceive. This couple will undoubtedly experience feelings of frustration and disappointment if a pregnancy is not easily achieved. Labeled as having a fertility problem may result in a severe insult to self-esteem, body image, and self assessed masculinity or femininity. Despite the fact that various studies have demonstrated the importance of the mind-body connection and fertility, the psychosocial aspects of infertility have not been adequately addressed. Chapter IX describes the development and evaluation of a brief, cognitive-behavioral group therapy approach offered to both members of a couple while they were undergoing in vitro fertilization. Couples who have difficulty conceiving a child frequently seek extensive, costly medical solutions to their infertility. Such treatments often involve the use of medication, surgery, and other high technology interventions and can involve the sharing of intimate personal details of one's sexual activities with medical personnel. Psychologically, infertility can be associated with the experience of stress, anxiety, and depression, and may result in relationship difficulties, and even divorce. Couples were recruited from an infertility center at a military hospital and either volunteered to participate in the groups and complete two sets of surveys, or to serve as controls by completing the two surveys but not attending the group sessions.

The objective of Chapter X is to investigate perceptions and perceived stress experience by women undergoing mammographic follow-up for probably benign lesions (registered category 3 according to Breast Imaging-Reporting And Data System of the American College of Radiology). Women report a good informative medical support and a right comprehension of the short follow-up mammography. They are reassured by the medical care, but the evaluation of the stress level is high, probably due to the uncertainty of the diagnosis.

In: Stress and Health: New Research
Editor: Kimberly V. Oxington, pp. 1-41
ISBN 1-59454-244-9
©2005 Nova Science Publishers, Inc.

Chapter I

PARENTAL STRESS AND CHILD BEHAVIORAL ADJUSTMENT IN CHILDREN WITH CONGENITAL HEART DISEASE

Karen J. Visconti
Department of Cardiac Surgery Children's Hospital Boston
Boston, Massachusetts

ABSTRACT

The birth of a child can be stressful enough for many parents, but when the child is born with a medical complication, the experience can take on a whole new level of fear and anxiety. Congenital heart disease is the most common birth defect affecting children. Advances in cardiovascular diagnostic and surgical techniques have reduced the mortality rate of these children. Concurrent with the increased survival rate, there is growing appreciation of the effects that a cardiac disorder may have on the emotional development of children and the impact the disease has on the family. Many parents seem to adjust successfully, but research has suggested that the anxiety of having a child with heart disease may affect the way they relate to the child and eventually compromise the social and emotional adjustment of the child. The following chapter will provide a review of research on the behavioral and emotional adjustment of children with cardiac disorders as well as factors that may affect child adjustment, such as parental stress, family social support, child intelligence, and child language development.

Findings from research conducted at Boston Children's Hospital will be presented and will demonstrate a favorable outcome for parents and children with transposition of the great arteries.

INTRODUCTION

About 1 in 100 live births, or about 1% of children born each year, make up the patient population requiring pediatric cardiology services in the United States (Fyler, 1992).

Researchers have become aware that pediatric heart surgery can affect the family (Goldberg, Morris, Simmons, Fowler & Levinson, 1990; Goldberg, Washington, Morris, Fischer-Fay, & Simmons, 1990). Many parents are able to cope with the demands of having a child with a cardiac disorder, but in some parents the anxiety of having a chronically ill child may affect the way they relate to their child (DeMaso, Campos, Wypij, Bertam, Lipshitz & Freed, 1991). For example, mothers of children with cardiac disorders have been reported to overprotect, to overindulge, and to limit the activities of their children (Glaser, Harrison & Lynn, 1964; Linde, Rasof, Dunn, & Rabb, 1966; Rozansky & Linde, 1971). As a result, restricted leisure-time activities and parental overprotectiveness may lead to poor psychological adjustment and low levels of social competence in children (Kramer, Awiszus, Sterzel, van Halteren, & Claben, 1989; Spurkland, Bjornstad, Lindberg, & Seem, 1993). The implication of the research noted above is that parenting stress and anxiety may compromise the social and emotional adjustment of children.

The following review of the literature provides a background of research that has been conducted on the behavioral and emotional adjustment of children, with a particular focus on children with cardiac disorders. Studies specifically investigating the incidence of behavioral and emotional adjustment of children with cardiac disorders are presented initially.

Further, in their quest to understand why children with cardiac disorders manifest behavior problems, investigators have examined factors that may affect child adjustment. Several of these areas will also be reviewed. First, studies examining the incidence of parental stress as well as the relation between stress and child behavior problems are presented. Next, studies that examine how social support is associated with parent perceptions of stress and child behavior are reviewed. In addition, studies examining the association between child intelligence and behavior problems are presented. Finally, studies examining the impact of language deficits in non-cardiac children are reviewed.

Behavioral and Emotional Adjustment of Children with Cardiac Disorders

Children with chronic health problems are 2.4 times more likely to have a behavior disorder than their healthy peers (Cadman, Boyle, Szatmari, & Offord, 1987). Congenital heart disease (CHD) is one of the most common birth defects, putting this group of children at risk for behavioral disturbances. Numerous studies have been conducted to examine the behavioral and emotional adjustment of children with CHD (DeMaso, Campis, Wypij, Bertam, Lipshitz & Freed, 1991; Linde, Rasof & Dunn, 1970; Goldberg, Morris, Simmons, Fowler & Levinson, 1990; Oates, Turnbull, Simpson & Cartmill, 1994; Utens et al., 1993). Researchers who have found behavioral disturbances in their samples of children with CHD have explored factors that may help to clarify their findings. Investigators have considered that the severity of the disease may influence the occurrence of behavior problems (Alden, Gilljam, & Gillberg, 1998; Brandhagen, Feldt, & Williams, 1991; DeMaso et al., 1990; Gupta, Giuffre, Crawford, & Waters, 1998). For instance, perhaps children who are sicker manifest greater disturbances. Based on the health of the child, limitations may be placed on his or her physical activities. Researchers have examined whether restricted physical ability in children may be related to behavioral adjustment (Spurkland, Bjornstad, Lindberg, & Seem, 1993; Bjornstad, Spurkland, & Lindberg, 1995). In addition, consideration has been given as to whether gender differences exist in the incidence of behavior problems in children with CHD (DeMaso et al., 1990; Spurkland et al., 1993).

To assess emotional adjustment, many studies have relied on the Achenbach Child Behavior Checklist (CBCL) (Achenbach, 1991). When this questionnaire was administered to parents and teachers of CHD children and healthy, non-surgical children, differences in perceptions of child behavior problems were found (Oates et al., 1994). Parents of the surgical children perceived a greater number of behavior problems than parents of healthy controls. This difference was particularly noted for internalizing behavior, suggesting that parents of CHD children viewed their children as more fearful and inhibited. However, unlike parents, teacher reports indicated no differences in behavior between the surgical and non-surgical children. Because a period of 4 to 8 years existed between the surgery and this study, it was believed that the majority of teachers were not aware of the cardiac status of the children and did not treat them differently from the healthy children. It was also believed that the differences were not the result of children behaving differently at home and at school, since differences were reported only by mothers of children with CHD and not by mothers of healthy children.

Three explanations have been put forth to explain the differences between parent and teacher ratings of behavior problems in CHD children. First, Oates et al. (1994) suggested that the differences may be the result of neurological impairment that occurred during repair. The increased prevalence of central nervous system (CNS) impairment in children with CHD has been reported by Silbert, Wolff, Mayer, Rosenthal and Nadas (1969). Central nervous system impairment may be subtle enough to be detected only by parents because they spend more time with their children. Second, parents may still harbor some of the anxiety resulting from having a child who underwent cardiac surgery and this may be shown by over-interpreting some of their children's behavior. Third, it might be that these children do act differently at home because they have learned that they can capitalize on their parents' concerns with behaviors that are of no advantage to them at school. For example, Linde (1982) reported that children have been known to use symptoms of fatigue to control their parents.

Reports of behavioral disturbances have been presented in studies of families from low socioeconomic backgrounds (Utens et al.,1993). Similar to the findings of Oates et al. (1994) noted above, Utens et al. (1993) also found a higher number of behavior problems in children with CHD compared to same-aged peers from a normative reference group. However, Utens et al. also reported that parents of a lower socioeconomic status (SES) rated their children as having more problem behaviors, especially on the internalizing scale, such as the anxious and depressed sub-scales, than did parents of higher SES groups. In the same study, a group of adolescents also completed the Youth Self-Report (YSR) (Achenbach, 1991). Like parent ratings of behavior, adolescents with CHD also reported more internalizing behavior problems than normative groups.

These results suggest that both parents' reports and children's self-reports of problem behaviors indicated unfavorable outcomes for children and adolescents with CHD. This is consistent with results found by Brandhagen, Feldt and Williams (1991) in their 25-year follow-up of 168 adults who, as children, underwent surgical repair of various types of CHD. These researchers found significant differences between CHD adults and standardized normative data used as the reference group. Thus, despite success in educational achievement and occupational level, adults with CHD reported high levels of distress.

Also using normative data as a comparison, Gupka, Giuffre, Crawford, and Waters (1998) reported that their group of CHD children as a whole was rated by mothers on the CBCL as having higher total problem behavior, internalizing, and anxiety scores. However, these researchers found that when they compared the children in their sample with cyanotic (less oxygen in the blood) forms of heart disease to those with acyanotic forms, group differences appeared on the delinquent scale, with the cyanotic group receiving higher scores. The incidence of delinquent behavior may appear surprising, since many studies have reported greater internalizing behavior. However, the incidence of conduct disorders, often viewed as an early form of delinquent behavior, has also been reported (Kong, Tay, Yip, & Chay, 1986).

Not all CHD patients report unfavorable outcomes. More positive self-report behavior has been presented by pediatric heart transplant recipients. In a study by Uzark et al. (1992), heart recipients completed questionnaires pertaining to self-concept, anxiety, and coping techniques. Compared to same-aged peers from the normative population, these patients did not differ significantly on measures of anxiety and self-concept. In terms of coping, heart transplant recipients were more likely than the normative population to cope by ventilating their feelings. Parents of these children completed the CBCL. Consistent with findings by Oates et al. (1994) and Utens et al. (1993), the heart recipient group exhibited significantly more behavioral problems, compared to the normative population, specifically on the Depression scale of the CBCL. Scores on the Depression scale were significantly related to increased patient anxiety and low self-concept. A significant inverse relation was found between ventilating feelings and behavior problems on the CBCL, suggesting that the ability to express feelings leads to better adaptation.

Additional favorable outcomes have been presented by Goldberg et al. (1997), who failed to find significant group differences on either the Total Problem Behavior or Internalizing scales of the CBCL in their sample of children with CHD, cystic fibrosis (CF) and healthy children. Interestingly, there was a higher proportion of children with CHD and CF, compared to healthy children, who scored in the deviant range (score >60) on the Internalizing scale.

To summarize, studies examining behavior problems in CHD children have reported a high incidence of behavioral disturbance, particularly in the area of internalizing behavior. The reason for this remains unclear and is further complicated by conflicting studies that fail to find group differences on behavior scales (Goldberg et al., 1997). Therefore, investigators have considered other factors in their research that may be associated with behavioral adjustment. Such factors include the severity of the cardiac condition, the physical capacity of the children, and gender differences.

Cardiac Severity

Congenital heart disease is composed of a spectrum of lesions that range in complexity. Researchers have considered whether children with more severe defects, and who may experience greater sickness, are subject to increased difficulties in adjustment. Gupta,

Giuffre, Crawford, & Waters (1998) reported that mothers who perceived their child's heart condition as "severe" compared to mothers who viewed their child's condition as "mild" reported higher internalizing behavior scores. Alden, Gilljam and Gillberg (1998) also found that the children in their study with the poorest heart function were at the greatest risk for developing psychiatric and behavioral problems compared to normative data. On the other hand, studies by DeMaso et al. (1990) and Brandhagen, Feldt, and Williams (1991) failed to find a relation between the severity of the cardiac lesion and later psychological distress. These discrepant results suggest that medical severity alone may not account for the incidence of behavioral disturbances.

Physical Capacity

In addition to cardiac severity, physical capacity, or physical fitness, has also been considered in understanding the behavioral disturbances of children with CHD. Spurkland et al. (1993) compared adolescents with severe congenital heart disease to those diagnosed with an atrial septal defect (ASD), who were considered to be physically fit. Additional support for the relation between cardiac severity and adjustment problems was provided. A higher frequency of psychiatric problems was found in the severe CHD group, mostly anxiety and depression, compared to the ASD group. In fact, the frequency of major psychiatric problems found in the ASD group was comparable to that found in the general population. When minor and moderate disturbances were taken into account, the ASD group also presented with more psychiatric problems than a normative reference group. The adolescents in the complex CHD group were less physically fit than the ASD group. A significant relation was found between psychosocial functioning and physical capacity, suggesting that the more reduced the physical capacity of the adolescent, the higher the risk for developing psychiatric disorders.

Gender Differences

In addition to cardiac severity and physical capacity, gender has also been considered in understanding the behavioral disturbances of children with CHD. There is, for example, a tendency for boys to be rated higher on externalizing behaviors (e.g., "fighting", "can't concentrate", "impulsive") and for girls to be rated higher on internalizing behavior items (e.g., "cries a lot", "too fearful or anxious", "shy or timid") (Achenbach et al., 1990; Achenbach, Hensley, Phares & Grayson, 1989). DeMaso et al. (1990) failed to find gender differences in their sample of children with CHD, but, in a study of adolescents, more females than males with complex CHD were reported to have psychiatric problems (Spurkland et al., 1993). Based on the relation that was found between psychiatric problems and physical capacity, Spurkland et al. speculated that poor psychosocial functioning in females may be the result of parents placing greater restrictions on physical activities and exercise on females than on males.

Parenting Stress

As previously noted, children with chronic health problems are at risk for behavioral disorders (Goldberg et al., 1997; Nolan & Pless, 1986). Research on children with CHD suggests that this is the case. Many studies have reported behavior problems, particularly internalizing behavior. These findings have prompted investigators to consider factors that may explain the reason for these disturbances. Although it appears that the risk for emotional disturbances is exacerbated by gender differences and by factors related to health problems, such as increased cardiac severity and reduced physical capacity, not all studies have found support for these associations (DeMaso et al., 1990). Thus, researchers have continued to explore other areas that may influence child behavior problems. Oates et al. (1994) speculated that parent reports of child behavior problems may be the result of parents still harboring some of the anxiety of having a child who underwent cardiac surgery. This may result in parents over-interpreting children's behavior. Investigators have considered this possibility by examining the impact of family variables, such as parenting stress, on child adjustment.

Medically compromised infants convey different cues to parents, making it difficult for parents to respond consistently and appropriately to their infants' needs (Goldberg, Washington, et al., 1990). For example, mothers of infants with CHD have reported difficulties in feeding (Lobo, 1992) and establishing social interactions with their infants (as cited in Goldberg et al., 1991). Difficulty coping with having a sick infant may lead to heightened stress, which in turn, may impair the quality of parent-infant interactions (Webster-Stratton, 1988) and affect later child adjustment (DeMaso et al., 1991). Researchers have examined the occurrence of stress in parents of children with medical conditions, such as CHD, as well as the impact stress has on child behavior (DeMaso et al., 1991; Goldberg, Morris et al., 1990; Uzark et al., 1992).

It is widely accepted that the birth of an infant is stressful in and of itself. The diagnosis of a heart defect can be expected to intensify this already stressful period for the parents (Goldberg, Morris, et al., 1990). The research suggests that this is the case. As part of a prospective, longitudinal study examining the impact of having an infant with CHD, Goldberg, Morris, et al. initially compared the responses on the Parenting Stress Index (PSI; Abidin, 1986) for parents of infants with cystic fibrosis (CF), parents of children with CHD and parents with healthy infants. It was predicted that the three groups would differ primarily in factors related to the child. The authors anticipated differences between the CF and the CHD groups in stress associated with child care, reasoning that, even though the CHD group requires medication and undergoes surgery, infants with CF require ongoing daily treatments of therapy. Group differences were found mainly on the Child domain scale with parents of ill infants reporting more stress. Specifically, parents of infants with CHD reported the highest amount of stress on the Acceptance, Mood, and Reinforcement to Parents subscales (e.g., "My child rarely does things that make me feel good.", "My child is not able to do as much as I expected."). High levels of stress on the Child Demandingness scale for parents of children with CF is consistent with the daily ongoing treatment required to maintain the health of these children. There were few differences on the Parent domain scale, however. Parents of ill infants reported more problems with depression and lowered sense of competence when compared to parents of healthy children (e.g., "Being a parent is harder than I thought it would be.").

A high incidence of stress in mothers of infants with CHD compared to mothers of non-cardiac infants is not uncommon and has been reported to continue to exist for months after surgical repair (Gardner et al., 1996; Rogers et al., 1984). In an investigation examining stress across time, for example, mothers of infants undergoing heart surgery (heart surgery group) were compared to mothers of infants admitted to the hospital as non-surgical patients (inpatient group) and mothers of infants attending well-baby visits (outpatient) on questionnaires pertaining to maternal adaptation and functioning (Rogers et al., 1984). Questionnaires assessing maternal distress were completed by mothers of cardiac infants preoperatively, 7 days postoperatively, and 2 months post discharge and by mothers of the comparison groups at comparable points in time. Unexpected results were found in that the heart surgery group did not differ from the outpatient group on the day of admission. It is conceivable that the time the heart surgery group spent planning and preparing for the surgery provided parents with the support needed to adjust to the situation. As predicted, however, the heart surgery group differed significantly from the outpatient group 7 days post surgery, particularly in the amount of depression mothers were reporting. Although it was hypothesized that the three groups would not differ 2 months after the initial contact, the mothers of infants who underwent heart surgery 2 months earlier reported more distress relative to the other two groups. These results suggested that stress associated with having a child with CHD may continue to exist months after surgical repair of the lesion.

Consistent with the findings by Rogers et al. (1984), the lingering effects of stress have been observed by others. For example, Gardner et al. (1996) found that mothers of cardiac infants reported more distress than mothers of healthy infants 6 months post repair. In contrast to the findings of Rogers et al. (1984), however, they also found that the cardiac group reported more stress prior to surgery than the healthy group, who completed questionnaires at comparable times. In addition, these researchers also considered the impact stress has on mother-infant interactions by conducting face-to-face observations of cardiac infant-mother dyads compared to non-cardiac infant-mother dyads both prior to surgery and 6 months post operatively for the cardiac group and at comparable times for the control group. Results from the interactions revealed that both cardiac infants and mothers showed less positive affect and engagement than the comparison group at both sessions (preoperative and postoperative). Cardiac infants showed significantly more positive engagement at the second session, but there were no differences in positive affect. There was a significant increase in the amount of positive affect between sessions for the cardiac mothers, but there was no difference in positive engagement. It appeared that some mothers had difficulty adapting to their infants, leading to disordered interactions.

Taken together, the literature suggests that parents of cardiac infants report heightened levels of stress compared to parents of non-cardiac infants. Studies that have examined stress across time revealed that stress is not limited to the period around repair but has the potential to linger for months post-operatively. The deleterious effects of stress have become an interest to researchers, as it appears that early mother-infant interactions may be affected by stress related to having an ill infant.

Parent Stress and Child Behavior

Consideration has also been given as to the influence of parental stress on later child behavior problems. Difficulties in parent-infant interactions resulting from stress (Gardner et al., 1996) may lead to child behavior problems. It is conceivable that parents who experience stress may be less tolerant of aberrant behaviors in their children, which may result in parents over-reporting behavior problems. It could also be that parents of children with CHD overcompensate by pampering or by demonstrating permissive parenting, thus leading to behavioral disturbances as children grow older (Linde et al., 1966). In an attempt to understand the occurrence of behavior problems in cardiac children, researchers have considered the influence of parent perceptions on reports of child behavior.

Of the various parent perception measures (e.g., Parenting Stress Index, Parental Locus of Control Scale, Mother's Perception of Medical Severity), stress appears to have the greatest impact on child behavior. DeMaso et al. (1990) asked mothers of cardiac children to complete parent perception questionnaires. These researchers found that child's age was negatively correlated with the Parent domain scores on the PSI, suggesting that parent stress was lower in the mothers with older children. No other demographic variables (e.g. sex, SES) were significantly correlated to maternal perception measures. The PSI child domain scores were positively correlated with a measure of medical severity. Children with increased illness severity tended to be less reinforcing to their mothers. The significant relation between the PSI and children's emotional adjustment, as assessed with the CBCL, indicated that mother-child systems under stress were associated with child maladjustment.

Further support of a relation between family stress and behavior problems was also found in a group of children who underwent heart transplantation (Uzark et al., 1992). In addition, the researchers also examined the role of family resources, which included social support. Parents of pediatric heart transplant recipients and parents of healthy children completed questionnaires that measured child adaptation, family stress, and family resources. Similar to the results presented by Goldberg, Morris et al. (1990) noted previously, parents of heart transplant recipients reported more stress than parents of children with no chronic illness. Behavior problems in children were associated with greater family stress as well as decreased family resources. Level of stress was also inversely related to family resources. Although family resources were related to lower SES, there was no correlation between SES and family stress, as was also found in the study by DeMaso et al. (1990). Thus, it appears that the assessment of both stress and resources is necessary to encourage positive psychosocial outcomes of children.

Optimal behavioral adjustment in children may also be achieved by identifying early predictors of later child behavior problems. However, despite the heightened levels of stress reported by parents of infants with CHD and the association that exits between stress and child behavior, few prospective, longitudinal studies have investigated the impact of early stress and later child adaptation. In order to evaluate predictors of later behavior, Goldberg et al. (1997) continued their initial research on the impact of having an infant with CHD. Children with cystic fibrosis, CHD, and healthy children were evaluated over the first three years of their lives on measures of child health, parent-child attachment, temperament, and family environment (PSI-Total domain score). When children were four years of age, parents completed the CBCL. In the CHD group, parenting stress was the best predictor of total behavior problems and internalizing scores, suggesting that children of parents who consistently reported high levels of stress were at a higher risk for behavior problems. Because measures at 1 year of age contributed significantly to behavior problems at 4 years, it appeared that early parent reports of difficulties in child rearing predict later reports of behavior problems.

Overall, it appears that parents of children with CHD experience higher amounts of stress relative to parents of non-cardiac children. Stress does not dissipate after surgical repair of a cardiac lesion, and the impact of having a sick child may encourage parents to pamper and to overindulge their children, thus leading to possible child behavior problems. It has been suggested that high parent stress, which may occur as early as the infancy period, may result in greater child behavior problems in preschoolers. Although early identification of stress is crucial in assisting in the prevention of child behavior problems, a more critical question is what may alleviate stress. Uzark et al. (1992) reported that families with greater resources experienced less stress. One family resource that has been examined is social support.

Social Support

In addition to parenting stress affecting the adjustment of children with CHD, social support is also a factor. It is conceivable that stress may be reduced or alleviated with the assistance of a social support network. Because of the heightened levels of stress in families of chronically ill children, the influence of social support in this group is especially pertinent. Studies on the influence of perceived social support have been conducted on families, including those with children with cancer (Nixon-Speechley & Noh, 1992; Varni, Katz, Colegrove, & Dolgin, 1994) and asthma (Hamlett, Pellegrini, & Katz, 1992). Less adequate social support in families of children with an illness or a disability compared to families with healthy children is not uncommon (Hamlett, Pellegrini, & Katz, 1992; Pearson & Chan, 1993). This section will review studies that assess whether more social support in families leads to better adjustment for parents and children. This will be followed by an examination of studies that deal with the moderating effect of social support. Finally, the section will review studies that have looked at the influence of social support in families of children with CHD.

Social Support and Adjustment

The belief that social support helps to reduce parental distress has been supported. For example, in a sample of children with cancer, parent psychological distress was inversely related to social support (Nixon-Speechley & Noh, 1992). Parents of cancer survivors did not report significantly higher levels of depression or anxiety compared to the matched sample of parents with healthy children. However, among the families who reported low levels of support, parents of children with cancer were more depressed and anxious than the comparison group. Similarly, in a study of mothers of children with phenylketonuria, Kazak,

Reber, and Carter (1988) also found an inverse relation between larger social networks and decreased psychological distress.

Although many studies have focused on the impact of family social supports on parental adjustment, the role of a social support system in the psychological and social adjustment of children coping with illness has also been given consideration (Varni et al., 1994). Children with newly diagnosed cancer were asked to complete questionnaires that assessed social support (parent, teachers, classmates, and close friends), depression, anxiety, and self-esteem. Perceived classmate support significantly predicted depressive symptoms and anxiety. Specifically, children who perceived more classmate social support reported fewer depressive symptoms, lower anxiety, and higher self-esteem. Children with more self-perceived classmate support were also rated by their parents on the CBCL as having fewer behavior problems.

Fewer child behavior problems were also reported by mothers who perceived their own social support system to be optimal (Hamlett, Pellergrini, and Katz,1992). Consistent with previous research, mothers of chronically ill children compared to mothers of healthy children reported a greater number of internalizing behavior problems. Mothers of ill children also reported fewer adequate social supports than mothers with healthy children. A relation was found to exist between child behavior problems and maternal reports of less adequate social support.

High levels of social support have been reported to reduce distress and anxiety. Parents who perceive their social support system as positive report fewer problem behaviors in their children. Since social support is related to both stress and child behavior, consideration has been given as to how it may moderate the adverse effects of stress on behavior problems.

Social Support as a Moderator

Studies on the joint impact of parent stress and social support have come into consideration in examining the moderating role of support on outcomes such as parent functioning and child behavior (Crnic et al., 1983; Ievers et al., 1998; Wertlieb, Weigel, & Feldstein, 1987). For example, in one study, stress and support both significantly predicted maternal satisfaction with parenting at 1 year and child behavior during 4 year interactions (Crnic et al., 1983). Social support also moderated the adverse effects of stress on mother's life satisfaction. Specifically, of mothers with high stress, those with more support reported greater life satisfaction. In addition, mothers with more stress and less support were less positive in their interactions and behavior and less sensitive to their children's needs, while mothers with more social support, particularly intimate support, were more positive. Social support moderated the effects of stress on child responsiveness during interactions at 4 years. Infants appeared to react to parent stress by being less responsive and less clear in the cues they provided. These results provided evidence of the importance of stress and support in parenting as well as the role of support in moderating adverse effects of stress on the parent-child relationship.

Further evidence of the moderating role of social support was presented by Wertlieb, Wiegel, and Feldstein (1987). In this study, the relation between stress and behavior problems in a group of healthy children was examined to determine whether social support buffered stressed parents in their perceptions of child behavior problems. The significant interactions found between stress and social support in predicting behavior problems supported the role of social support as a moderator. Specifically, parents with low support and high stress reported more child behavior problems.

Social Support in Families of Children with Cardiac Disease

The influence of social support on parenting stress and child behavior problems in families of children with CHD has not been frequently studied. In one of the few studies investigating this issue, social support was inversely related to parent stress and child behavior (Uzark et al., 1992). That is, families with more stress reported fewer resources. Low SES was also associated with decreased resources. A higher number of behavior problems were reported in families with more stress and fewer resources. The significant relation between family resources and behavior problems suggested that this is a factor that should be further considered in families of children with CHD.

These results suggest that, for many families, the stress associated with having a chronically ill child is reduced through social support. Studies examining the buffering role of support reported that it may moderate the adverse effects of stress on child behavior. Families with more support also reported fewer child behavior problems. Although few studies on children with CHD have examined the role of social support, the significant influence that support has on parent and child adjustment warrants further investigation.

Intelligence

In addition to parenting stress and social support affecting the adjustment of children with CHD, intelligence may also be a factor. An association between intelligence and behavior problems has been observed in children (Cook, Greenberg, & Kusche, 1994; Dietz, Lavigne, Arend, & Rosenbaum, 1997; Konstantareas & Homatidis, 1989; Sonuga-Barke, Lamparelli, Stevenson, Thompson, & Henry, 1994). Studies have shown that low intelligence may affect the emotional well being of children. For example, Sonuga-Barke et al. (1994) found that preschoolers diagnosed as hyperactive had lower intelligence test (IQ) scores than non-hyperactive peers. In another study examining the relation between psychopathology and intelligence in a nonclinical group of children, lower general, verbal, and performance IQ scores on the McCarthy Scales of Children's Abilities were associated with higher ratings on the Total Problem Behavior, Internalizing, and Externalizing scales of the CBCL (Dietz et al., 1997).

The role of intelligence in the behavioral adjustment of children with cardiac lesions has also been explored. Despite mean intelligence in the average range, children with CHD tend to have lower IQ scores than comparison groups and normative samples (Alden, Gilljam & Gillberg, 1998; DeMaso et al., 1990). It stands to reason that the increased frequency of behavior problems in this group of children may be the result of lower cognitive ability. DeMaso et al. (1990) considered this in their study comparing the psychological functioning of children with CHD compared to a group of children originally diagnosed with CHD, but who spontaneously recovered without surgery. Compared to children who experienced spontaneous recovery, children with continued heart disease had poorer emotional adjustment, greater CNS impairment scores, and lower IQ scores. However, when the effects of IQ and CNS impairments were controlled, there was no difference between groups, suggesting that a heart lesion, by itself, does not appear to be associated with an emotional disorder.

Consistent with the findings by DeMaso et al. (1990), Alden, Gilljam, and Gillberg (1998) also reported lower IQ scores in a group of cardiac children compared to the general population. In addition, more cardiac children than expected exhibited clinically significant psychiatric problems, mostly of an internalizing nature. Unfortunately, the researchers failed to carry out correlational analyses to examine the association between IQ and behavior, making comparisons between studies difficult.

On the other hand, however, the findings by DeMaso et al. (1990) conflict with Utens et al. (1993), who continued to find significantly more behavior problems reported by parents of children with CHD even when the sample was limited to those with IQ scores above 85. Similarly, Kramer, Awiszus, Sterzel, van Halteren, and Claben (1989) also found that IQ was not associated with behavior problems in a sample of cardiac children with physical limitations compared to healthy controls. Cardiac children with physical limitations received IQ scores below those of the healthy children. Surprisingly, however, the CHD children with physical limitations were not reported by parents as exhibiting greater behavioral disturbances than the control group.

This latter finding conflicts with Spurkland et al. (1993) who reported that physical functioning was related to psychosocial functioning in children with CHD. These divergent findings may, in some part, be related to differences in methodology. Kramer et al. (1989) used the Marburg Behaviuor List to assess behavior, which according to the investigators, contains items that are not very alarming to parents and could possibly underestimate true behavioral disturbances. Spurkland et al. administered the CBCL, which has been widely-used in identifying behavior problems.

To summarize, in the continuing search to explain why children with CHD are reported by parents as exhibiting more behavior problems than non-cardiac children, researchers have considered the role of intelligence. Because many children with CHD have lower IQ scores relative to the normative population, it would appear possible that lower cognitive ability may increase the risk of behavioral maladjustment. The work by DeMaso et al. (1990) supports this possibility, as they reported that, after controlling for intelligence, differences in behavior no longer existed in their sample of children with and without CHD. However, it is difficult to conclude that intellectual ability may explain why children with CHD are reported to have behavior problems as some findings have continued to report behavioral differences between cardiac and healthy children in samples of children with IQ scores in the average range. These discrepant findings highlight the need to further explore the role of intelligence in behavioral problems of children with CHD as well as to consider other factors for behavioral disturbances.

Language

Language ability is an additional factor to consider when examining the adjustment of children with CHD. Children with speech and language delays are also at risk for psychiatric disorders and behavioral disturbances (Beitchman, Nair, Clegg, Ferguson, & Patel, 1986; Beitchman et al., 1996; Cantwell, Baker, & Mattison, 1979; Carson, Klee, Perry, Donaghy, & Muskina, 1986; Carson, Klee, Perry, Muskina, & Donaghy, 1996). It is conceivable that children who have difficulties either verbally expressing themselves or understanding the intent of others may result in them either becoming self-conscious and withdrawn or acting out and misbehaving. Thus, the frustration and humiliation children experience because of poor language skills may result in a high frequency of either internalizing or externalizing behavior problems. For example, in a study of children, ages 2 to 13 years, visiting a speech and language clinic, over half were diagnosed with a psychiatric disorder (Cantwell, Baker, & Mattison, 1979). The most common diagnosis was Attentional Deficit Disorder followed by Oppositional Disorder.

The incidence of behavior problems in children with speech and language disorders has been presented in numerous studies, including prospective projects that have examined the association between early language deficits and later behavior problems. As part of a longitudinal investigation, Beitchman et al. (1986) confirmed a relation between language deficits and behavior problems. Their sample of 5-year-old children with a speech and language disorder were more likely than a control group to be rated by parents and teachers as having behavior problems, particularly in the area of anxious-passive problems. In fact, when these children were evaluated again at 12 years of age, a significant association was found between speech and language classification at 5 years and behavior ratings 7 years later (Beitchman et al., 1996). Contrary to findings by Beitchman et al., (1986) in which children with the lowest language skills showed the highest rates of behavior problems, Benasich, Curtis, & Tallai (1993) failed to find an association between early language at 4 years and behavior at 8 years in their sample of language impaired and non-impaired children. These researchers also measured intelligence at both 4 and 8 years, and although the children in both groups were matched on IQ at 4 years, the children in the language impaired group had significantly lower mean IQ scores than the control group at age 8. The decline in IQ in the language impaired children significantly predicted behavior ratings at age 8, suggesting the importance of considering the role that IQ plays in the etiology of behavior problems. Less cognitively advanced children may be unable to respond to the demands placed on them, and as a result, act out frustrations in an aggressive manner.

Lower IQ scores in a sample of language-delayed children compared to non-impaired children were also found by Silva, Williams, and McGee (1987). At ages 7 and 9 years, children with a language delay had significantly lower IQ scores than non-impaired children. At age 11, children with receptive and expressive language delays had lower verbal IQ and full-scale IQ scores, whereas the children with a general language delay also had lower performance IQ scores than the comparison group. This research is limited because the researchers failed to assess child behavior. Therefore, it is unknown whether IQ would predict behavior, as has been presented in studies by Dietz, Lavigne, Arend, and Rosenbaum (1997) and Sonuga-Barke, Lamparelli, Stevenson, Thompson, and Henry (1994).

Not all children with speech and language difficulties are at risk for behavior problems, however. The type of language delay a child is diagnosed with may affect the extent of the problem. Children with either pervasive speech/language or receptive language deficits have been reported to be at the greatest risk for behavioral disturbances in the areas of both internalizing and externalizing behaviors (Beitchman et al., 1996; Silva, Williams, & McGee, 1987). On the other hand, children with poor articulation early in childhood have not been reported to exhibit increased behavior problems, suggesting that these children, because of their intact receptive language skills, are capable of understanding the intent of others, and are less subject to frustrations (Beitchman et al., 1996).

Caulfield, Fischel, DeBaryshe, and Whitehurst (1989) reported that children with expressive-language delays were also not at an increased risk for parent reported behavior problems. Parents of children with expressive language delays did not report more behavior problems on questionnaires than parents of normally developing children. However, group differences in behavior were found during parent interviews and direct observation, with the expressive language delayed children exhibiting more negative behaviors. During interviews, parents also rated these children as more shy and exhibiting more problems at bedtime than did parents of matched controls. Results from the observation suggested that children with expressive language delays exhibited more behavior problems than children with normally developing language skills. The discrepancy between observational measures and questionnaire ratings of behavior is interesting. The researchers speculated that parents, when completing questionnaires about their child's behavior, may take into account the child's language, and, as result, not rate certain behaviors as aberrant. Thus, it is conceivable that questionnaire data may underestimate the extent of the problem.

In aggregate, these studies suggest that children with certain types of language disorders may be at an increased risk for behavior problems. Early delays may be associated with behavioral disturbances later in childhood. However, the intellectual level of the child is an important factor to consider. There is a tendency for children with speech and language delays to have low IQ scores, even on non-verbal IQ tests, and behavior problems may be a result of cognitive deficits rather than language deficits. It is also important to consider the nature of the delay, since not all types of deficits result in behavior problems. The relation between speech and behavior has not been widely studied in children with CHD. Research that has examined this relation in non-cardiac children lends support for the importance of examining the relation in other samples, such as children with CHD, who are at risk for behavior problems.

PURPOSE OF THE PRESENT RESEARCH

The specific purpose of this research was to examine the joint role of parental stress and social support in the emotional adjustment of children with transposition of the great arteries. Transposition of the great arteries (TGA) is a cardiac anomaly that afflicts one in every ten children born with CHD. In a healthy heart, the pulmonary artery arises from the right ventricle and the aorta arises from the left ventricle. In a heart with TGA, the pulmonary artery arises from the left ventricle and the aorta arises from the right ventricle. This is the complete opposite from normal circulation.

There are two major techniques used to support patients during the repair of complex congenital heart lesions in infancy. These include deep hypothermia with circulatory arrest and deep hypothermia with continuous low flow bypass. The advantage of circulatory arrest is that it allows surgeons to work free of blood in the operative field which can hamper exposure as well as free of cannulas which can distort cardiac structures. This procedure assumes that there is a safe duration of time in which the body can be deprived of oxygen. The organ with the shortest duration of safe time is the brain. The maximal duration of circulatory arrest that will not result in central nervous system damage is uncertain. An alternative to circulatory arrest is low-flow cardiopulmonary bypass. With this support technique, circulation is maintained throughout the surgery. However, concern has arisen as to whether prolonged extracorporeal oxygenation increases exposure to known pump related sources of brain injury (Newburger et al., 1993). To investigate the occurrence of brain injury in children undergoing both types of support techniques, a randomized, prospective study (The Boston Circulatory Arrest Study) was conducted at Children's Hospital in the late 1980's with ongoing follow-up of this cohort of children.

Research on the behavioral adjustment of children with CHD has yielded contradictory findings, from emotional disturbance (Oates et al., 1994; Utens et al., 1993; Casey et al., 1996) to healthy adjustment (DeMaso et al., 1991). It remains unclear why some children with CHD exhibit behavioral problems, particularly internalizing behaviors. Few studies have taken into account the influence of maternal perceptions of stress on child adjustment (DeMaso et al., 1991; Goldberg et al., 1997). A positive relation has been shown to exist between maternal perceptions of parenting stress and child behavior problems in children with CHD (DeMaso et al., 1991). Only recently has the relation between early parenting stress and later child behavior been examined across time (Goldberg et al., 1997). The present study was designed to provide additional information of the relation between parenting stress and child behavior problems as well as to examine the impact of stress across time on later child behavior

Stress in parents of children who are ill or who are born with disabilities is not uncommon. High levels of stress related to having a child born with CHD has been reported (Casey et al., 1996; Goldberg, Morris, et al., 1990; Rozansky & Linde, 1971). It is unknown whether parents continue to experience stress as their children with CHD grow older. DeMaso et al. (1991) reported a negative correlation between child's age and Parent domain scores on the PSI, suggesting that parent stress was lower in mothers with older children, but they did not examine the question longitudinally. Consequently, nothing can be said about the stability of stress across time. This led to the present study asking whether parents whose children underwent cardiac surgery during infancy would continue to experience feelings of stress when their children are preschoolers or whether stress would be limited to the period of time surrounding the surgery.

As previously noted, a relation has also been observed between social support and parenting stress in parents of children with cancer (Nixon-Speechley & Noh, 1992) as well as between maternal social support and child adjustment in families of children with asthma (Hamlett, Pellergrini, & Katz, 1992). There is, however, limited research available on the effects of social support on families of children with CHD. It is important to determine whether social support is an important contributor to parenting stress and maternal perceptions of child behavior. Stability of social support has been demonstrated in patients with depression and the general population (Flaherty, Gaviria, & Pathak, 1983). The present study addressed the question as to whether social support remained stable across time among families of children with CHD.

Despite mean intelligence in the average range, children with CHD tend to have lower scores compared to normative samples and comparison groups. Children with low intelligence have been found to be at risk for behavioral disturbances (Alden, Gilljam, & Gillberg, 1998). Thus, it was important to consider the cognitive ability of children in the present research. Analysis of the relation between intelligence and behavior was conducted to add resolution to previous findings. Also, the relation between child intelligence and parental stress has rarely been examined in children with heart disease. Since it is conceivable that parents of children with low intellectual ability may experience heightened stress, this relation was also examined in the present study. Similarly, children with delays in language skills are also at risk for behavior problems. It is also possible that parents experience increased stress if they are having difficulty communicating with their children. Therefore, the impact of language deficits in children with CHD on child behavior and parent stress was examined.

METHODS

Participants

Between April 1988 and February 1992, neonates and infants less than 3 months of age with TGA with or without a ventricular septal defect were randomized to undergo an arterial switch repair using either circulatory arrest or continuous low-flow cardiopulmonary bypass at the Boston Children's Hospital. One-hundred and seventy-one infants were enrolled in the trial, and 155 returned for the one-year developmental evaluation. Of the infants who returned for evaluation, 143 families (92%) completed the Parenting Stress Index (PSI) and 144 families (93%) completed the Social Support Network Inventory (SSNI). For one family, the SSNI score at one year was set to missing in the analysis because it was an outlier (>4 SD).

At 4 years, 158 of the initially-enrolled infants returned for a second evaluation. One-hundred and fifty-three families (97%) completed the PSI and 145 families (92%) completed the SSNI. At the 4 year assessment, 15 families who did not complete questionnaires when their children were 1 year agreed to do so. Demographic statistics for the group are provided in Table 1. Families were predominantly intact, Caucasian, and middle-class. The children in the sample consisted predominantly of males. At 1 year, there were 107 males (75%) and 36 females (25%). At 4 years, there were 116 males (76%) and 37 females (24%). This is consistent with the expected male-female ratio (3:1) in children with TGA (Fyler, 1992).

Table 1. Demographic Characteristics of the Sample

	Year 1				Year 4			
Demographic Variable	n	%	M	SD	n	%	M	SD
Race								
Caucasian	127	88.8			138	90.2		
Other	16	11.2			15	9.8		
Marital Status								
Yes	128	89.5			129	84.3		
No	15	10.5			24	15.7		
Maternal Occupation[a]	143		3.67	3.35	153		3.92	3.17
Maternal Education[b]	143		4.99	1.11	153		5.05	1.11
Maternal IQ[c]	133		95.98	12.89	137		96.7	12.7
Paternal Occupation[a]	134		5.56	2.30	135		5.78	2.27
Paternal Education[b]	134		4.92	1.36	135		5.21	1.23
Social Class[d]	143		42.4	14.5	153		42.6	14.48

Note. [a] On a scale from 1 (laborer) to 9 (professional). [b] On a scale of 1 (7th grade) to 7 (Graduate degree). [c] Score on the Peabody Picture Vocabulary Test (revised). [d] Score on the Hollingshead Four factor Index of Social Status, with higher score indicating higher social status.

MEASURES

1 And 4 Years of Age

The Parenting Stress Index (PSI; Abidin, 1986)

The PSI is a 101-item measure that identifies mother-child systems under excessive stress and at risk for development of dysfunctional parenting behaviors or child behavior problems. In addition to a Total Stress score, separate Parent and Child scales are obtained. For the Parent and Child scales, items are scored on a 5-point Likert scale ranging from 1 (strongly agree) to 5 (strongly disagree). The Parent and Child scales are further divided into seven and six subscales, respectively. The Parent scale evaluates parents' personal characteristics and social supports systems as they correspond to the demands and tasks of parenting (e.g., "I feel trapped by my responsibilities as a parent.", "I feel I cannot handle things well.). Subscales include Depression, Attachment, Role Restrictions, Sense of Competence, Social Isolation, Relationship with Spouse, and Parent Health. The Child scale assesses aspects of child temperament and the extent to which these child characteristics are stressful to the parent (e.g., "My child seems harder to care for than most.", "My child seems to cry more than most children."). This includes subscales for Adaptability, Acceptability, Demand, Mood, Distractibility/Hyperactivity, and Reinforces Parent. A Total Score is derived from adding the Parent and Child scales together. High scores on both the Parent and Child scales are indicative of greater stress.

The PSI has been shown to have a high degree of reliability, with alpha coefficients ranging in magnitude from .62 to .70 for the subscales of the Child Domain and from .55 to

.80 for the subscales of the Parent Domain. The coefficients for the two domains are .89 and .93, respectively, suggesting a high degree of internal consistency for these measures.

A considerable number of studies have been conducted to demonstrate the validity of the PSI. Construct validity of the PSI has been supported by examining the relationship between the PSI and the CBCL in a sample of children with otitis media (as cited in Abidin, 1986). Significant correlations have been found between the CBCL Total score and the PSI Child Domain score (r = .56, p < .001) and between the CBCL Total score and the PSI Parent Domain score (r = .40, p < .001). The predictive validity of the PSI has also been demonstrated by using the PSI in a longitudinal study of child adjustment at 5 years (as cited in Abidin, 1986). Although the range of correlation coefficients were not present in the PSI Manual, the authors indicated that significant correlations for 11 of the 16 PSI scores were reported for male children on the Total Adjustment Score of the Child Behavior Problem Checklist and five significant correlations were reported for the females.

The Social Support Network Inventory (SSNI; Flaherty, Gaviria, & Pathak, 1983)

The SSNI asks informants to list 4 individuals and one group that they are closest to in their lives. Subjects are asked to rate each of the 4 individuals and 1 group on 11 questions using a 5-point Likert scale ranging from 1 (no support) to 5 (high support). Questions address issues such as availability, reciprocity, practical support, emotional support, and event-related support (e.g., "How available is person?", "To what extent does person provide practical support?". Scores from each source are summed across each question (range = 5 to 25). Totals from each of the 11 questions are added to derive a total score (range = 55 to 275). Higher scores reflect greater social support.

The SSNI has demonstrated that it is a reliable measure. Previous research with the SSNI has found internal consistency reliabilities ranging from .76 to .90 (Flaherty, Gaviria, & Pathak 1983). Two week test-retest reliability was .87 (Flaherty, Gaviria, & Pathak, 1983).

In a clinical sample, the SSNI was significantly correlated with clinicians' ratings of patients' social support systems (r=.68), thus providing evidence of convergent validity (Flaherty, Gaviria, & Pathak, 1983). The SSNI has also demonstrated that it is construct valid in that, as would be predicted, members of a religious commune (mean=4.44) had higher social support scores than individuals from an urban community (mean=3.93).

4 Years of Age

The Achenbach Child Behavior Checklist 4-18 (CBCL/4-18; Achenbach, 1991)

This questionnaire, designed to obtain parents' reports of their children's behavioral and emotional problems, yields a Total Problem Behavior score, 2 broad-band scale scores (Internalizing, Externalizing), and 8 narrow-band scores (Withdrawn, Somatic Complaints, Anxious/Depressed, Social Problems, Thought Problems, Attention, Delinquent, Aggressive). Parents are presented with 118 items and requested to rate each item as either 0 (not true), 1 (somewhat or sometimes true), or 2 (very true or often true) (e.g., "cries a lot", "demands a lot of attention", "shy or timid").

One-week test-retest correlations for the behavior scales ranged from .82 to .95 (Achenbach, 1991). Over 1- and 2-year periods, correlations ranged from .41 to .87 and from .39 to .87, respectively (Achenbach, 1991). Interparent agreement ranged from .65 to .75 (Achenbach, 1991).

The ability of the CBCL items to discriminate between nonreferred and referred children has provided evidence for content validity (Achenbach, 1991). Evidence for construct validity has been provided by correlations between the CBCL and the Conners syndrome scales (1973), which ranged from .59 for the CBCL Attention Problems with Conners Impulsive-Hyperactive to .86 for CBCL Aggressive Behavior with Conners Conduct Problems.

The Wechsler Preschool and Primary Scale of Intelligence-R (WPPSI-R; Wechsler, 1989)

The WPPSI-R is a standardized measure used to assess intelligence in children aged 3 years through 7 years, 3 months. It is composed of five verbal subtests (Information, Comprehension, Arithmetic, Vocabulary, Similarities), which yield a verbal score (VIQ); five performance subtests (Object Assembly, Geometric Design, Block Design, Mazes, Picture Completion), which yield a performance score (PIQ); and 2 supplemental tests (Sentences, Animals Pegs). A full scale score (FSIQ) is derived from the verbal and performance scores. The mean IQ score is 100, with a standard deviation of 15.

This measure has well documented reliability and validity. With respect to test-retest reliability, over a period of 4 to 7 weeks (mean=4 weeks), the VIQ, PIQ, and FSIQ coefficients were .90, .88, and .91, respectively (Wechsler, 1989). Concurrent validity has been demonstrated by examining the relation between the WPPSI-R and other measures of intelligence and achievement (Phillips, Paseark, & Tindall, 1978, as cited in Wechsler, 1989). The correlation between the FSIQ and the Kauffman Assessment Battery for Children Mental Processing Composite was .49. The Mental Processing Composite correlated with VIQ (r=.42) and PIQ (r=.41). The WPPSI-R has also shown predictive validity in predicting later intelligence and academic achievement (White & Jacobs, 1979, as cited in Wechsler, 1989). For example, WPPSI-R scores correlated with reading scores (FSIQ, r=.58; PIQ, r=.51; VIQ, r=.54)

The Expressive One-Word Picture Vocabulary Test (EOWPVT-R; Gardner, 1990)

The EOWPVT-R is a standardized and well normed instrument used to assess expressive vocabulary skills in children 2 years to 12 years. The mean standard score is 100, with a standard deviation of 15. The authors have demonstrated that the measure is reliable and valid. Internal consistency has been established. For 4-year-old children, the reliability coefficient is .89. Concurrent validity has been established by the high correlations between the EOWPVT and tests of intelligence (r=.69), achievement (r=.46),and receptive language (r=.61) (Gardner, 1990)

RESULTS

Attrition Effects

Of the families who completed questionnaires at one year, 7 did not participate in the 4 year follow-up evaluation, and therefore, questionnaires were not available. Of these 7 families, 3 families did not return because they lived too far away, 1 child was untestable (i.e., autistic), 2 families refused participation, and 1 family spoke Spanish as the primary language. The Spanish- speaking family was initially included in the study because the parents were proficient enough in English to complete questionnaires at 1 year. However, because language constraints prevented the child from completing developmental testing at 4 years, questionnaire data were not collected from the parents at that time. To assess the effects of attrition on the representativeness of the sample, the families who completed questionnaires at 4 years were compared to those who did not on the following variables: occupational level of parents, education level of parents, maternal IQ, socioeconomic status (SES), Parent and Child scores on the PSI, and the SSNI. The families who did not complete questionnaires when their children were 4 did not differ significantly from those who did in terms of sociodemographic factors (e.g., occupation, education, IQ, and SES) or the SSNI. However, these non-participating families reported significantly more parent and child-related stress when their children were one year of age than families who participated at both time points (Parent PSI: $\underline{M}_{\text{non-participants}}$=127.3 $\underline{SD}$=4.9, $\underline{M}_{\text{participants}}$=114.9 $\underline{SD}$=22.2; $\underline{t}(25)$=4.7, $\underline{p}$=.0001; Child PSI: $\underline{M}_{\text{non-participants}}$ =116.1 $\underline{SD}$=18.6, $\underline{M}_{\text{participants}}$=96.7 $\underline{SD}$=13.9; $\underline{t}(141)$=3.6, $\underline{p}$=.0005, respectively).

Normative Data

The present sample was compared to normative data to determine how representative this sample is of the general population. Table 2 presents normative scores and mean scores from the present sample on measures of the PSI, CBCL, and SSNI. Normative data for the PSI came from a sample of 534 parents of children visiting pediatric clinics and parents of children visiting clinics for special problems (Abidin, 1986). The children from the normative sample ranged in age from one month to 19 years with a mean age of 14 months (SD=23.2) and a median age of 9 months. In the present sample, parents reported significantly less parent-related stress than the normative sample at both 1 and 4 years (Year 1: M=115.5; Year 4: M=112.9). Consistent with previous findings (Goldberg, Morris et al., 1990), parent scores on the Child domain scale did not differ significantly from parents in the normative sample at 1 and 4 years (Year 1: M=97.6; Year 4: M=99.1).

The normative sample for the CBCL was composed of parental ratings of 2,368 non-clinical children with ages ranging from 4 to 18 years (Achenbach, 1991). Of these children, there were 581 males and 619 females between the ages of 4 and 11. Comparison with norms indicated that the present sample did not differ significantly from the normative sample in terms of Total Problem Behavior or Externalizing scores (M=50.7; M=50.7, respectively). However, the parents in the present sample perceived significantly fewer problems than did parents in the normative sample on Internalizing behavior (M=46.5). The CBCL was the only measure used that included gender norms. Patterns of results were similar for parents of male and female children.

Table 2. Scores on Parent Perception Measures of tress, Social Support, and Child Behavior Problems

	Normative Sample		Year 1					Year 4				
Scale	M	SD	n	M	SD	t	p	n	M	SD	t	p
PSI[a]												
Parent	122.7	24.6	143	115.5	21.8	-3.9	.0001	153	112.9	22.3	-5.4	.0001
Child	98.4	19.2	143	97.6	14.7	-.63	.53	153	99.1	19.1	.43	.67
SSNI[b]	212.9	-[d]	143	224.9	24.6	5.87	.0001	145	226.1	27.1	5.86	.0001
CBCL[c]												
Total	50.1	9.9						152	50.7	9.3	.79	.43
Internalizing	50.1	9.7						152	46.5	8.5	-5.3	.0001
Externalizing	50.0	9.8						152	50.7	9.7	.93	.36

Note. [a]PSI =Parenting Stress Index Parent and Child Scores. Normative scores are from Abidin, 1986. [b]SSNI=Social Support Network Inventory. Normative scores are from Flaherty, Gaviria, & Pathak, 1983. [c]CBCL=The Child Behavior Checklist. Scores are T scores. Normative scores are from Achenbach, 1991. [d]Information is not provided.

The SSNI provides normative data from 207 nonpatients: medical students, members of an urban community, and a religious commune community (Flaherty, Gaviria, & Pathak, 1983). The age of these participants ranged from 18 to 80 years. The present sample was compared to the urban community, as this group appeared to be the most comparable to the present sample. Comparison with established norms indicated that scores from the present sample were significantly higher than those from the normative sample from an urban community at both 1 and 4 years (Year 1: $\underline{M}$=224.9; Year 4: $\underline{M}$=226.1, respectively).

Relations between Contemporaneous Measurements of Parent Perceptions of Stress and Social Support at 1 and 4 Years of Age

It was predicted that parents who reported more social support would also report less stress. Support for this hypothesis was found. At both ages, there were significant negative correlations between parent perceptions of stress (Parent PSI and Child PSI) and social support (SSNI) (Table 3). Parent PSI scores and Child PSI scores were also significantly related at both ages, suggesting that parents who perceived their child's temperament and characteristics as stressful also viewed disturbances in their own functioning as parents. The pattern of correlations was similar for parents of male and female children.

Table 3. Correlations Between Parent Perceptions of Stress and Social Support at 1 and 4 Years of Age

Perception Variable	Year 1 r	Year 4 r
PSI Parent[a]-SSNI	-.43***	-.41***
PSI Child[b]-SSNI[c]	-.23**	-.31***
PSI Parent-PSI Child	.51***	.60***

Note. [a] Parenting Stress Index Parent Scale. [b] Parenting Stress Index Child Scale. [c] Social Support Network Inventory.
*p<=.05. **p<=.01. ***p<=.001.

Relations Between Parent Perceptions of Stress at 1 and 4 Years and Child Behavior at 4 Years of Age

Parents who report higher levels of stress were predicted to perceive a greater number of child behavior problems. To address this issue, correlational analyses were conducted to examine associations between the 1 and 4 year measures of parent and child-related stress and child behavior problems at age 4 (Table 4). As expected, parents who reported higher parent and child-related stress, at both 1 and 4 years, also reported more child behavior problems at age 4, as indicated by the positive correlations between the following variables: Parent PSI at 1 year and Total Problem Behavior, Internalizing, and Externalizing scores; Parent PSI at 4 years and Total Problem Behavior, Internalizing, and Externalizing scores; Child PSI at 4 years and Total Problem Behavior, Internalizing, and Externalizing scores. Child PSI at 1 year was positively correlated with Total Problem Behavior and Externalizing scores, but the relation between Child PSI at 1 year and Internalizing score did not reach significance (p=.10). Again, the present pattern of correlations was similar for parents of male and female children.

Table 4. Correlations Between 1 and 4 Year Measures of Parent Perceptions of Stress and Social Support with Parent Perceptions on the Child Behavior Checklist at 4 Years

Perception Variable	CBCL[a] Total Problem Behavior	Internalizing Score	Externalizing Score
Year 1			
PSI Parent[b]	.31***	.23**	.23**
PSI Child[c]	.22**	.14	.19*
Year 4			
PSI Parent	.53***	.39***	.44***
PSI Child	.68***	.51***	.59***

Note. [a] CBCL=The Child Behavior Checklist. [b] PSI Parent=Parenting Stress Index Parent Score. [c] PSI Child=Parenting Stress Index Child Score. *p<=.05. **p<=.01. ***p<=.001.

Parent Perceptions of Stress and Child Behavior Problems in the Clinical Range

It was questioned whether levels of stress would differ for parents who rated their children as having behavior problems in the clinical range compared to those who reported child behavior problems in the average range. A clinical cutpoint of ≥ 60 for the Total Problem Behavior score and the Internalizing and Externalizing scales of the CBCL is suggested (Achenbach, 1991). Twenty-five (16 %) of the children received Total Problem Behavior Scores in the clinical range. Eleven (7 %) of the children were rated in the clinical range on Internalizing behavior and twenty-eight (18 %) children fell within the clinical range for Externalizing behaviors. Table 5 presents a comparison of Parent PSI and Child PSI scores, at 1 and 4 years, between the children in the clinical and non-clinical range of behavior problems. Compared to parents of children who scored in the average range in terms of behavior problems, parents of children rated in the clinical range for Total Problem Behaviors reported significantly more parent-related stress at both 1 and 4 years. Parents of children in the clinical range also reported significantly more child-related stress than parents of children in the average range in terms of total problem behaviors at 4 years but not at 1 year. Parents of children with scores in the clinical range on internalizing problems reported significantly more parent stress at 4 years but not at 1 year. Similarly, parents reported significantly more child stress at 4 years but not at 1 year. Parents of children rated in the clinical range on externalizing problems reported significantly more parent stress at 4 years, however, stress at 1 years approached significance ($p=.05$). Parents reported significantly more child stress at both 1 and 4 years.

Relations Between Social Class and Parent Perception Measures

Research has documented that children of a lower socioeconomic background are rated as exhibiting more problem behaviors (Utens et al., 1993). To investigate this issue, correlational analyses were conducted to examine associations between socioeconomic status (SES), Parent PSI, Child PSI, social support, and child behavior measures (Table 6). At 1 year, parents from lower SES backgrounds reported more parent and child stress. At 4 years, parents from a lower SES background also reported more child-related stress but not more parent-related stress. Social support and SES were not significantly related at either age. In support of previous findings (Utens et al., 1993), parents from a lower SES background reported more Total Problem Behaviors, Internalizing, and Externalizing behaviors at 4 years.

Table 5. Scores on Parent Perceptions of Stress at 1 and 4 Years and Clinically Rated Child Behavior Problems

	CBCL[a]					
	Clinical		Non-Clinical			
Perception Variable	M	SD	M	SD	t	p
Total Problem Behavior						
Parent PSI[b]						
Year 1	124.3	22.5	112.8	21.9	-2.24	.03
Year 4	130.7	19.8	108.9	20.6	-4.87	.0000
Child PSI[c]						
Year 1	100.6	11.8	95.9	14.2	-1.46	.15
Year	121.2	16.4	94.7	16.5	-7.33	.0000
Internalizing						
Parent PSI						
Year1 1	123.9	17.9	114.0	22.5	-1.28	.20
Year 4	134.5	15.5	110.8	21.5	-3.60	.0004
Child PSI						
Year 1	102.0	11.3	96.3	14.0	-1.19	.23
Year 4	121.5	13.6	97.3	18.5	-4.22	.0000
Externalizing						
Parent PSI						
Year 1	122.9	22.3	112.9	22.0	-1.97	.05
Year 4	127.6	23.0	109.1	20.3	-4.25	.0000
Child PSI						
Year 1	101.5	9.8	95.6	14.4	-2.39	.02
Year 4	118.9	16.8	95.6	16.8	-6.90	.0000

Note. [a]CBCL=The Child Behavior Checklist. [b]PSI Parent=Parenting Stress Index Parent Score. [c]PSI Child=Parenting Stress Index Child Score.

Table 6. Correlations of Parent Perceptions of Stress, Social Support, and Child Behavior at 1 and 4 Years with Socioeconomic Status at 4 Years

Perception Variable	Year 1 r	Year 4 r
PSI Parent[a]	-.23**	-.12
PSI Child[b]	-.20*	-.24**
SSNI[b]	.07	.01
CBCL[d]		
Total Problem Behavior		-.31***
Internalizing		-.21**
Externalizing		-.30***

Note. [a]PSI Parent=Parent Stress Index Parent Scale. [b]PSI Child=Parenting Stress Index Child Scale. [c]SSNI=Social Support Network Inventory. [d]CBCL=Child behavior Checklist.
*p<=.05. **p<=.01. ***p<=.001.

Prediction of Child Behavior from Parent Stress

It was predicted that parent stress at age 1 and parent stress at age 4 would each contribute uniquely to the prediction of child behavior at age 4. Separate multiple linear regression analyses were conducted for each of the CBCL scales (Total Problem Behavior, Internalizing, Externalizing) using the Parent PSI and Child PSI at 1 and 4 years as the predictor variables. Because SES was related to both the predictor (Parent PSI, Child PSI) and outcome (CBCL) variables, SES was added into the regression models to adjust for confounding effects. The results are presented in Table 7. In multiple regression analyses, only measures of parent and child stress at 4 years contributed significantly in predicting Total Behavior Problems, Internalizing, and Externalizing scores.

Because both parent and child stress at 4 years predicted behavior problems in their separate models, an additional multiple linear regression analysis was conducted for each of the CBCL scales (Total Problem Behavior, Internalizing, and Externalizing) to see if Parent and Child PSI at 4 uniquely predicted behavior problems. Again, SES was added to adjust for confounding effects. For Total Problem Behaviors, both Parent and Child PSI were unique predictors. However, Child PSI, but not Parent PSI, significantly predicted Internalizing and Externalizing scores. Behavior problems, such as internalizing or externalizing, may be predicted by child stress because the Child PSI assesses qualities similar to the CBCL, such as demandingness, distractibility, and mood. On the other hand, the Total Problem Behavior scale is a global measure that takes into account both internalizing and externalizing problems. It is possible that child behavior problems of a global nature may be so overwhelming that they impinge on parents experiencing emotional closeness to their children and leave parents feeling more depressed and less competent in their parenting skills. Thus, both parent and child stress are important predictors of Total Problem Behaviors.

Table 7. Regression Analysis of Variables in Relation to Behavioral Problems at 4 Years of Age

Variable	Total Problem Behavior Score			Internalizing[a]			Externalizing[a]		
	B	t for Ho (parameter =0)	P	B	t for Ho (parameter =0)	p	B	t for Ho (parameter =0)	p
PSI Parent 1[b]	-.04	-1.12	.27	-.02	-.40	.69	-.07	-1.56	.12
PSI Parent 4	.24	6.42	.0001	.16	3.96	.0001	.23	5.51	.0001
SES	1.95	3.23	.002	.80	1.26	.21	2.29	3.44	.001
PSI Child 1[c]	-.02	-.49	.63	-.01	-.35	.73	-.03	-.55	.58
PSI Child 4	.32	9.73	.0001	.22	5.84	.0001	.29	7.77	.0001
SES[d]	1.26	2.29	.02	.36	.59	.56	1.61	2.56	.01
PSI Parent 4	.08	2.43	.02	.06	1.53	.13	.06	1.49	.14
PSI Child 4	.26	6.69	.0001	.18	4.17	.0001	.25	5.54	.0001
SES	.96	1.83	.07	.07	0.13	.89	1.28	2.16	.03

Note. [a]CBCL=The Child Behavior Checklist. [b]PSI Parent=Parenting Stress Index Parent Score. [c]PSI Child=Parenting Stress Index Child Score. [d]SES was calculated from the Hollingshead Four Factor Index of Social Status.

Relations Between Social Support at 1 and 4 Years and Child Behavior Problems at 4 Years

Because a significant relation between stress and social support was found, additional analyses were conducted to examine the relation between social support and child behavior problems at 4 years (Table 8). Social support at age 1 was not significantly related to CBCL (Total Problem Behavior, Internalizing, Externalizing) at age 4. However, there was a contemporaneous relationship between social support and CBCL at age 4. Specifically, the significant negative correlation between SSNI and Total Behavior Problem and SSNI and Externalizing behavior indicates that parents who reported more social support tended to have children with lower Total Problem Behavior and Externalizing scores.

Table 8. Correlations Between 1 and 4 Year Measures of Parent Perceptions of Social Support with Parent Perceptions on the Child Behavior Checklist at 4 Years

Perception Variable	CBCL[a] Total Problem Behavior	Internalizing Score	Externalizing Score
Year 1			
SSNI[b]	-.13	-.11	-.12
Year 4			
SSNI	-.21**	-.12	-.21**

Note. [a]CBCL=The Child Behavior Checklist. [b]SSNI=Social Support Network Inventory.
*p<.05. **p<.01. ***p<.001.

Does Social Support Moderate the Relationship Between Stress and Behavior Problems?

Social Support and Stress at 1 Year

It was predicted that a significant interaction would exist between stress and social support at age 1 in predicting child behavior problems at age 4. To investigate this issue, multiple regression analyses were conducted to examine interactions between the PSI (parent and child, separately) and SSNI at 1 year in predicting child behavior problems at 4 years (Table 9). There was a significant interaction between Parent PSI and social support in the prediction of Total Problem Behavior Score (p=.04). The impact of stress at 1 year on child adjustment at 4 years was a function of social support. When parent-related stress was low, families with high levels of social support reported fewer behavior problems than families with low levels of social support. Surprisingly as stress increased, particularly when it exceeded the mean amount of stress for this sample (M= 115.5), families with high levels of social support reported more child behavior problems than families with low levels of social support (Figure 1). Although this significant interaction suggests a moderating role of social support in the relation between stress and child behavior problems, caution is taken in interpreting this finding. Because of the series of analyses conducted to examine interactions, this finding may be the result of chance.

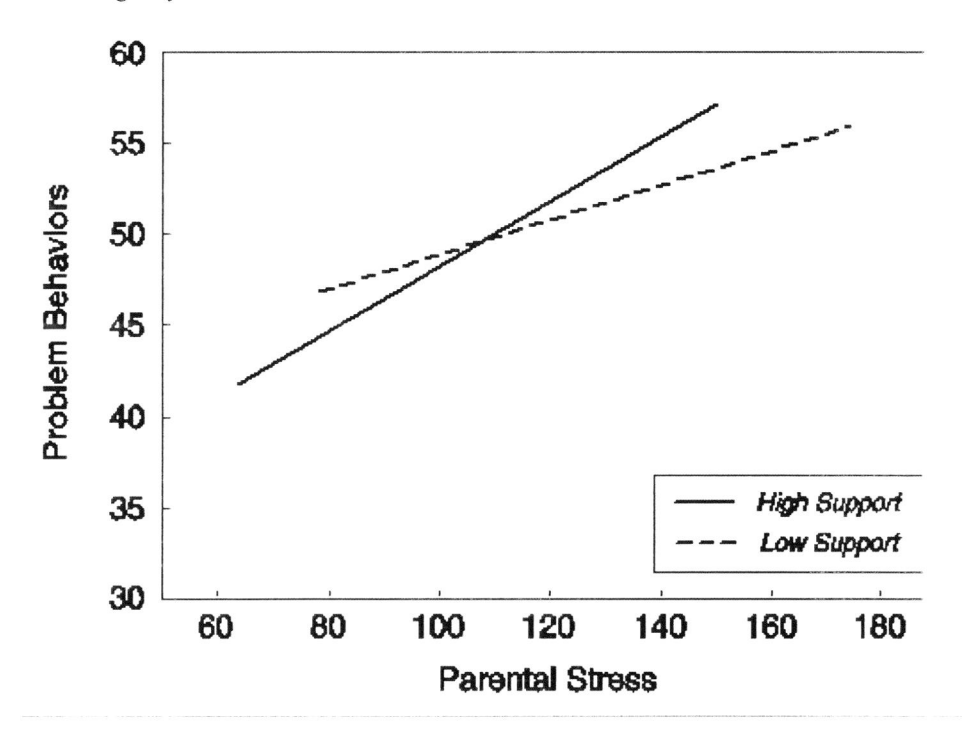

Figure 1. Social Support as a moderator in the relationship between parent stress at 1 year and total problem behavior at 4 years.

Table 9. Summary of Multiple Regression Analysis of 1 Year Parent Perception Variables in Relation to Behavioral Problems at 4 Years of Age

	Total Problem Behavior Score[a]			Internalizing[a]			Externalizing[a]		
Perception Variable	B	t for Ho (parameter =0)	p	B	t for Ho (parameter =0)	p	B	t for Ho (parameter= 0)	p
PSI Parent 1[b]	.24	3.28	.0001	.15	2.14	.03	.15	1.95	.05
SSNI 1[c]	.34	2.34	.02	.18	1.31	.19	.23	1.44	.15
PSI Parent 1 x SSNI 1	-.003	-2.03	.04	-.001	-1.15	.25	-.001	-1.07	.29
PSI Child 1[d]	.32	2.4	.02	.15	1.13	.26	.29	2.02	.05
SSNI 1	.46	1.8	.08	.20	.80	.43	.40	1.45	.15
PSI Child 1 x SSNI 1	-.004	-1.63	.11	-.001	-.67	.51	-.003	-1.35	.18

Note. [a]Subscales of the Child Behavior Checklist. [b]PSI Parent=Parenting Stress Index Parent Score. [c]SSNI=Social Support Network Inventory. [d]PSI Child=Parenting Stress Index Child Score.

Social Support and Stress at 4 Years

It was predicted that social support at age 4 would moderate the adverse effects of stress at age 4 on behavior problems at age 4. Multiple regression analyses were conducted to examine interactions between stress (parent and child, separately) and social support at 4 years in predicting behavior problems at age 4. The results are presented in Table 10. No significant interactions were found between Parent PSI and SSNI or Child PSI and SSNI with respect to the outcome variables (Total Problem Behavior, Internalizing, and Externalizing). Thus, concurrent social support does not appear to buffer the effects of stress on child adjustment.

Long Term Continuity and Change in Stress and Social Support

Stability of Stress and Support

To examine long-term stability in parent perceptions of stress and social support over time, Pearson product-moment correlations were calculated at year 1 and year 4 on measures of Parent PSI, Child PSI, and SSNI. As expected, there was a moderate degree of stability for all three measures ($r=.63$, $p=.0001$; $r=.33$, $p=.0001$; $r=.63$, $p=.0001$, respectively).

Table 10. Regression Analysis of 4 Year Parent Perception Variables in Relation to Behavioral Problems at 4 Years of Age

	Total Problem Behavior Score[a]			Internalizing[a]			Externalizing[a]		
Perception Variable	B	t for Ho (parameter r=0)	p	B	t for Ho (parameter =0)	p	B	t for Ho (parameter =0)	p
PSI Parent 4[b]	.32	4.85	.0001	.19	2.86	.005	.21	2.89	.004
SSNI 4[c]	.21	1.54	.13	.07	.54	.59	.05	.36	.72
PSI Parent 4 x SSNI 4	-.002	-1.59	.11	-.001	-.63	.53	-.003	-.29	.77
PSI Child 4[d]	.39	6.97	.0001	.29	4.80	.0001	.28	4.35	.0001
SSNI 4	.15	1.41	.16	.14	1.23	.22	-.02	-.13	.89
PSI Child 4 x SSNI 4	-.001	-1.36	.15	-.001	-1.36	.18	.0002	.20	.84

Note. [a]Subscales of the Child Behavior Checklist. [b]PSI Parent=Parenting Stress Index Parent Score. [c]SSNI=Social Support Network Inventory. [d]PSI Child=Parenting Stress Index Child Score.

Relations Between Developmental Measures and Parent Stress Measures

Infant Development

The development of the children in this sample was evaluated at 1 year with the Bayley Scales of Infant Development (Bayley, 1969), and the results revealed that scores on the Psychomotor Development Index were significantly lower for children assigned to the circulatory arrest group than to those assigned to low-flow cardiopulmonary bypass (p=.01). On the Mental Development Index, scores were lower among children assigned to the circulatory arrest group than to the cardiopulmonary bypass group, although differences were not significant (p=.10) (Bellinger et al., 1995). To examine whether a relation exists between early development and parent perceptions of stress at 1 and 4 years, correlations were calculated (Table 11). The Mental Development Index at 1 year did not significantly correlate with either the Parent PSI or the Child PSI at ages 1 and 4. Similarly, the Psychomotor Development Index did not significantly correlate with either the Parent PSI or the Child PSI at ages 1 and 4.

Table 11. Correlations Between Parent Perceptions of Stress at 1 and 4 Years and Infant Development at 1 Year

Bayley Scales of Infant Development Perception Variable	MDI	PDI
Year 1		
PSI Parent[a]	-.04	.05
PSI Child[b]	-.05	.06
Year 4		
PSI Parent	-.07	-.03
PSI Child	-.12	-.05

Note. [a]PSI Parent=Parenting Stress Index Parent Score. [b]PSI Child=Parenting Stress Index Child Score. *p<.05. **p<.01. ***p<.001.

Intelligence at 4 Years

Because parents of children with learning disabilities report greater child behavior problems (Sonuga-Barke et al., 1994), the relation between intelligence and behavior problems was examined in this sample. It was also questioned whether parent reports of stress would be related to child intelligence. Table 12 provides correlations between full scale IQ (Wechsler, 1989) at 4 years and Parent PSI and Child PSI at 1 and 4 years and the CBCL at 4 years. The only significant correlation was the negative correlation between Child PSI at 4 years and FSIQ indicating that parents of children with lower IQ scores perceived more child-related stress.

Table 12: Correlations of Parent Perception Measures at 1 and 4 Years with Child Intelligence at 4 Years

	FSIQ[a]	
Perception Variable	Year 1	Year 4
PSI Parent[b]	.03	-.03
PSI Child[c]	.05	-.21**
CBCL[d]		
Total Problem Behavior		-.15
Internalizing		-.06
Externalizing		-.09

Note. [a]FSIQ=Wechsler Preschool and Primary Scale of Intelligence-Revised Full Scale IQ.
[b]PSI Parent=Parenting Stress Index Parent Scale. [c]PSI Child=Parenting Stress Index Child Scale.
[d]CBCL = Child Behavior Checklist
*p<=.05. **p<=.01. *** p<=.001.

Speech at 4 Years

The relation between speech delays and parent stress or child behavior problems was also examined. Speech Apraxia, the difficulty with motor components of speech production, was diagnosed in 34 (32%) of the children during the 4 year evaluation. T-tests were conducted to examine whether children diagnosed with apraxia would differ from those not diagnosed with apraxia on parents' ratings of stress and child behavior problems. At 4 years, parents of children with apraxia reported more parent-related stress ($M_{apraxia}$=119.5 SD=17.9, $M_{non-apraxia}$=110.0 SD=23.3;t(138)=1.95, p=.05) and more child-related stress ($M_{apraxia}$=108.1 SD=16.7, $M_{non-apraxia}$=96.2 SD=19.2; t (138)=3.22, p=.002). In support of research that has reported greater behavior problems in children with speech and language disorders (Beitchman et al., 1986), the children with speech apraxia in the present study were reported by their parents as having higher Total Problem Behavior scores ($M_{apraxia}$=55.2 SD=7.1, $M_{non-apraxia}$=49.3 SD=9.5; t (137)=3.32, p=.001) and more Internalizing behavior problems ($M_{apraxia}$=49.4 SD=7.1; $M_{non-apraxia}$=45.4 SD= 8.8; t (137)=2.34, p=.02, but not externalizing behavior problems ($M_{apraxia}$=53.0 SD=9.1, $M_{non-apraxia}$=50.1 SD=10.2; t (137)=1.51, p=.13).

Language at 4 Years

The Expressive One Word Picture Vocabulary Test (EOWPVT) (Gardner, 1990) was also administered during the year 4 evaluation to assess expressive vocabulary ability. The relation between expressive vocabulary and parenting stress and child behavior was examined in the present analysis. Scores on the EOWPVT did not correlate significantly with parent and child stress at 1 or 4 years. However, expressive vocabulary scores were inversely related to Total Problem Behavior score (r=-.19, p=.02), and the relation between language and Internalizing or Externalizing scores approached significance (r=-.15, p=.08; r=-.15, p=.07, respectively). It appears that children with difficulties in expressive language are perceived by their parents as having greater problem behaviors.

DISCUSSION

Children with congenital heart disease are at risk for behavior problems. It has been speculated in the literature that child behavior problems may be the result of parents experiencing the stress associated with having a child who underwent cardiac surgery. Few studies, however, have examined the impact of parenting stress on child behavior. The specific aim of the present study was to examine the joint role of parent stress and social support in the emotional adjustment of children with congenital heart disease.

The findings from the present study provide evidence for a favorable outcome for parents and children with congenital heart disease. Compared to normative samples, parents in the current study experienced low stress and high social support. In addition, parents rated children as exhibiting fewer child behavior problems at age 4. Parents with more stress at both ages reported more behavior problems. Families with less social support reported more stress at both 1 and 4 years. Further, families with less support at 4 years reported more child behavior problems. Social support, however, did not moderate the relationship between stress and child behavior problems.

The following discussion of the findings is organized to consider each area of interest. First, the impact of parenting stress associated with caring for a child with TGA is presented. Second, the occurrence of behavior problems in this sample and the association between behavior problems and parenting stress is reviewed. Third, the role of social support in this sample is discussed.

Parenting Stress

Although it has been suggested in the literature that parents of children with CHD experience higher amounts of stress compared to parents of healthy children, the parents in this study reported significantly less parent-related stress than the normative sample on the PSI. In addition, they did not differ significantly from the normative sample in terms of child-related stress. These findings suggest that the parents in the present sample viewed their children as being no different temperamentally than the normative sample. Parents found interactions with their children to be positive and reinforcing. Further, they saw themselves as less depressed and more competent parents. It appears that the parents in this study were capable of coping with having a sick child more effectively than what has been presented in the literature.

Findings of low levels of stress in families of children with CHD are in accordance with those presented by Demaso et al. (1990) and Goldberg, Morris, et al. (1990). Specifically, Goldberg, Morris, et al. found that scores on the PSI were not significantly different between parents of infants with CHD and the normative sample. Although Goldberg, Morris, et al. used a sample of children with various types of cardiac lesions, they reported that parents of children who underwent repair of TGA in their study were encouraged by cardiologists to view their children's condition as "fixed". Parents may be able to adapt to having a chronically ill child if they perceive the problem as resolved. Similarly, positive encouragement by physicians in the present sample may also explain the low levels of stress. Another possible explanation for the lack of differences between the present sample and normative samples on levels of stress is the fact that the initial measure of stress was collected approximately 9 months after surgical repair. It is possible that this was sufficient time for parents to adapt to and cope with having a child with CHD. Consistent with this, Crnic et al. (1983) speculated that their failure to find group differences in their sample of premature infants and healthy infants on measures of stress was related to the duration of time the infants had been at home after hospitalization. It was believed that the month the premature infants had been home before the questionnaires were administered was sufficient time for the crisis to stabilize.

Few studies have been conducted examining the long-term impact of caring for an infant with CHD. The present study addressed whether stress would continue as children grew older or whether it would be limited to the period around surgery. Few data have been collected on the stability of stress across time in samples of children with CHD. In the present sample, levels of parent and child-related stress were both stable from the time children were 1 to 4 years of age, suggesting that levels of stress remain constant as children grow older. As previously mentioned, the present study initially assessed parenting stress 9 months after surgical repair, and while amount of stress was close to or less than normative levels, it is possible that parents may have experienced heightened levels of stress around the time of surgery. Therefore, it is not known whether stress dissipated from time of surgery to the time parents completed questionnaires or whether stress was always low for these families. It is possible that the stress reported by parents from 1 and 4 years refers to daily life stress and not the lingering effects of stress associated with having a child who underwent cardiac surgery. The lingering effects of stress across time have, however, been reported by Rogers et al. (1984), who found that parents of children who underwent cardiac repair continued to exhibit more distress up to 2 months after the surgery compared to parents of non-surgical patients. The present study did not use a control group to compare parent stress levels. It is possible, as was found by Goldberg, Morris, et al. (1990), that parents of infants with CHD may report more stress than parents of healthy infants, despite levels of stress being no different from normative scores.

Levels of child stress differed depending upon the social class of the family. It appears that parents from lower SES backgrounds tended to experience more stress. These parents viewed their children as more demanding and distractible than parents from higher social class backgrounds. They experienced fewer positive interactions with them. These findings are in accordance with other studies that have reported that families of a low social class background experience more stressful life events (Cohen, Kapla, & Salonen, 1999; Wamala, Wolk, & Orth-Gomer, 1997).

Surprisingly, the inverse relation between stress and SES in the present study conflicts with findings presented by DeMaso et al. (1990) and Uzark et al. (1992) who failed to find associations between SES and stress in their samples of cardiac children. Differences on measures of SES may help to explain the divergent findings. DeMaso et al. used only parent occupation as an indication of SES, while Uzark et al. used family income as a measure of SES. In the present study, the Hollingshead Four Factor Index of Social Status was used, which takes into account both parent occupation and educational level.

There are few data available examining the impact of child cognitive development on parent stress in families of children with CHD. Parents of children with lower FSIQ scores perceived more child-related stress when their children were four years of age. Less cognitively advanced children may have difficulty responding to the demands placed on them, and as a result, exhibit behaviors such as distractibility, demandingness, or difficulty adapting to changes. These qualities have the potential to result in less positive and reinforcing interactions between parents and children. High child-related stress scores may also suggest that parents experience difficulty accepting a child with lower intelligence, since their child may not match their hoped for expectations.

Parents of children with speech apraxia reported more parent and child stress than parents of non-apraxic children. Children who have difficulty with the motoric components of speech may be difficult for parents to understand. This may lead to poor interactions between parent and child. Parents may also have difficulty accepting this disability in their child. Providing assistance to a child with speech apraxia may be an overwhelming challenge for parents, which may result in many parents feeling depressed and questioning their abilities and competencies as parents.

The lack of association between child expressive vocabulary ability and parent or child stress, on the other hand, may stem from the fact that despite low expressive vocabulary attainment, children are still capable of communicating with others. Children may also still have an intact receptive language ability that allows them to understand the intent of others and to interact appropriately with their parents. Expressive vocabulary delays do not appear to prevent parents from experiencing emotional closeness to their children.

Stress and Behavior Problems

As previously noted, few studies have taken into account the impact of parent perceptions of stress and child adjustment. Surprisingly, the children in this sample were not rated by parents as being significantly different from the normative sample in terms of total problem behavior and externalizing behaviors on the CBCL. In fact, they were perceived by parents as demonstrating significantly fewer internalizing problems. This is consistent with the results of the present sample at 2 ½ years when parents were also asked to complete the CBCL 2-3 (Bellinger et al., 1997). It also supports previous studies that did not find children with CHD to be significantly different from comparison groups (DeMaso et al., 1990) or normative groups in terms of behavior (Goldberg et al., 1997). Studies reporting increased frequency of behavior problems have examined older children, with ages ranging from 7 to 17 years (Oates et al., 1994; Utens et al., 1993; Uzark et al., 1992; Casey et al., 1996). The children in this study were 4 years of age when the behavior measure was administered. It is possible that parents of cardiac children do not perceive behavior problems in children this young, and it may not be until children enter school and receive reports from teachers that parents are able to identify disturbances. It may also be the case that the parents, when completing the CBCL, take into account the fact that the child has been sick and do not rate behaviors as aberrant. This has been reported as a possible factor as to why parents reported fewer problems than expected in their children with expressive language delays (Caulfield et al., 1989).

Children with both speech apraxia and lower expressive language abilities were rated by parents as having more behavior problems, specifically total problem behaviors and internalizing problems. Behavior problems that manifest as internalizing are conceivable.

Children who have difficulty communicating may become frustrated and embarrassed and, in turn, become quiet and withdrawn. The increased risk of behavioral disturbances in children with speech and language delays has been presented in numerous studies, although data examining the association in cardiac children are lacking (Beitchman et al., 1986; Benasich, Curtis, & Tallai, 1993).

In the present study, parents of children with TGA who experienced greater amounts of parent and child-related stress at 4 years also reported more child behavior problems at 4 years. This finding is in accordance with research by DeMaso et al. (1990) and Uzark et al. (1992), who also reported that parents of children with CHD who perceived stress associated with both themselves and their children also rated their children as exhibiting more child behavior problems. The present study extends these findings by reporting that parents who perceive higher levels of stress also rate their children as exhibiting more internalizing and externalizing behaviors in addition to having higher total problem behavior scores. These findings suggest that parents of well-adjusted children experienced a greater sense of emotional closeness to their children. They reported fewer depressive tendencies and a greater sense of competence. They perceived children as meeting their expectations and found interactions with the child to be rewarding.

In addition to providing further support of the concurrent relation between stress and behavior problems, this study was also designed to explore this relation across age, as few data are available on this association. The more stress parents reported when their infants were 1 year of age, the more behavior problems they reported when their children were 4 years. Although both stress at 1 and 4 years were related to child behavior problems, it was found that contemporaneous stress was a better predictor of behavior problems than past stress. Parent and child stress measured at 4 years were better predictors of child behavior problems at 4 years than were parent and child stress measured at 1 year.

The predictability of stress has only recently been examined by Goldberg et al. (1997), who reported that scores on the PSI at 1, 2, and 3 years were consistent predictors of later behavior problems at 4 years, with the predictive value of the PSI increasing for measures closer to the outcome variable at 4 years. Although Goldberg et al. studied the predictability of stress longitudinally, the present study extends this research by examining stress both longitudinally and contemporaneously. Providing a measure of stress at 4 years, as the present study did, adds resolution to the findings by Goldberg et al. that found that measures as early as 1 year predict later behavior problems. The findings from the present study suggest that the association between stress at 1 year and behavior problems at 4 years is based on the relation between stress at 1 year and stress at 4 years. As previously noted, stress at 1 year is not a unique predictor of behavior problems. Rather, it appears that stress at 1 year, because of its stability, predicts stress at 4 years, which uniquely predicts behavior problems. That is, stress at 1 year is a proxy for stress at 4 years. From a longitudinal standpoint, it does, however, remain important to know early stress, because it has the potential to predict levels of stress later in life. If stress is initially elevated in parents of infants with CHD, it is important to reduce it early in order to limit later stress and to decrease the occurrence of child behavior problems.

Social Support

Another topic of interest in the present study was the joint impact of parenting stress and social support on the behavioral adjustment of children with TGA. Social support is a resource that has been found to help reduce stress in families. However, there is limited research available on the effects of social support on families of children with CHD. Although it has been reported that families of children with chronic illness often experience less support, the parents in this sample reported more social support than a normative group of families from an urban community. Thus, it appears that these parents are capable and willing to seek out sources of support. In fact, social support in these families remained stable from the time children were 1 to 4 years.

Social support was not related to family SES. In the present study, families from lower social class backgrounds did not have fewer social supports. This is inconsistent with findings by Uzark et al. (1992) who found that families of lower SES backgrounds had fewer resources. These authors administered the Family Inventory of Resources for Management questionnaire, which assessed resources, one of which was social support. It is possible that the positive relation between resources and social class in their study was in part the result of the overlap between family finances, as a resource, and social class levels.

Parents who reported more social support experienced less parent and child stress at both 1 and 4 years. The relation between social support and parenting stress in families with children with CHD has not been frequently examined. Uzark et al. (1992) also found that families who experienced more stress reported fewer resources, including social support, to deal with stress. This finding provides further evidence of the importance of social support in reducing feelings of stress.

An association between social support and child behavior problems was found. Parents with more social support at 4 years rated their children as having fewer total behavior problems and fewer externalizing problems at 4 years. Again, in one of the few studies examining this relation in cardiac children, Uzark et al. (1992) also reported that families with fewer resources reported more child behavior problems. However, the analysis of behavior problems by Uzark et al. was limited to the Total Problem Behavior score and did not specifically examine if problems tended to be of the internalizing or externalizing nature.

Because of the impact both stress and social support have on child behavior, it was hypothesized that social support would buffer the effects of stress on child behavior. It was speculated that the effects of stress on behavior problems would differ across levels of social support. This does not appear to be the case in this sample, as the only significant interaction that emerged was between parent stress and support at 1 year which predicted total problem behavior at 4 years. When parent-related stress was low, families with high levels of social support reported fewer behavior problems than families with low levels of social support. Surprisingly, as stress increased, families with high levels of social support reported more child behavior problems than families with low social support. Taking into consideration that the present sample reported higher social support than a normative sample, it is plausible that the high functioning status of this sample attenuated the results. Of the families who completed the SSNI, only 27% and 31% had scores below the mean of the normative sample at 1 and 4 years, respectively. Many families in the present study who scored on the low end of the range of social support scores were still close to the normative mean, suggesting that even these families were sufficiently functioning in terms of social support.

An alternative explanation as to why parents with high social support reported more child behavior problems is that these parents may have sought out more support to help them cope with their children's behavioral maladjustment. Because of the high support, they may have been more comfortable acknowledging the problems. In addition, high social support may not always be associated with positive outcomes. For example, Belle (1982) reported that high social support may be associated with an overload of responsibilities and heightened distress, particularly if support is not reciprocated. Furthermore, it has also been found that for adolescents of a depressed or arthritic parent, compared to adolescents with healthy parents, more social support was related to poorer adjustment (Hirsch & Reischl, 1986).

Limitations

Because the present study was a secondary analysis of the data, there are several limitations associated with the study. First, families who discontinued participating in the study after 1 year reported more stress than those who participated at both time points. It is possible that the data underestimate parental stress. Had these families continued with the project, the overall level of stress in this sample as a whole may have been higher than that reported by parents of a normative sample. High levels of stress would be consistent with other studies examining stress in parents of children with cardiac disease (Casey et al., 1996; Uzark et al., 1992).

Second, stress was not measured at the time of repair. The first measure of stress for these families was obtained approximately 9 months after surgical repair. Although these families reported less stress than the normative sample at 1 and 4 years, it is unknown whether their level of stress at time of repair, when it is conceivable that stress may reach its peak, was higher than norms.

Third, no comparison group was included in the present study. Scores on parenting stress, social support and child behavior were compared to scores from normative samples. It is possible that findings may have been altered by using a comparison group of healthy children from the community. For instance, Goldberg et al. (1990) reported that, although the parents in their sample appeared similar to the normative group in terms of stress levels, their scores were higher than the parents of healthy infants from the community.

Fourth, the generalizability of the study may be questioned. The present sample reported lower levels of stress, higher amounts of social support, and fewer reports of child behavior problems than what has been reported in the literature. It is questioned whether this optimal outcome is specific to children with TGA or if it is common in families of children with other types of heart lesions. Congenital heart disease involves a spectrum of lesions ranging in severity. Transposition of the great arteries, although a serious heart defect that requires early repair for survival, generally involves one operation and parents are encouraged to consider the problem as corrected. Some lesions necessitate a series of procedures during infancy and early childhood while other lesions are not repaired until children are older. Because of the uncertainties involved in caring for a child with these types of cardiac disorders, it may be that levels of parent stress would be heightened. It is also questioned whether more stress may result in parents reporting more behavioral adjustment difficulties in their children.

Fifth, the amount of parental stress, social support, and child behavior problems was evaluated through self-report questionnaires completed by one parent. It is possible that reporting tendencies of the respondents affected the results. For example, some parents may take into consideration the fact that their child has been sick and may be more tolerant of aberrant behavior in their children. This may result in parents may under reporting behavior problems. It is also possible that parents who experience high stress may be less tolerant and over reporting behavior problems. Multiple respondents may assist in providing an accurate assessment of behavior problems in children.

Implications

Despite limitations, this study presents some noteworthy contributions. In general, this study provides support for the favorable outcomes of parents and children with CHD. Parents demonstrated a resilience that has not often been presented in the literature. They experienced low stress and their children had optimal behavioral adjustment. This study also found certain associations that are important to consider in understanding the impact of parental stress on the adjustment of children. Although both stress at 1 and 4 years were related to behavior problems, it is contemporaneous stress that best predicts behavior problems. Stress at 1 year should not be dismissed, however, as it is a stable measure that may predict later stress levels. This finding has clinical importance because it suggests that early detection of distressed families may allow for early interventions and a reduction of later child behavior problems. One such approach to alleviate stress is social support. The parents in this study who experienced the lowest levels of stress also reported the highest amount of social support. This finding provides evidence of the benefits of social support for families of children with medical conditions.

REFERENCES

Abidin, R.R. (1986). *Parenting Stress Index.* Charlottesville, VA: Pediatric Psychology Press.

Achenbach, T.M. (1991). *Manual for the Child Behavior Checklist/4-18.* University of Vermont, Department of Psychiatry: Burlington, VT.

Achenbach, T.M. (1991). *Integrative Guide for the 1991 CBCL/4-18, YSR and TRF Profiles.* University of Vermont, Department of Psychiatry: Burlington, VT.

Achenbach, T.M., Bird, H.R., Canino, G., Phares, V., Gould, M.S., & Rubio-Stipec, M (1990). Epidemiological comparisons of Puerto Rican and U.S. mainland children: Parent, teacher, and self-reports. *Journal of the American Academy of Child and Adolescent Psychiatry, 29,* 84-93.

Achenbach, T.M., Hensley, V.R., Phares, V. & Grayson, D. (1989). Problems and competencies reported by parents of Australian and American children. *Journal of Child Psychology and Psychiatry, 31,* 265-286.

Alden, B. Gilljam, T., & Gillberg, C. (1998). Long-term psychological outcome of children after surgery for transposition of the great arteries. *Acta Paediatrica, 87,* 405-410.

Bayley, N. (1969). *The Bayley Scales of Infant Development.* New York: The Psychological Association.

Beitchman, J.H., Nair, R., Clegg, M., Ferguson, B., & Patel, P.G. (1986). Prevalence of psychiatric disorders in children with speech and language disorders. *Journal of the American Academy of Child Psychiatry, 25,* 528-535.

Beitchman, J.H., Wilson, B., Brownlie, E.B., Walters, H., Inglis, A., & Lancee, W.(1996). Long-term consistency in speech/language profiles: II. Behavioral, emotional, and social outcomes. *Journal of the American Academy of Child and Adolescent Psychiatry, 35,* 815-825.

Belle, D. (1982). The stress of caring: Women as providers of social support. In L. Goldberger & S. Breznitz (Eds.), *Handbook of stress: Theoretical and clinical aspects* (pp. 496-505). New York: Free Press.

Bellinger, D.C., Rappapport, L.A., Wypij, D., Wernovsky, G., & Newburger, J.W. (1997). Patterns of developmental dysfunction after surgery during infancy to correct transposition of the great arteries. *Developmental and Behavioral Pediatrics, 18,* 10-18.

Bellinger, D.C., Jonas, R.A., Rappaport, L.A., Wypij, D., Wernovsky, G., Kuban, K.C.K, Barnes, P.D., Holmes, G.L., Hickey, P.R., Strand, R.D., Walsh, A.Z., Helmers, S.L., Constantinou, J.E., Carrazana, E.J., Mayer, J.E., Hanley, F.L., Castaneda, A.R., Ware, J.H., & Newburger, J.W. (1995). Developmental and neurological status of children after heart surgery with hypothermic circulatory arrest or low-flow cardiopulmonary bypass. *New England Journal of Medicine, 332,* 549-555.

Benasich, A.A., Curtiss, S., & Tallal, P. (1993). Language, learning, and behavioral disturbances in childhood: A longitudinal perspective. *Journal of the American Academy of Child and Adolescence Psychiatry, 32,* 585-594.

Bjornstad, P.G., Spurkland, I., & Lindberg, H.L. (1995). The impact of severe congenital heart disease on physical and psychosocial functioning in adolescents. *Cardiology in the Young, 5,* 56-62.

Brandhagen, D.J., Feldt, R.H., & Williams, D.E. (1991). Long-term psychologic implications of congenital heart disease: A 25-year follow-up. *Mayo Clinic Proceedings, 66,* 474-479.

Cadman, D., Boyle, M.H., & Offord, D.R. (1988). The Ontario Child Health Study: Social adjustment and mental health of siblings of children with chronic health problems. *Journal of Developmental and Behavioral Pediatrics, 9,* 117-121.

Campis, L.K., Lyman, R.D., & Prentice-Dunn, S. (1986). The parental locus of control scale: Development and validation. *Journal of Clinical Child Psychology, 15,* 260-267.

Cantwell, D.P., Baker, L., & Mattison, R.E. (1979). The prevalence of psychiatric disorder in children with speech and language disorder. Journal of the American Academy of Child Psychiatry, 18, 450-461.

Carson, D.K., Klee, T., Perry, C.K., Donaghy, T., & Muskina, G. (1997). Measures of language proficiency as predictors of behavioral difficulties, social and cognitive development in 20 year-old children. *Perceptual and Motor Skills, 84,* 923-930.

Carson, D.K., Klee, T., Perry, C.K., Muskina, G., & Donaghy, T. (1998). Comparisons of children with delayed and normal language at 24 months of age on measures of behavioral difficulties, social and cognitive development. *Infant Mental Health Journal, 19*, 59-75.

Casey, F.A., Sykes, D.H., Craig, B.G., Power, R., & Mullholland, H.C. (1996). Behavioral adjustment of children with surgically palliated complex congenital heart disease. *Journal of Pediatric Psychology, 21*, 335-352.

Caulfield, M.B., Frischel, J.E., DeBaryshe, B.D., & Whitehurst, G.J. (1989). Behavioral correlates of developmental expressive language disorder. *Journal of Abnormal Child Psychology, 17*, 187-201.

Cohen, S., Kaplan, G.A., & Salonen, J.T. (1999). The role of psychological characteristics in the relation between socioeconomic status and perceived health. *Journal of Applied Social Psychology, 29*, 445-468.

Conners, C.K. (1973). Rating scales for use in drug studies with children. *Psychopharmacology Bulletin, 3*, 24-29.

Cook, E.T., Greenberg, M.T., & Kusche, C.A. (1994). The relations between emotional understanding, intellectual functioning, and disruptive behavior problems in elementary-school-aged children. *Journal of Abnormal Child Psychology, 22*, 205-219.

Crnic, K.A., Greenber, M.T., Ragozin, A.S., Robinson, N.M., & Basham, R.B. (1983). Effects of stress and social support on mothers and premature and full-term infants. *Child Development, 54*, 209-217.

DeMaso, D.R., Campis, L.K., Wypij, D., Bertram, S., Lipshitz, M., & Freed, M. (1991). The impact of maternal perceptions and medical severity on the adjustment of children with congenital heart disease. *Journal of Pediatric Psychology, 16*, 137-149.

DeMaso, D.R., Beardslee, W.R., Silbert, A.R., & Fyler, D.C. (1990). Psychological functioning in children with cyanotic heart defects. *Developmental and Behavioral Pediatrics, 11*, 289-294.

Dietz, K.R., Lavigne, J.V., Arend, R., & Rosenbaum, D. (1997). Relation between intelligence and psychopathology among preschoolers. *Journal of Clinical Child Psychology, 26*, 99-107.

Flaherty, J.A., Gaviria, F.M., & Pathak, D.S. (1983). The measurement of social support: The support network inventory. *Comprehensive Psychiatry, 24*, 521-529.

Fyler, D.C. (1992). Trends. In D.C. Fyler (Ed.), *Nadas' Pediatric Cardiology* (pp. 273-280). Philadelphia, PA: Hanley & Belfus, Inc.

Fyler, D.C. (1992). D-Transposition of the great arteries. In D.C. Fyler (Ed.), *Nadas' Pediatric Cardiology* (pp. 557-575). Philadelphia, PA: Hanley & Belfus, Inc.

Gardner, M.F. (1990). *The Expressive One Word Picture Vocabulary Test- Revised.* Novato, California: Academic Therapy Publications.

Gardner, F.V., Freeman, N.H., Black, A.M.S., & Angelini, G.D. (1996) Disturbed mother-infant interaction in association with congenital heart disease. Heart, 76, 56-59.

Glaser, H.H., Harrison, G.S., & Lynn, D.B. (1964). Emotional implications of congenital heart disease in children. *Pediatrics, 3*, 367-379.

Goldberg, S., Janus, M., Washington, J., Simmins, R.J., MacClusky, I., & Fowler, R.S. (1997). Prediction of preschool behavioral problems in healthy and pediatric samples. *Developmental and Behavioral Pediatrics, 18*, 304-313.

Goldberg, S. (1991). Recent developments in attachment theory and research. *Canadian Journal of Psychiatry, 36,* 393-400.

Goldberg, S., Morris, P., Simmons, R.J., Fowler, R.S., & Levinson, H. (1990). Chronic illness in infancy and infant stress: A comparison of three groups of parents. *Journal of Pediatric Psychology, 15,* 347-358.

Goldberg, S., Washington, J., Morris, P., Fischer-Fay, A., Simmons, R. (1990). Early diagnosed chronic illness and mother-child relationships in the first two years. *Canadian Journal of Psychiatry, 35,* 726-733.

Gupka, S., Giuffre, R.M., Crawford, S., & Waters, J. (1998). Covert fears, anxiety and depression in congenital heart disease. *Cardiology in the Young, 8,* 491-499.

Hamlett, K.W., Pellergrini, D.S., Katz, K.S. (1992). Childhood chronic illness as a family stressor. Journal of Pediatric Psychology, 17, 33-47.

Henderson, S., Duncan-Jonas, P., Bryne, D.G., & Scott, R. (1980). Measuring social relationships: The interview schedule for social interaction. *Psychological Medicine, 10,* 732-734.

Heller, A., Ratman, S., Zvagulis, I, & Pless, I.B. (1985). Birth defects and psychosocial adjustment. *American Journal of Diseases of Children, 139,* 257-263.

Hirsch, B.J., & Reischl, T.M., (1985). Social networks and developmental psychopathology: A comparison of adolescent children of a depressed, arthritic, or normal parent. *Journal of Abnormal Psychology, 94,* 272-281.

Hollingshead, A. (1975). *Four Factor Index of Social Status.* New Haven, CT: Department of Sociology, Yale University.

Ievers, C.E., Brown, R.T., Lambert, R.G., Hsu, L., & Eckman, J.R. (1998). Family functioning and social support in the adaptation of caregivers of children with sickle cell syndromes. *Journal of Pediatric Psychology, 23,* 377-388.

Kazak, A.E., Reber, M., & Carter, A. (1988). Structural and qualitative aspects of
social networks in families with young chronically ill children. *Journal of Pediatric Psychology, 13,* 171-182.

Kong, S.G., Tay, S.H., Yip, W.C., 7 Chay, S.O. (1986). Emotional and social effects of congenital heart disease. *Australian Paediatric Journal, 22,* 101-106.

Konstantareas, M.M. & Homatidis, S. (1989). Parental perception of learning-disabled children's adjustment problems and related stress. *Journal of Abnormal Child Psychology, 17,* 177-186.

Kramer, H.H., Awiszus, D., Stersel, U., van Halteren, A., & Clafsen, R. (1989). Development of personality and intelligence in children with congenital heart disease. *Journal of Child Psychology and Psychiatry, 30,* 299-308.

Linde, L.M. (1982). Psychiatric aspects of congenital heart disease. *Psychiatric Clinics of North America, 2,* 399-406.

Linde, L.M., Rasof, B., & Dunn, O.J. (1970). Longitudinal studies of intellectual and behavioral development in children with congenital heart disease. *Acta Paediatrica Scandinavica, 59,* 169-176.

Linde, L.M., Rasof, B., Dunn, O.J., & Rabb, E. (1966). Attitudinal factors in congenital heart disease. *Pediatrics, 38,* 92-101.

Lobo, M.L. (1992). Parent-infant interaction during feeding when the infant has congenital heart disease. *Journal of Pediatric Nursing, 7,* 97-105.

Newburger, J.W., Jonas, R.A., Wernovsky, G., Wypij, D., Hickey, P.R., Hickey, P.R., Kuban, K.C.K, Farrell, D.M., Holmes, G.L., Hickey, P.R., Helmers, S.L., Constantinou, J.E., Carrazana, E.J., Barlow, J.K., Walsh, A.Z., Lucius, K.C., Share, J.C., Wessel, D.L., Hanley, F.L., Mayer, J.E., Castaneda, A.R., Ware, J.H., & Ware, J.H. (1993). A comparison of the perioperative neurological effects of hypothermic circulatory arrest versus low-flow cardiopulmonary bypass in infant heart surgery. *New England Journal of Medicine, 329,* 1057-1064.

Nolan, T. & Pless, I.B. (1986). Emotional correlates and consequences of birth defects. *The Journal of Pediatrics, 109,* 201-216.

Nixon-Speechley, K. & Noh, S. (1992). Surviving childhood cancer, social support, and parents' psychological adjustment. *Journal of Pediatric Psychology, 17,* 15-31.

Oates, R.K., Turnbull, J.A., Simpson, J.M., & Cartmill, T.B. (1994). Parent and teacher perceptions of child behavior following cardiac surgery. *Acta Paediatrica, 83,* 1303-1307.

Pearson, V. & Chan, T.W.L., (1993). The relationship between parenting stress and social support in mothers of children with learning disabilities: A Chinese experience. *Social Science and Medicine, 37,* 267-274.

Rogers, T.R., Forehand, R., Furey, W., Baskin, C., Finch, A.J., & Jordan, S. (1984). Heart surgery in infants: A preliminary assessment of maternal adaptation. *Children's Health Care, 13,* 52-58.

Rozansky, G. I., & Linde, L.M. (1971). Psychiatric study of parents of children with cyanotic congenital heart disease. *Pediatrics, 48,* 450-451.

Silbert, A., Wolff, P.H., Mayer, B., Rosenthal, A., & Nadas, A.S. (1969). Cyanotic heart disease and psychological development. *Pediatrics, 43,* 192-200.

Silva, P.A., Williams, S., & McGee, R. (1987). A longitudinal study of children with developmental language delay at age three: Later intelligence, reading, and behavior problems. *Developmental Medicine and Child Neurology, 29,* 630-640.

Sonuga-Barke, E.J.S., Lamparelli, M., Stevenson, J., Thompson, M., & Henry, A. (1994). Behaviour problems and pre-school intellectual attainment: The associations of hyperactivity and conduct problems. *Journal of Child Psychology and Psychiatry, 35,* 949-960.

Spurkland, I., Bjornstad, P.G., Lindberg, H., & Seem, E. (1993). Mental health and psychosocial functioning in adolescents with congenital heart disease. A comparison between adolescents born with severe heart defect and atrial septal defect. *Acta Paediatrica, 82,* 71-76.

Stein, R.E.K., & Reissman, C.K. (1980). The development of an impact-on-family scale, preliminary findings. *Medical Care, 18,* 465-472.

Utens, E.M.W.J, Verhulst, F.C., Meijboom, F.J., Duivenvoorden, H.J., Erdman, R., Bos, E., Roelandt, J., & Hess, J. (1993). Behavioral and emotional problems in children and adolescents with congenital heart disease. *Psychological Medicine, 23,* 415-424.

Uzark, K.C., Sauer, S.N., Lawrence, K.S., Miller, J., Addonizio, L., & Crowley, D.C. (1992). The psychosocial impact of pediatric heart transplantation. *Journal of Heart and Lung Transplant, 11,* 1160-1167.

Varni, J.W., Katz, E.R., Colegrove, R., & Dolgin, M. (1994). Perceived social support and adjustment of children with newly diagnosed cancer. *Developmental and Behavioral Pediatrics, 15,* 20-26.

Wamala, S.P., Wolk, A., & Orth-Gomer, K. (1997). Determinants of obesity in relation to socioeconomic status among middle-aged Swedish women. *Preventive Medicine, 26,* 734-744.

Wechsler, D. (1989). *Wechsler Preschool and Primary Scale of Intelligence-Revised.* New York: The Psychological Corporation.

Wertlieb, D., Weigel, C., & Feldstein, M. (1987). Stress, social support, and behavior symptoms in middle childhood. *Journal of Clinical Child Psychology, 16,* 204-211.

In: Stress and Health: New Research
Editor: Kimberly V. Oxington, pp. 43-60

ISBN 1-59454-244-9
©2005 Nova Science Publishers, Inc.

Chapter II

STRESS, CARDIOVASCULAR DISEASE AND HYPERTENSION

Pedro Armario[*], Raquel Hernández del Rey, Pere Castellanos, Mari Cruz Almendros and Montserrat Martín-Baranera

Unit of Hypertension and Vascular Risk. Department of Internal Medicine. Hospital General de L'Hospitalet. Barcelona. Spain

ABSTRACT

Psychosocial factors could be important determinants of cardiovascular disease. Exposure to such factors may influence health directly through neuroendocrine mechanisms or indirectly, through their association with unhealthy behavior. Anger, hostility, depression, anxiety and other personality factors and character traits have been related to an increased risk of cardiovascular disease. A high level of anger in response to stress is associated in young men with an increased risk of subsequent premature cardiovascular disease, especially myocardial infarction. Chronic psychosocial stress can lead to exacerbation of coronary artery atherosclerosis, probably by excessive sympathetic nervous activation, manifested by exaggerated heart rate and blood pressures responses, as well as to transient endothelial dysfunction and even necrosis.

Sudden life stressors, such earthquakes, or war can precipitate cardiac events such as acute myocardial infarction or sudden cardiac death. Mental stress triggers myocardial infarction in patients with coronary artery disease. Studies have shown that mental stress induced in the laboratory triggers ischemia in 40-70% of stable coronary patients who have positive exercise tests. In these patients with coronary artery disease and exercise-induced ischemia, the presence of mental stress-induced ischemia predicts subsequent death. The mechanisms by which stress causes vascular injury are not very well known, but some studies have demonstrated that mental stress induces endothelial dysfunction. Research from animals demonstrates that acute stress triggers myocardial ischemia,

---

[*] Unit of Hypertension and Vascular Risk. Department of Internal Medicine. Hospital General de L'Hospitalet. Avda Josep Molins 29-41 08906 L'Hospitalet de Llobregat. Barcelona. Spain email: pedro.armario@sanitat integral.org , parmario@ub.edu

promotes arrhytmogenesis, stimulates platelet function, and increases blood viscosity through hemoconcentration. In the presence of underlying atherosclerosis, acute stress also causes coronary vasoconstriction. The existing literature on the association between stress and the risk of stroke is inconclusive, with some studies showing that there is a relation and others indicating that there is not.

The risk of hypertension is linked to several psychosocial factors, in particular, symptoms of depression and or anxiety predicted risk of hypertension development. Cardiovascular hyper-reaction to different physical or mental stress tests or to acute emotional stress have been shown as predictors of future hypertension. When different mental stress tasks are investigated in the laboratory, people with greater increases in heart rate and or blood pressure, have been observed to have greater risk of developing chronic hypertension.

PSYCHOSOCIAL RISK FACTORS FOR CARDIOVASCULAR DISEASE

In addition to the standard risk factors for coronary heart disease, psychosocial factors have been implicated in the pathogenesis of coronary hearth disease. Evidence supporting the adverse effects of stress on cardiovascular disease began to emerge more than forty years ago by Friedman and Roseman [1-2]. They showed that men with type A behavior had greater of risk of coronary heart disease [3]. In a later study carried out in 2,289 patients with documented coronary atherosclerosis, type A behavior was involved in the pathogenesis of coronary artery disease, but only in younger age groups [4]. In this study the effect of type A pattern was small relative to that of both smoking and hyperlipidemia. The type A behavior is characterized by extremes of competitiveness, a chronic sense of time urgency, and easily evoked hostility. Subsequent research demonstrated that of the 3 components of global type A behavior, hostility was the one most reliably associated with increased coronary heart disease risk [5]. There is abundant evidence that anger, hostility, depression or anxiety increase the risk of cardiac events in patients with coronary heart disease. More recently, Yan et al [6] have observed that not only hostility, but another type A component, time urgency/impatience are both independently associated with 2-fold increase in hypertension incidence.

There is probably no single biobehavioral pathway whereby psychosocial factors can influence the development of cardiovascular disease [7]. An association between anger and an increased cardiovascular reactivity has been observed. Chronically, anger may influence risk through established cardiovascular risk factors, such as hypertension or depression. Chang et al [8] have observed that high level of anger in response to stress in young men is associated with an increase risk of subsequent premature cardiovascular disease, particularly myocardial infarction. In the ARIC Study, individuals with high trait anger were at an increased risk of coronary heart disease in comparison with their low anger counterparts. The multivariate-adjusted hazard ratio of coronary heart disease in high versus low anger was 2.20 (95% IC 1.36 to 3.55) [9].

It is not clear that all negative emotions affects all patients and all cardiac end points in the same way or to the same degree. Although numerous studies have established a link between hostility and anger and coronary heart disease, there is little evidence that anger has prognostic significance after myocardial infarction [10].

In contrast with the high numbers of studies implicating psychological stress as risk factor or precursor of coronary heart disease and death, little attention has been paid to psychosocial factors in relation to stroke. One prospective study published more than ten years ago, showed a positive association between psychological stress and stroke [11]. Perceived mental stress has been associated with increased mortality from stroke for women and with coronary heart disease for men and women [12]. Everson et al [13] examined the association between blood pressure reactivity to the anticipation of bicycle exercise and subsequent incidence of stroke in 2303 men from the Kuopio Ischemic Heart Disease Risk Factor Study in Finland. Men with elevated systolic blood pressure greater or equal to 20 mmHg had a 72% greater risk of any stroke and 87% greater risk of ischemic stroke relative to less reactive men. The results of the Copehangen City Heart Study, study performed in a total de 55604 men and 6970 women, after 13 years of follow-up [14], have found an association between self-reported high stress intensity and weekly stress with a higher risk of fatal stroke compared with no stress.

It is well established that behavioral stimuli often evoke substantial responses of the autonomic and neuroendocrine systems [15]. The evidence from animal research, basically in the cynomolgus monkey, Macaca fascicularis, reveals that chronic psychosocial stress can lead to exacerbation of coronary atherosclerosis, probably by excessive sympathetic nervous system activation as well as transient endothelial dysfunction [16]. On the other hand, behavioral and psychological factors can promote coronary artery disease development, exacerbating lifestyles that can increase the risk of coronary heart disease as eg, smoking.

CHRONIC AND ACUTE LIFE STRESS AND CARDIOVASCULAR DISEASE

Work-related stress is the most widely studied chronic life stress relative to cardiovascular disease, basically coronary heart disease and hypertension [17,18]. Most interest has focused on models of job strain, as the model defined by Karasek et al, as jobs with high demand but low decision latitude [19]. In one prospective study of 1928 male workers followed-up for 6 years, job strain was associated with a 4-fold increase in the risk of cardiovascular death [19]. Subsequent studies have supported the relationship between job strain and coronary artery disease risk [20,21] but negative studies have also been reported [22,23].

More recently, research focusing on other forms of work-related stress has been published, such as the model of high work demand and low reward. This model predicts cardiac events [23,24] and has been correlated with progression of carotid atherosclerosis [25].

Like other psychosocial factors, chronic stress appears to cause direct pathophysiological effects, including elevation of arterial blood pressure and neurohumoral arousal [16]. Stress engages the central nervous system and activates behavioral and physiological response patterns, such as the "defense" and "defeat" reactions, which have been beneficial for the survival of the individual and the species but may become maladaptive when stress is chronic [26-27]. Stress activates the sympathoadrenal system and the hypothalamic-pituitary-adrecortical axis. Defense reactions involve catecholamine release, vagal withdrawal, cortisol secretion, and activation of the renin-angiotensin system: The defeat reaction is les well characterized but it is a stimulus for cortisol production [26,27].

The effects of acute stress on heart disease are well supported by epidemiological studies regarding natural life stressors [28], such as after bereavement [29], during earthquakes [30-32], wars [33] or even during important sporting events [34]. In one study of 95 647 subjects followed-up for 4 to 5 years, the highest relative mortality occurred immediately after bereavement, with a more than 2 fold higher risk for men and 3-fold higher risk for women [29]. On January 17, 1994, at 4:31 a.m., an earthquake occurred in Los Angeles. Millions of people were awakened simultaneously at this time by a life-threatening situation, providing a rare opportunity to investigate features of the relation between emotional stress and sudden death due to cardiac diseases [30]. In the day of the earthquake, there was a sharp increase in the number of sudden death from cardiac causes that were related to atherosclerotic cardiovascular disease, from a daily average of 4.6 ± 2.1 in the preceding week to 24 on the day of the earthquake. Only 3 of the 24 deaths were related to physical effort. During the six days after the earthquake, the number of sudden death declined to below the base-line values. The increased rate of cardiovascular mortality during an earthquake has been ascribed to the impact of emotional stress on the heart, mediated through an increase in cardiac sympathetic activity [31]. Some studies have demonstrated a substantial increase in the blood pressure levels after a major earthquake [35]. Parati et al [36] had the opportunity to directly record in a patient by 24-hour ambulatory blood monitoring, the acute blood pressure and heart rate changes induced by an earthquake in Italy in March 1998. The previous blood pressure levels were restored only one hour later, but blood pressure presented a pronounced variability throughout the following 6 hours.

MENTAL-STRESS INDUCED MYOCARDIAL ISCHEMIA

Mental stressors can provoke ischemia in patients with coronary artery disease. Structured mental stress testing using standardized simulated stress tasks has been used in the laboratory to provoke myocardial ischemia in cardiac patients [37]. A recent systematic review of 34 studies have demonstrated that mental stress induces transient myocardial ischemia in about 30% of patients with coronary artery disease, using electrocardiographic criteria, and 37-41% of patients with coronary heart disease based on decreased ejection fraction or wall motion abnormalities, while more than 75% of patients have perfusion abnormalities measurable by scintigraphy or PET scanning [38]. Ischemia mental stress-induced occurs primarily among patients with evidence of exercise-inducible ischemia and is frequently silent. In these patients, the presence of mental stress-induced ischemia is associated with significantly higher rates of subsequent fatal and nonfatal cardiac events, independent of age, baseline left ventricular ejection fraction, and previous myocardial infarction [39], and predicts subsequent death [40].

Blumenthal et al [41], carried out a study in one hundred thirty-two patients with documented coronary disease and recent evidence of exercise-induced myocardial ischemia underwent 48-hour ambulatory monitoring and radionuclide ventriculography during exercise and mental stress testing. They observed that patients who displayed mental stress-induced ischemia in the laboratory were more likely to exhibit ischemia during daily life, and patients who exhibited ischemia during ambulatory monitoring presented higher diastolic blood pressure, heart rate and rate-pressure product responses during mental stress. Results of this study also suggested that patients who exhibit myocardial ischemia during mental stress testing and daily life responded with increased hemodynamic responses to laboratory mental stress. Because mental stress-induced ischemia is more likely to be associated with ambulatory ischemia than exercised-induced ischemia, mental stress testing may help to identify patients at risk for exhibiting transient myocardial ischemia during daily life, and may be helpful in guiding therapeutic efforts to reduce myocardial damage.

Several mechanisms can contribute to mental stress-induced ischemia. The hemodynamic and neuroendocrine responses to stress are characterized by release of catecholamines and corticosteroids, and concomitant increases in heart rate, cardiac output, and blood pressure changes. Stress-induced autonomic nervous system activation might also predispose to clinical cardiovascular events by promoting atherosclerosis and/or by directly triggering arrhythmias [42]. Some mental stress-induced abnormalities in hemostasis and thrombosis can contribute to cause ischemia [42,43]. On the other hand, mental stress can induce a paradoxical arterial vasoconstriction in diseased coronary vessels with damaged coronary endothelium [44]. Spieker et al [45] have demonstrated that mental stress induces prolonged endothelial dysfunction. Findings of this study are in consonance with the concept of an atherogenic effect of mental stress [16].

STRESS AND BLOOD PRESSURE

Psychosocial Factors and Hypertension

Acute stress is typically associated with increased blood pressure [46-47], but the hypothesis that chronic stress exposure could lead to hypertension is of major interest but still remains debated. Clinical, epidemiological and laboratory research does provide increasing evidence that psychological factors may be important in the pathogenesis of hypertension. Although a typical hypertensive personality does not exist as a characteristic behavioral pattern, hypertensive patients have been reported to commonly exhibit abnormal levels of assertiveness and suppression of hostile impulses [48]. In some studies symptoms of depression and/or anxiety have predicted a 1.59 to 3.24 increase of risk for hypertension development across 5 to 20 years [49-50], but results are not consistent across age groups, race, gender and setting. In a prospective study carried out in initially healthy normotensive middle-aged women, followed- by an average of 9.2 years, a high level of anxiety throughout the follow-up, an increase of feelings of anger, and a decrease in the level social support were significant predictors of hypertension [51]. In another study performed in Japanese men, the results suggested that subjects who do not express their anger might have an increased risk of high blood pressure [52]. An alternative explanation for the personality of hypertensive subjects is that at least some behaviors could represent consequences rather than be a cause of hypertension [53].

In summary, we can say that hypertensive subjects has a personality pattern typified by behaviors of anger inhibition, passivity, and avoidance of confrontation [53], and other personality factors such as depression, anxiety could influence in hypertension development [53-56].

Job Stress and Hypertension

Whether or not repeated exposure to environmental stress, particularly in the workplace might lead to sustained hypertension has been an issue of debate for some years [56-57]. One reason for the discrepant views is the methodological difficulties when trying to precisely assess and quantify the effects of stress on cardiac and vascular targets in humans [48]. The workplace is a useful setting for studying the role of chronic stress in the pathogenesis of hypertension. Two different models of work stress have been used in research: The first one is the job strain model of Karasek [19] that proposes that job demand in combination with low levels of decision latitude (control over one's work situation), increases risk of disease and the second one is the effort-reward imbalance model of Siegrist [24]. This model proposes that high levels of effort combined with low perceived rewards are a risk factor for cardiovascular disease. This model proposes that effort is produced by both extrinsic factors such as external job demands and intrinsic factors related to motivation and attitudes [58,59].

The results of the studies designed to assess the long-term effect of job strain on blood pressure have produced controversy. Some studies have found a positive relationship between work stress and hypertension, but the results of other studies have been negative. Schnall et al [60,61] conducted a case-control study at seven urban work sites of employed men aged 30 to 60 years without evidence of coronary heart disease. They found that job strain, defined as high psychological demands and low decision latitude on the job, was associated with increased workplace diastolic blood pressure and the left ventricular mass index. The results of another study confirmed the previous findings of Schnall et al showing that high job strain is associated with higher blood pressure in the job in working men [62]. Cesana et al [63] carried out a cross-sectional study in a population-based sample of 527 normotensive or mild untreated hypertensive men 25 to 64 year old residents of Monza (Italy), ant they found that job strain affected blood pressure.

Other prospective studies have confirmed this association between job strain and hypertension [64,65]. In a recently published study, a relationship between job strain and blood pressure was observed in men, but not in women [65], and the results of other studies have been negative [66-67].

Fauvel et al [67] conducted a prospective study in a cohort of 292 healthy subjects aged 38±1 years old, followed-up during 5 years. The progression to hypertension was reached in 93 subjects (31.8%). In this study neither high strain (perceived job stress) (20.9% of the subjects) nor the highest blood pressure reactivity (20,9% of the subjects) increased the incidence of progression to hypertension. Steptoe et al [68-69] observed that ambulatory blood pressure and diastolic blood pressure were greater throughout the working day in men and women reporting low job control, but jobs demands and job strain had little association with blood pressure. The differences in blood pressure between high and low job control averaged 3.3/2.9 mm Hg over the day and evening (not recording at night were obtained, and hypertensive subjects were excluded of the analysis). These differences are probably not important, but may be indicative of moderate stress-induced neuroendocrine and sympathetic nervous system activation). This group has observed an interaction between work stress and cardiovascular stress reactivity [70-71].

Cardiovascular Reactivity and Hypertension

A model has hypothesized that repetitive exaggerated cardiovascular responses play a causal role in the development of hypertension, but in this model one assumption in that reactivity is a property of persons, unrelated to the circumstances in which the reactivity occurs. Increase in blood pressure in response to emotional arousal is very well know, but support for this hypothesis of reactivity in predicting future hypertension is limited.

In 1932, Hines and Brown published the first results about cardiovascular reactivity testing using the cold pressure test for measuring the reactivity of the blood pressure in normal and hypertensive subjects [72]. Only a few years later, a relationship was observed in persons who showed unusual blood pressure increase on routine examinations during prehypertensive stage and future hypertension [73]. More than forty years ago the circulatory changes underlying blood pressure elevation during acute emotional stress (mental arithmetic) in normotensive and hypertensive subjects were described [74-75]. Another interesting aspect is the stability of individual differences in cardiovascular reactivity, demonstrated by different authors, including the results of our group [76-81]. Kamarck et al [82] found that aggregating reactivity measures across three different stressors produced stronger test-retest associations (most of them being greater than 0.70) than had previously been observed.

Over the past half-century, hundreds of cardiovascular reactivity studies have been published. Although some studies show a relationship between reactivity and blood pressure level, or hypertension status, the observed relationships are not strong enough to allow us to make predictions on a case-by-case basis [83-85].

The traditional approach to this quantification is based on the use of laboratory stressors, which are believed to reproduce, in a controlled environment, the effects of psycho-emotional daily life challenges. Lucini et al [86] have observed that mild real-life stress, measured in university students, increases arterial pressure and impairs cardiovascular homeostasis.

The effect of stressors on the cardiovascular system involve two components: The first component is individual stress perception quantified by questionnaires, and the second one is individual cardiovascular reactivity to stress, assessed by the blood pressure increase in response to the stress tests. The most common mental stress tasks employed include mental arithmetic (administering subtractions of numbers of increasing complexity under pressure of time), mirror drawing test (reproduction of geometrical drawing by observing the pencil-carrying hand only as reflected by a mirror), the Stroop color-word test (computer-based test requiring the subject under examination to select a colored object while exposed to conflicting visual and auscultatory stimulation), public speaking, or stressful interview [87-91].

Sympathetic nervous system activation constitutes the major mechanism in mediating cardiovascular responses during psychological stress. Sherwood et al [92] measured cardiac output and arterial blood pressure using impedance cardiography during behavioral tasks. The results of their studies showed that there were increased cardiac responses during behavioral challenges and administration of propranolol, a beta adrenergic blocking agent reduced heart rate and cardiac output responses, indicating that beta adrenergic influences were an important cause of the cardiac responses during mental stress. Both mental and physical stress cause an increase in venous plasma epinephrine and norepinephrine levels, but the epinephrine response to psychological stressors was greater to the response to mild exercise [93]. Heart rate and blood pressure rise was attenuated and there was an increase in the total peripheral resistance during mental arithmetic. Thus, it means that beta-adrenergic influences affected peripheral vascular response as well as cardiac response to psychological stressors. In Figure 1, we can observe various integrated responses postulated to explain the pathophysiology of mental stress induced hypertension [94].

One of the limitations of the analysis of the cardiovascular responses during these mental tasks is that the correlation of the blood pressure responses during the mental tasks in the laboratory and the blood pressure levels obtained during 24-hour ambulatory blood pressure monitoring are only weak or intermediate [95-98]. However, left ventricular mass index or relative wall thickness have been correlated with laboratory stress blood pressure in some studies [99,100].

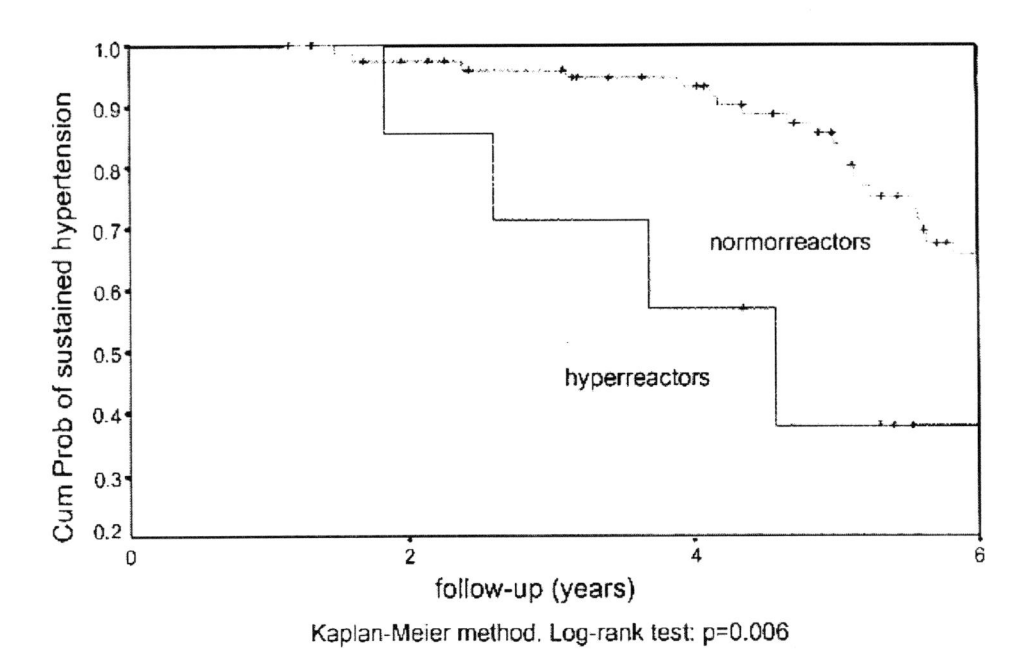

Figure 1: Various integrated responses postulated yo explain the pathophysiology of mental stress induced hypertension. Bedi et al. Ref 84

Role of Cardiovascular Reactivity to Mental Stress in Predicting Future Hypertension

Cardiovascular reactivity as a clinical index of future hypertension becomes a controversial issue [83-85]. Manuck et al [101] find that the reactivity hypothesis is strong on the basis of indirect evidence and as well the results of a few prospective follow-up studies. Several workers have found that high reactivity to different mental stress tasks is associated with greater incidence of future hypertension [102-113] (Table 1), but these results cannot be viewed as definitive [83,84]. The largest of these studies was based on 3,300 black and white young adults from the longitudinal CARDIA Investigation [109] and their results were mixed, indicating that after 5 years of follow-up, high systolic reactivity to the active coping video game was predictive of greater blood pressure rises and increased incidence of hypertension in men but not in women. Other studies have failed to obtain a predictive relation between cardiovascular stress responses and hypertension development. A good example is the analysis of the results of the Whitehall II Study, after nearly 5 years of follow-up in 1003 middle-aged men. In this study, the increases of blood pressure during mental stress was not an independent predictor of future hypertension [108]. In a recently prospective study published by our group, we observed in a small sample of 89 patients that an exaggerated response of blood pressure to mental stress task could identify a group with higher risk of sustained hypertension in comparison with subjects with less blood pressure response to the task (Fig 2) [113].

Table 1. Blood pressure response to mental stress tests and future hypertension

	n	average of follow-up	up predictor of future BP
Falkner et al (1981) ref 92	80	5 years	Yes
Borghi et al (1986,1996) ref 93,94	70	5-10 years	Yes
Light KC et al (1992) ref 95	51	10-15 years	Yes
Murphy et al (1992) ref 96	292	5 years	Yes
Matthews et al (1993) ref 97	206	6,5 years	Yes
Carroll et al (1995) ref 98	1003	4,9 years	No
Markovitz et al (1998) ref 99	3364	5 years	Yes
Newman et al (1999) ref 100	83	14-18 years	Yes
Light et al (1999) ref 101	103	18-22 years	Yes
Armario et al (2003) ref 103	89	5 years	Yes

Studies in animal models have provided direct confirmation that stress exposure play a causal role in the pathogenesis of hypertension, but each of the models demonstrate that stress exposure can be a critical factor leading to hypertension; however, hypertension only occurs in those animals with high susceptibility due to genetic and/or environmental factors [114-115].

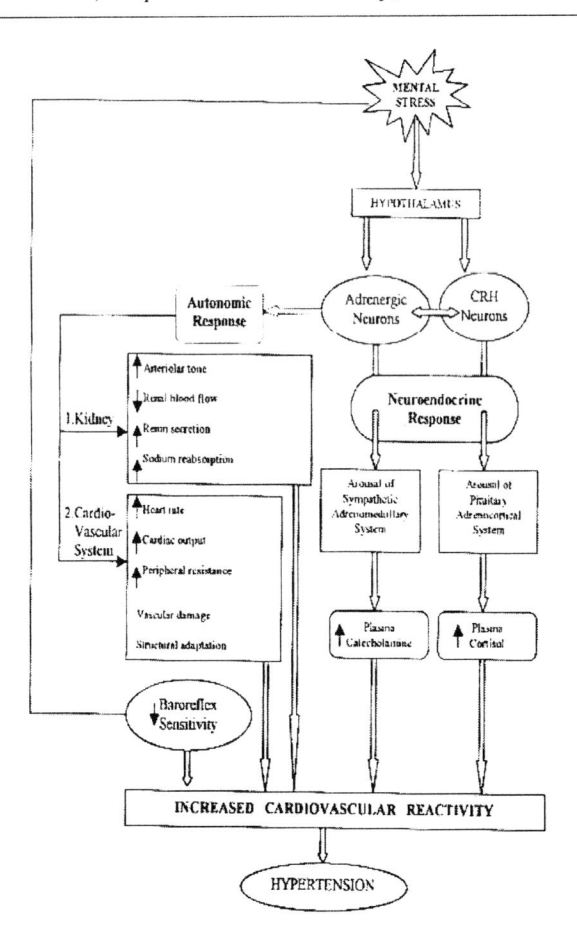

Figure 2: Cumulative probability of developing sustained hypertension over time. Comparison of hyperreactors and normoreactors. Armario et al. Ref 103

The results have been confirmed by those obtained by Light et al [111] in 103 men originally tested at age 18 to 22 years old and reassessed 10 years later: They observed that men with a combination of high stress response and hypertensive parents demonstrated higher systolic and diastolic blood pressure levels at follow-up, and they showed a 7-fold increase in relative risk of change in blood pressure status versus men with no family history of hypertension, and a 3-fold increase versus less stress-responsive men who also had hypertensive parents. These results suggest that stress response is a long-term predictor modulated by both genetic and environmental factors [111]. Some workers have studied the value of a delayed recovery of blood pressure after acute mental stress, hypertension and parental history of hypertension [116,117].

Finally, other findings supporting the importance of blood pressure response to mental stress are the results of a recently published prospective study. In this study, it was observed that blood pressure response to mental stress tasks improved the prediction of left ventricular mass index in comparison with causal blood pressure measurements [118].

REFERENCES

[1] Friedman M, Rosenman RH. Association of specific overt behavior pattern with blood and cardiovascular findings: blood cholesterol level, blood clotting time, incidence of arcus sinilis, and clinical coronary artery disease. *JAMA* 1959;169:1286-96

[2] Rosenman RH, Brand RJ, Jenkins D, Friedman M, Straus R, Wurm M. Coronary heart disease in the Westerm Collaborative Group Study. *JAMA* 1975;233:872-77

[3] Williams RB Jr, Haney TL, Lee KL, Kong YH, Blumenthal JA, Whalen RE. Type A behavior, hostility, and coronary atherosclerosis. *Psychosom Med* 1980;42:539-49

[4] Williams RB, Barefoot JC, Haney TL, Harrell FE Jr, Blumenthal JA, Pryor DB et al. Type A behavior and angiographycally documented coronary atherosclerosis in a sample of 2,289 patients. *Psychosom Med* 1988;50:139-52

[5] Miller TQ, Smith TW, Tuner CW, Guijarro ML, Hallet AJ. A metanalytic review of research on hostility and physical health. *Psychol Bull* 1996;119:322-48

[6] Yan LL, Liu K, Matthews KA, Daviglus ML, Ferguson TF, Kiefe CI. Psychosocial factors and risk of hypertension. The coronary artery risk development in young adults (CARDIA) Study. *JAMA* 2003;290:2138-48

[7] Williams RB, Barefoot JC, Scheneiderman N. Psychological risk factors for cardiovascular disease. More than one culprit at work. *JAMA* 2003;290:2190-2

[8] Chang PP, Ford DE, Meoni LA, Wang NY, Klag MJ. Anger in young men and subsequent premature cardiovascular disease. The Precursors Study. *Arch Intern Med* 2002;162:901-6

[9] Williams JE, Paton CC, Siegler IC, Eigenbrodt ML, Nieto FJ, Tyroler HA. Anger proneness predicts coronary heart disease risk. Prospective analysis from the Atherosclerosis Risk in Communities (ARIC) Study. *Circulation* 2000;101:2034-9

[10] Carney RM. Psychological risk factors for cardiac events. Could there be just one? *Circulation* 1998;97:128-9

[11] Harsmsen P, Rosengren A, Tsipogianni A, Wilhelmsen L. Risk factors for stroke in middle-aged men in Göteborg. Sweden. *Stroke* 1990;21:223-9

[12] Iso H, Date C, Yamamoto A, Toyoshima H, Tanabe N, Kikuchi S, et al. Perceived mental stress and mortality from cardiovascular disease among Japaneses men and women. The Japan Collaborative cohort Study for the evaluation of cancer Risk Sponsored by Monbusho (JAAC Study). *Circulation* 2002;106:1229-36

[13] Everson SA, Lynch JW, Kaplan GA, Lakka TA, Sivenious J, Salonen JT. Stress-induced blood pressure reactivity and incident stroke in middle-aged men. *Stroke* 2001;32:1263-70

[14] Truelsen T, Nielsen N, Boysen G, Gronbaek M. Self-reported stress and risk of stroke. The Copehangen City Heart Study. *Stroke* 2003;34:856-62

[15] Habib KE, Gold PW, Chrousos GP. Neuroendocrinology of stress. *End Metab Clin N Am* 2001;30:695-728

[16] Rozanski A, Blumenthal JA, Kaplan J. Impact of psychological factors on the pathogenesis of cardiovascular disease and implications for therapy. *Circulation* 1999;99:2192-2217

[17] Matthews KA, Cottington EM, Talbott E, Kuller LH, Siegel JM. Stressful work conditions and diastolic blood pressure among blue collar factory workers. *Am J Epidemiol* 1981;126:280-91

[18] Theorell T, De Faire U, Johnson J, Hall E, Perski A, Stewart W. Job strain and ambulatory blood pressur profile. *Scand J Work Environ Health* 1991;17:380-5

[19] Karasek RA, Baker D, Marxer F, Ahlbom A, Theorell T. Job decision latitude, job demands, and cardiovascular disease: a prospective study of Swedish men. *Am J Public Health* 1981;71:694-705

[20] Karasek RA., Theorell T, Schwartz JE, Schnall PL, Pieper CF, Michela JL. Job characteristics in relation to the prevalence of myocardial infarction in the US Health Examination Survey (HES) and the Health and Nutrition Examination Survey (HANES). *Am J Public Health* 1988;78:910-8

[21] Theorell T, Tsutsumi A, Hallquist J, Reuterwall C, Hogstedt C, Fredlund P et al. and the SHEEP Study Group. Decision latitude, job strain, and myocardial infarction : a study of working men in Stockolm. *Am J Public Health* 1998;88:382-8

[22] Hlatky MA, Lam LC, Lee KL, Clap-Channing NE, Williams RB, Pryor DB et al. Job strain and the prevalence and outcome of coronary artery disease. *Circulation* 1995;92:327-33

[23] Bosma H, Peter R, Siegrist J, Marmot M. Two alternative job stress models and the risk of coronary heart disease. *Am J Public Health* 1998;88:68-74

[24] Siegrist J, Peter R, Junge A, Cremer P, Seidel D. Low status control, high effort at work and ischemic heart disease: prospective evidence from blue-collar men. *Soc Sci Med* 1990;31:1127-34

[25] Lynch J, Krause N, Kaplan GA, Salonen R, Salonen JT. Work place demands, economic reward, and progression of carotid atherosclerosis. *Circulation* 1997;96:302-7

[26] Hjemdahl P. Stress and the metabolic syndrome. An interesting but enigmatic association. *Circulation* 2002;106:2634-6

[27] Folkow B. Physiological aspects of the "defense" and "defeat" reactions. *Acta Physiol Scand* 1997;161 (suppl 640):34-37

[28] McEwen BS. Prospective and damaging effects of stress mediators. *N Engl J Med* 1998;338:171-9

[29] Kaprio J, Koskenvuo M, Rita H. Mortality after bereavement: a prospective study of 95,647 persons. *Am J Public Health* 1987;77:283-7

[30] Trichopoulos D, Katsouyanni K, Zavitsanos X, Tzoriou A, Dalla-Vorgia P. Psychological stress and fatal heart attack: the Athens eartquake natural experiment, 1981. *Lancet* 1983;1:441-4

[31] Dobson AJ, Alexander HM, Malcolm JA, Steele PL, Miles TA. Heart attacks and the Newcastle eartquake. *Med J Aust* 1991;155:757-61

[32] Leor J, Polle WK, Kloner RA. Sudden cardiac death triggered by an earthquake. *N Engl J Med* 1996;334:413-9

[33] Meisel SR, Kutz I, Dayan KI, Pauzner H, Chetboun I, Arbel Y, et al. Effects of Iraqi missile war on incidence of acute myocardial infarction and sudden death in Israeli civilians. *Lancet* 1991;338:660-1

[34] Witte DR, Bots ML, Hoes AW, Grobbee DE. Cardiovascular mortality in Duth men during 1996 European football championship: longitudinal population study. *BMJ* 2000;321:1552-4

[35] Kario K, Matsuo T, Shimada K, Pickering TG. Factors associated with the occurrence and magnitude of earthquake-induced increases in blood pressure. *Am J Med* 2001;111:379-84

[36] Parati G, Antonicelli R, Guazzarotti F, Paciaroni E, Mancia G. Cardiovascular effects of an earthquake. Direct evidence by ambulatory blood pressure monitoring. *Hypertension* 2001;38:1093-5

[37] Rozanski A, Bairey CN, Krantz DS, Friedman J, Resser KJ, Morell M, et al. Mental stress and the induction of silent myocardial ischemia in patients with coronary artery disease. *N Engl J Med* 1988;318:1005-12

[38] Strike PC, Steptoe A. Systematic review of mental stress-induced myocardial infarction. *Eur Heart J* 2003;24:690-703

[39] Jiang W, Babyak M, Krantz DS, Waugh RA, Coleman RE, Hanson MM, et al. Mental stress-induced myocardial infarction ischemia and cardiac events. *JAMA* 1996;275:1651-6

[40] Sheps DS, MacMahon RP, Becker L, Carney RM, Freedland KE, Cohen JD, et al. Mental stress-induced ischemia and all-cause mortality in patients with coronary artery disease. Results from the Psychophysiological Investigations of Myocardial Ischemia Study. *Circulation* 2002;105:1780-4

[41] Blumenthal JA, Jiang W, Waugh RA, Frid DJ, Morris JJ, Coleman RE, et al. Mental stress-induced ischemia in the laboratory and ambulatory ischemia during daily life. *Circulation* 1995;92:2102-8

[42] Krantz DS, Sheps DS, Carney RM, Natelson BH. Effects of mental stress in patients with coronary artery disease. Evidence and clinical implications. *JAMA* 2000;283:1800-2

[43] Tomoda F, Takata M, Kagitani S, Kinuno H, Yasumoto K, Tomita S et al. Different platelet aggregability during mental stress in two stages of essential hypertension. *Am J Hypertens* 1999;12:1063-73

[44] Yeung AC, Vekshtein VI, Krantz DS, Vita JA, Ryan TJ Jr, Ganz P et al. The effect of atherosclerosis on the vasomotor response of coronary arteries to mental stress. *N Engl J Med* 1991;325:1551-6

[45] Spieker LE, Hürlimann D, Ruschitzka F, Corti R, Enseleit F, Shaw S et al. Mental stress induces prolonged endothelial dysfunction via endotlein-A receptors. *Circulation* 2001;105:2817-20

[46] Minami J, Kawano Y, Ishimitsu T, Yoshimi H, Takishita S. Effect of the Hanshin-Awaji earthquake on home blood pressure in patients with essential hypertension. *Am J Hypertens* 1997;10:222-5

[47] Lipsky SI, Pickering TG, Gerin W. World Trade Center disaster effect on blood pressure. *Blood Press Monit* 2002;7:249

[48] Esler M, Parati G. Is essential hypertension sometimes a psychosomatic disorder? *J Hypertens* 2004;22:873-6

[49] Jonas BS, Franks P, Ingram DD. Are symptoms of anxiety and depression risk factors for hypertension?: longitudinal evidence from the national health and nutrition examination survey, I: Epidemiologic Follow-up Study. *Arch Fam Med* 1997;6:43-9

[50] Davidson K, Jonas BS, Markovitz JH. Do depression symptoms predict early hypertension incidence in young adults in the CARDIA study? Coronary Artery Risk Development in Young Adults. *Arch Intern Med* 2000; 22:1495-500

[51] Markovitz JH, Matthews KA, Kannel WB, Cobb JL, D'Agostino RB. Psychological predictors of hypertension in the Framingham Study. Is there tension in hypertension? *JAMA* 1993;270:2439-43

[52] Raïkkönen K, Matthews KA, Kuller LH. Trajectory of psychological risk and incident hypertension in middle-aged women. *Hypertension* 2001;38:798-802

[53] Shapiro AP. *Hypertension and stress. Un unified concept*. Lawrence Erlbaum Associates, Mathwah, New Jersey, 1996.

[54] Johnson EH, Gentry WD, Julius S. *Personality, elevated blood pressure, and essential hypertension*. Hemisphere Publishing Corporation, Washington 1992.

[55] Ohira T, Iso H, Tanigawa T, Sankai T, Imano H, Kiyama M et al. The relation of anger expression with blood pressure levels and hypertension in rural and urban Japanese communities. *J Hypertens* 2002;20:21-7

[56] Pickering TG. Mental stress as a causal factor in the development of hypertension and cardiovascular disease. *Curr Hypertens Rep* 2001;3:249-54

[57] Knardhal S. Cardiovascular psychophysiology. *Ann Med* 2000;32:329-35

[58] Siegrist J, Peter R. Job stressors and coping characteristics in work-related disease: issues of validity. *Work & Stress* 1994;8:130-40

[59] Bosma H, Peter R, Siegrist J. Two alternative job stress models and the risk of coronary hear disease. *Am J Public Health* 1998;88:68-74

[60] Schnall PL, Pieper C, Schwartz JE, Karasek RA, Schlussel Y, Devereux RB et al. The relationship between 'job strain', workplace diastolic blood pressure, and left ventricular mass index. Results of a case-control study. *JAMA* 1990;263:1929-35

[61] Schnall PL, Schwartz JE, Landsbergis PA, Warren K, Pickering TG. *Hypertension* 1992;19:488-94

[62] Light KC, Turner JR, Hinderliter AL. Job strain and ambulatory work blood pressure in healthy young men and women. *Hypertension* 1992;20:214-8

[63] Cesana G, Ferrario M, Sega R, Milesi C, De Vito G, Mancha G et al. Job strain and ambulatory blood pressure levels in a population-based employed sample of men from northern Italy. *Scand J Work Environ Health* 1996;22:294-305

[64] Schnall PL, Schwartz JE, Landsbergis PA, Warren K, Pickering TG. A longitudinal study of job strain and ambulatory blood pressure: results from a three-year follow-up. *Psychosom Med* 1998;60:697-706

[65] Cesana G, Sega R, Ferrario M, Chiodini P, Corrao G, Mancia G. Job strain and blood pressure in employed men and women: a pooled analysis of four northern Italian population samples. *Psychosom Med* 2003;65:558-63

[66] Fauvel JP, Quelin P, Ducher M, Rakotomalala H, Laville M. Perceived job stress but not individual cardiovascular reactivity to stress is related to higher blood pressure at work. *Hypertension* 2001;38:71-5

[67] Fauvel JP, M'Pio I, Quelin P, Rigaud JP, Laville M, Ducher M. Neither perceived job stress nor individual cardiovascular reactivity predict high blood pressure. *Hypertension* 2003;42:1112-6

[68] Steptoe A, Roy MP, Evans O, Snashall D. Cardiovascular stress reactivity and job strain as determinants of ambulatory blood pressure at work. *J Hypertens* 1995;13:201-10

[69] Steptoe A, Willemsen G. The influence of low job control on ambulatory blood pressure and perceived stress over the working day in men and women from the Whitehall II cohort. *J Hypertens* 2004;22:915-20

[70] Steptoe A, Cropley M, Joekes K. Job strain, blood pressure and response to uncontrollable stress. *J Hypertens* 1999;17:193-200

[71] Steptoe A, Cropley M. Persistent high job demands and reactivity to mental stress predict future ambulatory blood pressure. *J Hypertens* 2000;18:581-6

[72] Hines EA, Brown GF. The cold pressor test for measuring the reactibility of the blood pressure: data concerning 571 normal and hypertensive subjects. *Am Heart J* 1936;11:1-9

[73] Hines EA. Range of normal blood pressure and subsequent development of hypertension: a follow-up of 1522 patients. *JAMA* 1940;115:271-8

[74] Brod J, Fencl V, Jirka J. Circulatory changes underlying blood pressure elevation during acute emotional stress (mental arithmetic) innormotensive and hypertensive subjects. *Clin Sci* 1959;18:269-79

[75] Brod J. Haemodynamic basis of acute pressor reactions and hypertension. *Br Heart J* 1963;25:227-45

[76] Manuck SB, Schaefer DC. Stability of individual differences in cardiovascular reactivity. *Physiology&Behavior* 1978;21:675-8

[77] Manuck SB, Garland FN. Stability of individual differences in cardiovascular reactivity: a thirteen month follow-up. *Physiology&Behavior* 1980;24:621-4

[78] Langewitz W, Rüddel H, Noack H, Wachtarz K. The reliability of psychological examinations under field conditions: results of repetitive mental stress testing in middle-aged men. *Eur Heart J* 1989;10:657-65

[79] Armario P, Hernandez del Rey R, Castellsagué J, Torres G, Navarro LA, Pardell H. Reproducibility of two mental stress tasks in subjects with borderline or mild hipertensión. *Am J Hypertens* 1995;8:84A

[80] Jern S, Wall U, Bergbrant A. Long-term stability of cardiovascular reactivity to mental stress in borderline hypertension. *Am J Hypertens* 1995;8:20-8

[81] Veit R, Brody S, Rau H. Four-year stability of cardiovascular reactivity to psychological stress. *J Behav Med* 1997;20:447-60

[82] Kamarck TW, Jennings JR, Debski TT, Glickman-Weiss E, Johnson PS, Eddy MJ et al. *Psychophysiology* 1992;29:17-28

[83] Pickering TG, Gerin W. Cardiovascular reactivity in the laboratory and the role of behavioural factors in hypertension: a critical review. *Ann Behav Med* 1990;12:3-16

[84] Gerin W, Pickering TG, Glynn L, Christenfeld N, Schwartz A, Carroll D, et al. An historical context for behavioural models of hypertension. *J Psychosom Resech* 2000;48:369-77

[85] Fredeerikson M, Matthews KA. Cardiovascular responses to behavioural stress and hypertension: a meta-analytic review. *Ann Behav Med* 1990;12:30-39

[86] Lucini D, Norbiato G, Clerici M, Pagani M. Hemodynamic and autonomic adjustements to real life stress conditions in humans. *Hypertension* 2002;39:184-8

[87] Adler PSJ, Ditto B. Psychophysiological effect of interviews about emotional events on offspring of hypertensive and normotensives. *Int J Psychophysiol* 1998;28:263-71

[88] Armario P, Hernández del Rey R, Torres G, Martin-Baranera M, Almendros MC, Pardell H. Relationship between cardiovascular reactivity to mental stress and early target-organ damage in untreated mild hypertension In Spanish). *Med Clin* (Barc) 1999;113:401-6

[89] Fichera LV, Andreassi JL. Cardiovascular reactivity during public speaking is a function of personality variables. *Int J Psychophysiol* 2000;37:267-73

[90] Saab PG, Llabre MM, Ma M, DiLillo V, McCalla JR, Fernander-Scott A et al. Cardiovascular responsivity to stress in adolescents with and without persistenly elevated blood pressure. *J Hypertens* 2001;19:21-7

[91] Hamer M, Boutcher Y, Boutcher SH. Cardiovascular and renal responses to mental challenge in highly and moderately active males with a family history of hypertension. *J Human Hypertens* 2002;16:319-26

[92] Sherwood A, Allen MT, Murell D, Obrist PA, Langer AW. Evaluation of betaadrenergic, influences on cardiovascular and metabolic adjustments to physical and psychological stress. *Psychophysiology* 1986;23:89-104

[93] Dimsdale JE, Moss J. Plasma catecholamines in stress and exercise. *JAMA* 1980;243:340-2

[94] Bedi M, Varshney VP, Babbar R. Role of cardiovascular reactivity to mental stress in predicting future hypertension. *Clin Exp Hypertens* 2000;22:1-22

[95] Parati G, Trazzi S, Ravogli A, Casadei R, Omboni S, Mancia G. Methodological problems in evaluation of cardiovascular effects of stress in humans. *Hypertension* 1991;17(suppl III):50-55

[96] Mattews KA, Owens JF, Allen MT, Stoney CM. Do cardiovascular responses to laboratory stress relate to ambulatory blood pressure levels?: Yes, in some of the people, some of the time. *Psychosom Med* 1992;54:686-97

[97] Linden W, Con A. Laboratory reactivity models as predictors of ambulatory blood pressure and heart rate. *J Psychosom Res* 1994;38:217-28

[98] Armario P, Hernández del Rey R, Pont F, Alonso A, Tresserrras R, Pardell H. Blood pressure response to mental stress in young subjects with high or slightly high blood pressure. Does it reflect the changes in blood pressure observed during out patient monitorization? (in Spanish). *Med Clin* (Barc) 1994;102:647-51

[99] Sherwood A, Gullette ECD, Hinderliter AL, Georgiades A, Babyak M, Waught RA et al. Relationship of clinic, ambulatory, and laboratory stress blood pressure to left ventricular mass in overweight men and women with high blood pressure. *Psychosom Med* 2002;64:247-57

[100] Al'Absi M, Devereux RB, Lewis CE, Kitzman DW, Rao DC, Hopkins P, et al. Blood pressure responses to acute stress and left ventricular mass (The Hypertension Genertic Epidemiology Network Study). *Am J Cardiol* 2002;89:536-40

[101] Manuck SB, Kasprowitz AL, Muldoon MF. Behaviorally-evoked cardiovascular reactivity and hypertension: Conceptual issues and potential associations. *Ann Behav Med* 1990;12:17-29

[102] Falkner B, Kushner H, Onesti G, Angelakos ET. Cardiovascular characteristics in adolescents who develop essential hypertension. *Hypertension* 1981;3:521-7

[103] Borghi C, Costa FV, Boschi S, Muchi A, Ambrosioni E. Predictors of stable hipertensión in young borderline subjects: A five-year follow-up study. *J Cardiovasc Pharmacol* 1986;8(Suppl 5): S138-S141

[104] Borghi C, Costa FV, Boschi S, Bacchelli S, Degli ED, Piccoli M et al. Factors associated with the development of stable hypertension in young borderline hypertensives. *J Hypertens* 1996;14:509-17

[105] Light KC, Dolan CA, Davis MR, Sherwood A. Cardiovascular responses to an active coping challenge as a predictors of blood pressure patterns 10 to 15 years later. *Psychosom Med* 1992;54:217-30

[106] Murphy JK, Alpert BS, Walker SS. Ethnicity, pressor reactivity, and children's blood pressure: five years of observation. *Hypertension* 1992; 20:327-32

[107] Matthews KA, Woodall KL, Allen MT. Cardiovascular reactivity to stress predicts future blood pressure status. *Hypertension* 1993;22:479-85

[108] Caroll D, Smith GD, Sheffield D, Shipley MJ, Marmot MG. Pressor reactions to psychological stress and prediction of future blood pressure: data from the Withehall II Study. *BMJ* 1995;310:771-6

[109] Markowitz JH, Raczynski JM; Wallace D, Chettur V, Chesney MA. Cardiovascular reactivity to video game predicts subsequente blood pressure increases in young men: the Cardia Study. *Psychosom Med* 1998;60:186-91

[110] Newman JD, McGarvey ST, Steele MS. Longitudinal association of cardiovascular reactivity and blood pressure in Samoan adolescents. *Psychosom Med* 1999;61:243-9

[111] Light KC, Girdler SS, Sherwood A, Bragdon EE, Brownley KA, West SG et al. High stress responsivity predicts later blood pressure only in combination with positive family history and high life stress. *Hypertension* 1999;33:1458-64

[112] Knox SS, Hausdorff J, Markovitz JH. Reactivity as a predictor of subsequent blood pressure. Racial differences in the Coronary Artery Risk Development in Young Adults (CARDIA) Study. *Hypertension* 2002;40:914-9

[113] Armario P, Hernandez del Rey H, Martín-Baranera M, Almendros MC, Ceresuela LM, Pardell H. Blood pressure reactivity to mental stress task as a determinant of sustained hipertensión after 5 years of follow-up. *J Hum Hypertens* 2003;17:181-6

[114] Mormede. Genetic influences on the responses to psychosocial challenges in rats. *Acta Physiol Scand* 1997;161(suppl 640):65-8

[115] Ely D, Caplea A, Dunphy G, Smith D. Physiological and neuroendocrine correlates of social position in normotensive and hypertensive rat colonies. *Acta Physiol Scand* 1997;161(suppl 640):92-95

[116] Gerin W, Pickering TG. Association between delayed recovery of blood pressure after acute mental stress and parental history of hypertension. *J Hypertens* 1995;13:603-10

[117] Schuler JL, O'Brien WH. Cardiovascular recovery from stress snf hypertension risk factors: a meta-analytic review. *Psychophysiology* 1997;34:649-59

[118] Jokiniitty JM, Tuomisto MT, Mahahalme SK, Kähönen NAP, Turjanmaa SK. Pulse pressure responses to psychological tasks improve the prediction of left ventricular mass: 10 years of follow-up. *J Hypertens* 2003;21:789-95

In: Stress and Health: New Research
Editor: Kimberly V. Oxington, pp. 61-79

ISBN 1-59454-244-9
©2005 Nova Science Publishers, Inc.

Chapter III

OF STRESS, MICE AND MEN: A RADICAL APPROACH TO OLD PROBLEMS

Rubina Mian[1], Graeme McLaren[2] and David W. Macdonald[2]

[1] Department of Physiology & Bioscience, School of Science & Environment, Coventry University, Cox St, Coventry CV1 5FB, U.K.
[2] Wildlife Conservation Research Unit, Department of Zoology, Oxford University, South Parks Road, Oxford OX1 3PS

ABSTRACT

The tremendous destructive capabilities of reactive oxygen species in stress related disorders has become apparent only recently, although in early historical times the ancients may have been aware of the devastating power of stress on well-being. This chapter explores ancient myths and modern techniques surrounding stress-induced immunosupression in species as diverse as mice and humans, investigating techniques and mechanisms, and speculating on possible therapeutic interventions.

CURSES AND PLAGUES: FACT OR FICTION?

A modern idiom speaks of people making themselves sick with worry. As with so many aphorisms that are casually used, this linkage of stress and illness embodies a deep truth, a truth that may already have been familiar to the ancients.

It is an archaeological fact that most tombs of the Pharaohs had a curse written above the door, to deter intruders, warning that whoever opened or entered the tomb would die.

'Death will slay with his wings whoever disturbs the peace of the Pharaoh.' (Budge 2001)

For centuries such curses have been dismissed as superstitious nonsense, but recent evidence shows that unwittingly or otherwise, the ancient Egyptians had harnessed a powerful tool: danger whether real or perceived can have devastating effect psychology can have on the immune system. Psychological stress may reduce the effectiveness of the immune system, thus increasing the risk of infection or disease (Dhabhar et al., 1996; Kang et al., 1996). The ancient Egyptians may have in fact been familiar with this. In 1999 the German microbiologist Gotthard Kramer analysed 40 mummies and found them contaminated with several varieties of potentially dangerous mould spores, which when exposed to air and a suppressed immune system could have caused fatal illness (Viegas 1999).

It is also tempting to speculate that the plague of boils mentioned in Book of Exodus 9:8-12, in the Old Testament, the sixth plague to hit Egypt would have been exacerbated by the psychological endured by those who had already experienced plagues of blood, gnats, flies and diseases of livestock. The psychological stress would have burdened only the Pharaoh and his people, thus automatically excluding those who firmly they were divinely protected.

Stress and Disease

Epidemiological studies show that those individuals who are more psychologically stressed are more prone to opportunistic infections (Clover 1989; Galinowski, 1997). For example stress associated with family dysfunction is significantly associated with increased incidence of upper respiratory tract infection and influenza B (Clover 1989) and work-related stress results in DNA damage in female workers (Irie 2001). Similarly persistent stress in elite athletes has been associated with chronic immunosupression and hence susceptibility to opportunistic infections (for review see Gleeson 2000). In animal models of stress, the spread of *Candida albicans* (an opportunistic fungal disease) is greater in stressed rats than non-stressed animals (Rodriguez et al., 2001). Results from studies associating psychological stress with an increased cancer are contradictory: some suggest an increased risk of developing cancer in those exposed to psychological stress (Irie et al 2001) others support no such link (Johansen et al 1998)and most are inconclusive (Kiecolt-Glaser 1999). Overall psychological and behavioural factors may well influence the progression of cancer through psychosocial influences on immune function.

Current Measures of Stress

Objective, quantitative and practicable measures of stress are pivotal to studies in many branches of vertebrate biology, including animal welfare (e.g. Dawkins, 1980; Bateson & Bradshaw, 1997). The stress response in animals is currently assessed using a variety of techniques, including cortisol measurement (e.g. Palme & Möstl, 1997; Creel, 2001), haematological values (e.g. Millspaugh et al., 2000) and behavioural observations (reviewed by Rushen, 2000). We have recently reported a novel technique to measure the stress response (McLaren et al., 2003), based on the capacity of circulating neutrophils to produce reactive oxygen species in response to an external stimulus..

Neutrophils as Indicators of Stress

Neutrophils can respond rapidly to a wide range of physical and psychological stressors, and these responses can affect the ability of the immune system to react to ongoing or potential challenge (Maes *et al* 1999; Dhabhar *et al.*, 1995; Gleeson & Bishop, 2000). Stress has been shown to influence the number, distribution and activation of neutrophils in the blood in a rapid and reversible manner (Dhabhar *et al.* 1995; Goebel & Mills, 2000; Ellard *et al.*, 2001; McLaren *et al.*, 2003; Montes *et al.*, 2003; Mian *et al.*, 2003). One component of the response of neutrophils to stress is the release of reactive oxygen species (Mian *et al.*, 2003; Montes *et al.*, in press). This response is strictly controlled; only a subpopulation of neutrophils is activated, and the size of the subpopulation is related to the intensity of the stressor (Montes *et al.*, in press).

Leukocyte Coping Capacity: Stress Revealed from a Drop of Blood

Leukocytes are exposed to diverse factors: endocrine factors in the plasma, changes in blood biochemistry, changes in red cell haemodynamics, cytokines and factors released from other cells both circulating and non-circulating cells such as endothelial cells and changes in the hypothalamic-pituitary-adrenal axis and the sympathetic nervous system. As stress affects each of these factors, leukocytes make ideal indicators of stress, being constantly exposed to a diverse range of stress stimuli.

We have used this fact to develop a novel approach to measuring stress. In summary, after a potentially stressful event, the capacity of circulating leukocytes to produce reactive oxygen species *in vitro* in response to challenge by phorbol myristate acetate (PMA) is measured, a measure called Leukocyte Coping Capacity (LCC). LCC is affected directly and rapidly by stress and the strengths of this technique, is: (1) the method can be used on whole blood (avoiding centrifugation); (2) it yields results within minutes and does not require baseline data from animals which have not been stressed and (3) it is practical to use in a wide variety of situations. Whole blood is used instead of fractionated centrifuged leukocyte subsets, as the primary aim is to produce a measure of cell activation that minimises *in vitro* manipulation of fresh blood, and to reflect as far as possible the *in vivo* condition of the cells. This method is of particular use in situations where a rapid assessment of the individual's ability to cope is required. The term LCC is used since a wide range of immune cells can respond to PMA, although neutrophils are responsible for most of the PMA response (Mian *et al.*, 2003), and represent the majority of leukocytes in the circulation. The aim of this chapter is to elucidate the mechanisms involved in the science underpinning this novel measure of stress.

The Leukocyte Coping Capacity reveals significant information about an animal's physiological status during and after stressful events (McLaren *et al.*, 2003). We have used it to demonstrate that even short-term psychological stressors can produce demonstrable physiological changes in neutrophil activation (Figure 1; Ellard *et al.*, 2001; McLaren *et al.*, 2003; Montes *et al.*, 2003; Mian *et al.*, 2003; Montes *et al.*, in press). For example, as a model for studying stress we used wild badgers (*Meles meles*) that were trapped and transported (10 minutes on a trailer pulled by an all-terrain quad bike) as part of a long-term ecological and behavioural study (Macdonald & Newman, 2002). Badgers that had been transported showed, in comparison to badgers that had not been transported, changes in circulating cell numbers and composition that were indicative of stress (McLaren *et al.*, 2003), and their circulating neutrophils showed a reduced responsiveness to PMA (McLaren *et al.*, 2003; Figure 1).

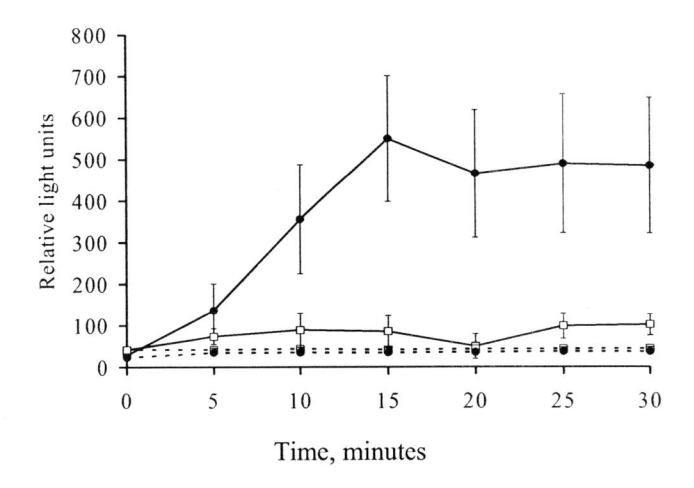

Figure 1 The response of circulating neutrophils to PMA (10^{-6} mol l^{-1}) stimulation in transported (lower solid line, n=8) and non-transported (upper solid line, n=8) badgers. Dashed lines represent unstimulated leukocyte activity levels (without PMA). The release of reactive oxygen species (measured here in relative light units) in response to PMA stimulation is much reduced by transport stress. That is LCC is diminished (McLaren *et al.* 2003).

The Importance of Reactive Oxygen Species

Reactive oxygen species (ROS) have an important role in immune defence, but can also potentially damage healthy tissue and organs (Weiss, 1989; Boxer & Smolen, 1998) and the activation of neutrophils is potentially detrimental to health (Weiss, 1989). Activated neutrophils and other phagocytic leukocytes can take up oxygen and make a range of ROS, such as O_2^-, H_2O_2 and $OH\cdot$, and these oxygen metabolites are potent microbicidal agents (Figure 2; Bokoch 2002). The potential for ROS to cause cellular damage is perhaps best demonstrated by the extensive antioxidant defence systems that are possessed by cells (Halliwell 1996; Kruidenhier & Verspaget 2002). Atanackovic et al., also reported (2003) reported that acute psychological stress reduced the capacity of human phagocytic leukocytes to produce basal levels of ROS. PMA used by McLaren et al (2003) measures the *capacity* of circulating neutrophils to release reactive oxygen species. Stress-induced immune alterations occur more or less in parallel to increases in hormonal & immunological markers of cells (Atanackovic et al 2003) but immune alterations remained long after these traditional measures of stress (changes in heart rate and blood pressure) had returned to basal values (Mian *et al.* 2003).

WATCHING A HORROR FILM: STRESS BY PROXY

Even short-term psychological stressors can produce demonstrable physiological changes in heart rate, blood pressure and the activation of neutrophils (Ellard *et al.,* 2001; Goebel 2000). Activated neutrophils release many mediators, which can potentially damage even healthy tissue and organs, so this activation of neutrophils is potentially detrimental to health (Weiss, 1989; Weiss *et al.,* 1989; Boxer *et al.,* 1998). The many biologically active compounds released by neutrophils when they are activated include: cationic proteins, myeloperoxidase, lysozyme, acid hydrolases, lactoferrin (an iron-binding protein), B12-binding protein, cytochrome b and collagenase (Abramson, 1993).

Individuals who are more psychologically stressed are more prone to opportunistic infections (Clover 1989; Galinowski, 1997).

Acute psychological stressors have also been shown to increase the number of circulating leukocytes, and significantly to affect erythron variables such as haematocrit, mean cell haemoglobin content and the number of red blood cells (Maes *et al* 1998).

Psychological stress comes in many guises. Some individuals deliberately expose themselves to a form of psychological stress by watching horror movies.

There have been no reported studies on the effect such a 'passive stressor' has on leukocyte activation. We asked whether passive observation of a stressful event, namely witnessing an emotionally disturbing movie, would result in leukocyte mobilisation and activation. The aim of this study was thus to investigate the effect of *observing* a stressful event, albeit fictitious, on leukocyte distribution and activation in otherwise healthy human subjects.

Blood samples were obtained from 32 healthy male and female subjects aged between 20-26 years before, during and after either watching an 83-minute horror film that none of the subjects had previously seen (The Texas Chainsaw Massacre, 1974) or by sitting quietly in a room (control group). Total differential cell counts, leukocyte activation as measured by the nitroblue tetrazolium test, heart rate and blood pressure measurements were taken at defined time points.

There were statistically significant increases in peripheral circulating leukocytes, the number of activated circulating leukocytes, haemoglobin concentration and haematocrit in response to the stressor (Mian *et a*l 2003). These were accompanied by significant increases in heart rate, systolic and diastolic blood pressure. The study reveals the importance of the perception of stress. Watching a psychosocial stressful event that by definition has no objective effect on survival can thus affect immune reactivity.

The role of the psychobiological characteristics of the individual has been shown to be an important in the response to stress, for example Interleukin -1 (an indicator of stress) production is greater in right than in left-pawed mice (Neveu 2003).

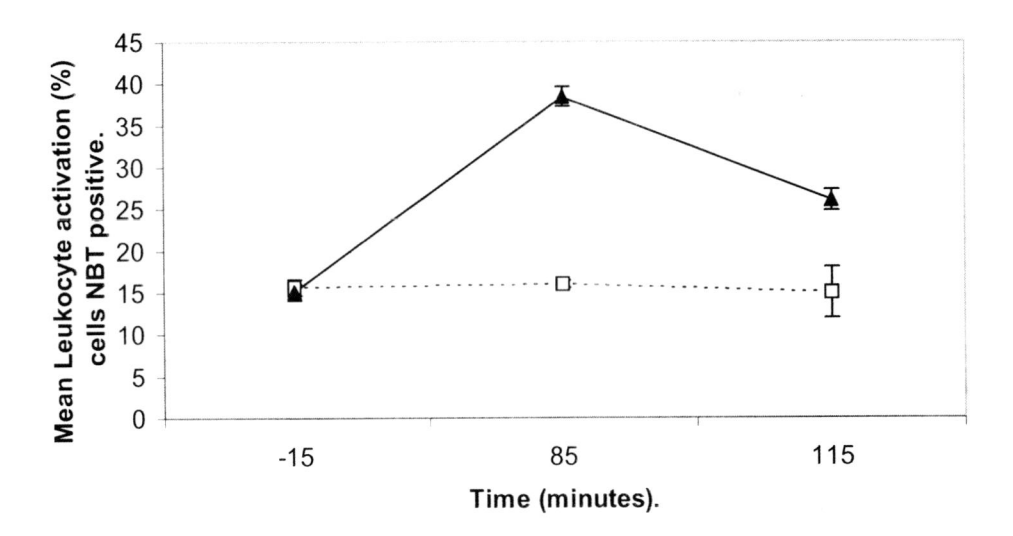

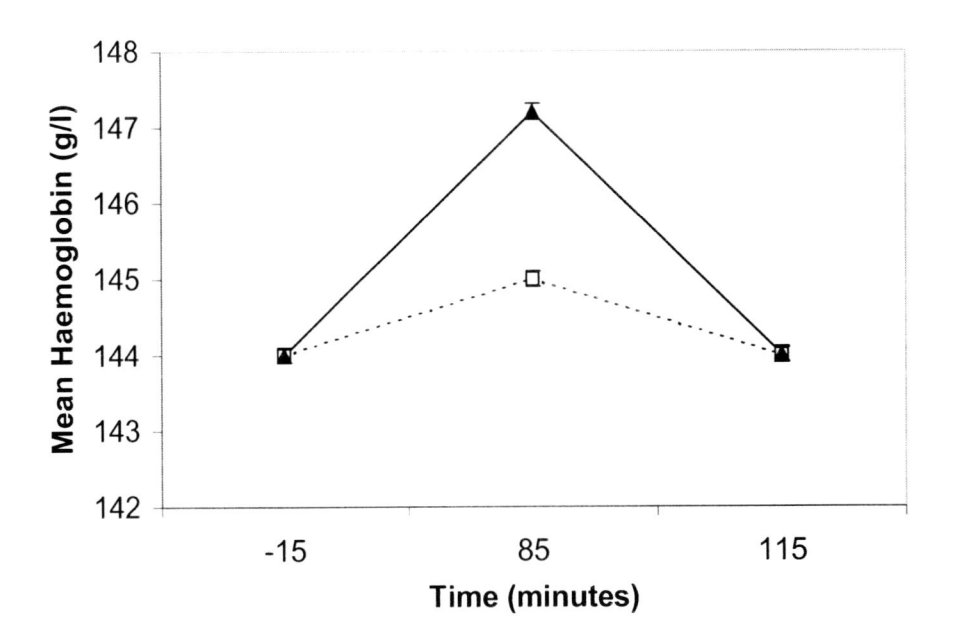

Figure 2. continued on next page

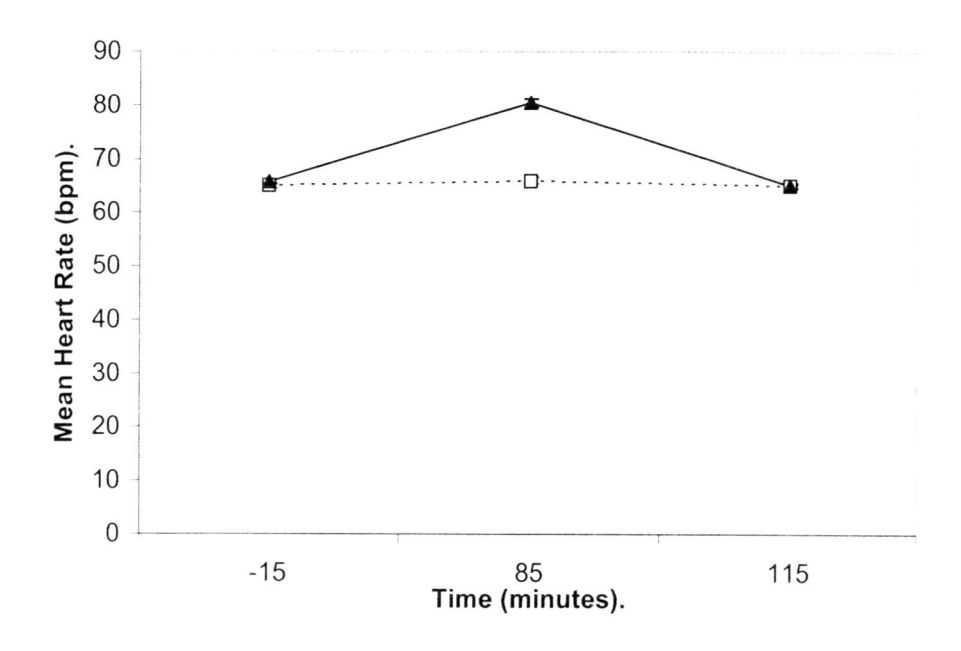

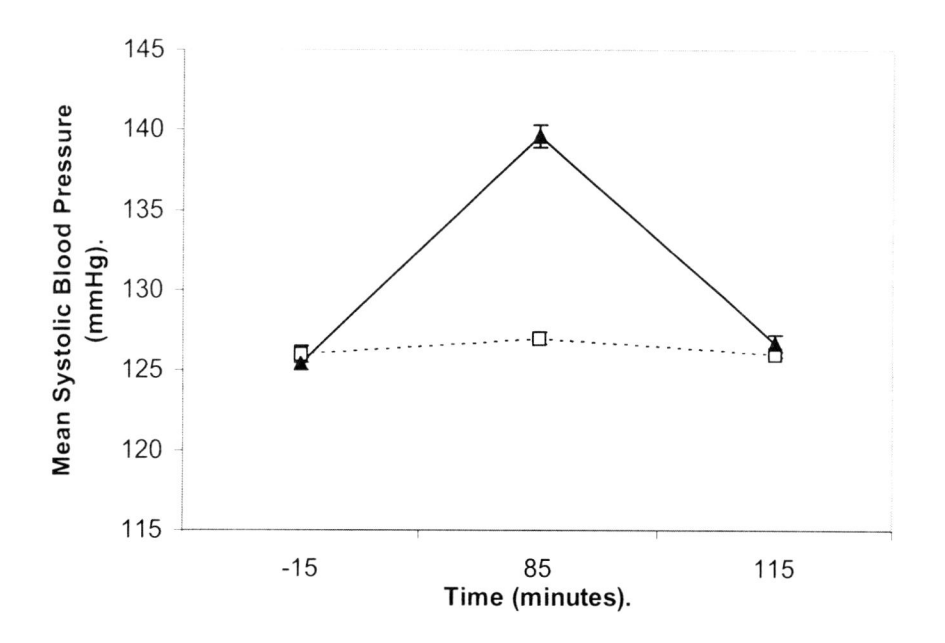

Of Stress, Mice and Men: A Radical Approach to Old Problems

Figure 2. continued on next page

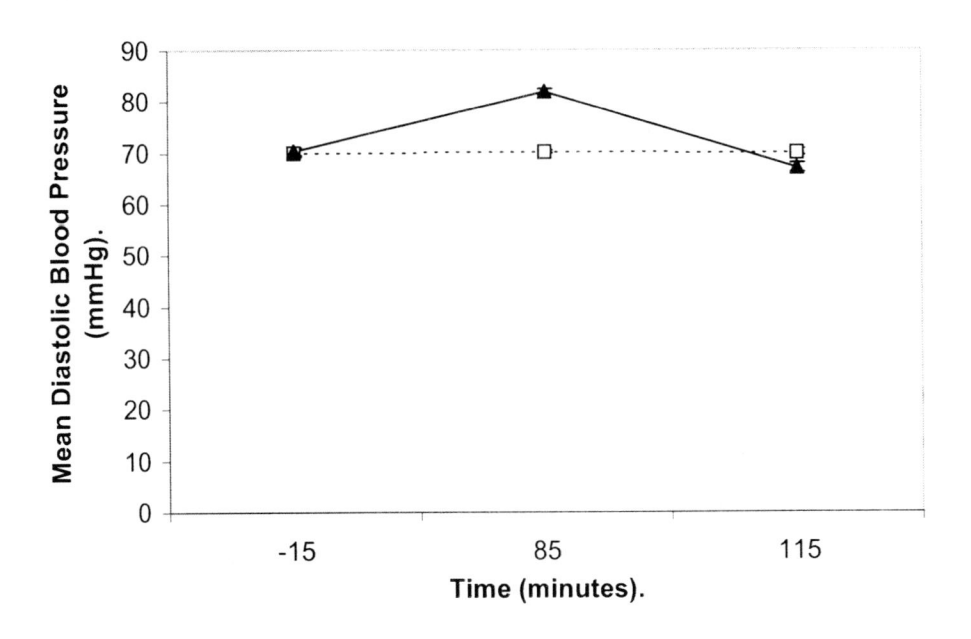

Figure 2. Haematological Variables: The effect of watching a horror film on subjects Open squares represents mean ± SEM from 16 control subjects Closed triangles represents mean ± SEM from subjects exposed to the horror film for all graphs.

The Mechanisms Involved

Watching a horror movie elicited psycho- physiological arousal which was comparable to Canon's fear –flight- fight- defence reaction, the so called 'stress response' which involves stimulation of the hypothalamus (Canon 1932; Folklaw 1982), a change in peripheral resistance (Brod 1972) and an increase in the release of stress hormones including catecholamines and cortisol (Seyle 1946) and increases in haematocrit and haemoglobin concentration (Maes et al., 1998).

The increase in the numbers of circulating leukocytes during the horror film is comparable to that reported by others. Changes in circulating cell numbers reflects the cell trafficking between reservoir sites including the liver, lungs, spleen, bone marrow and peripheral blood (Cruse 1995). This process is modified by receptors (Hou 1996; Ley 1996) on both the endothelium (P-selectin; Intracellular Adhesion Molecule-1; Vascular cell Adhesion Molecule-1) and leukocytes (L-selectin; integrins and P-Selectin Glycoprotein Ligand-1 PSGL-1). Modification of the receptors on either the endothelial cells or leukocytes can also dramatically alter the number of adherent (and thus the number of free flowing) leukocytes (Ley 1995; 1996).

PSGL-1 is constitutively expressed on all lymphocytes, monocytes, eosinophils and neutrophils Ley 1997. PSGL-1 has a glycosylation pattern enabling it to bind to endothelial P-selectin (Ley 1997). This interaction results in the margination of the leukocytes, which is the process by which leukocytes exit the central blood stream, and initiate mechanical contact with the endothelial cells (Cruse et al.,1995).

The margination process is enhanced in vessels of a particular size by the aggregation of erythrocytes, which tend to occupy the centre of microvessels and thus promote margination (Firrell et al., 1989). The increase in haematocrit and haemoglobin concentration observed in this and previous studies (Maes et al., 1998) could thus selectively promote margination in some vessels. Previous studies have demonstrated that margination of leukocytes is not a uniform process, and occurs in particular sized vessels within the microcirculation (Mian et al., 1993). In larger- sized vessels it is possible that the shear stress of flowing blood might be sufficient to dislodge marginated leukocytes, thus increasing the numbers of free-flowing leukocytes. The changes in shear stress likely to have been brought about by the increased haemoconcentration may also serve as a trigger mechanism for leukocyte activation (Schmid-Schonbeim et al., 2001).

It has been recognised for some time that physiological stressors such as exercise induce leukocytosis from marginal pools (Shephard & Shek, 1996; Gleeson et al., 1998). Current literature indicates that exposure to hostile conditions or other psychological stressors initiates the secretion of several hormones, including cortisol, catecholamines, prolactin, oxytocin and renin (Van de Kar & Blair, 1999; Toft et al., 1994)), any of which could alter adhesion receptors on circulating leukocytes and thus contribute to their altered distribution. Stimuli such as adrenaline that disrupt this process (Iversen et al., 1993) and increase the circulating numbers of leukocytes. Recent studies by Maes et al. (1999) have revealed that an increase in the levels of pro-inflammatory cytokines, such as interleukin-6 and tumour necrosis factor, result in the demargination of some leukocytes. It is thus possible that the stress -induced production of adrenaline and cytokines could orchestrate the increased numbers of leukocytes within the general circulation.

Non-physical stressors have now also been shown to influence the number and distribution of leukocytes in the blood. Kang et al., (1996, 1997) and Dhabhar (1996) reported that the mental stress of academic examinations stimulated increases in the number and distribution of leukocytes. These changes were found to be both rapid and reversible.

Nitroblutetrazolium (NBT) reduction is a measure of cell activation which minimises in vitro manipulation of fresh blood, and reflects the in vivo condition of the cells. Recent studies have demonstrated that the NBT reduction assay is a reliable measure of the activation of neutrophils in whole blood (Takase et al., 1999; Delano et al., 1997). Wikstrom et al., (1996) demonstrated a highly significant linear relationship between the % NBT – positive cells and chemiluminescence measurements of the same cell suspensions with and without chemical stimulation, supporting the idea that the NBT-test accurately measures oxidative metabolism. Thus the significant increase in the number of Nitroblue tetrazolium leukocytes after watching the horror film reflects an increase in the numbers of activated leukocytes. Activation of leukocytes has been reported by Kang et al., (1996) who found that superoxidase production in neutrophils increased in those undertaking examinations.

The Pathophysiological Consequences of Stress by Proxy

In a broader context, the pathophysiological relevance of the changes observed need to be explored. If the human mind cannot discriminate observation of fictional stressful situations from personal psychological experience, then the results have implications for anyone witnessing a stressful event. Witnessing a stressful event could well be sufficient to alter the number and activation state of circulating leukocytes. Indeed the percentage of activated leukocytes remained high even though many of the other variables such as the number of circulating leukocytes and haematocrit and haemoglobin concentration had returned to basal (pre-stress) values. In this state of activation, leukocytes are primed and ready for action. If however the leukocytes actually release the contents of their granules, then there will be a period of time, a 'window of opportunity', in which they will not be able to respond to opportunistic infections, having already degranulated. Such leukocytes would be unable to respond to opportunistic infections thus rendering the host more susceptible to disease, as well as to potential tissue damage from a host of proteolytic enzymes and oxygen free radicals.

Unlike other cardiovascular and immune measurements, leukocyte activation was sustained for at least 20 minutes after the stress exposure, suggesting that this condition of the leukocytes is not rapidly reversible. The potential long-term effects of repeatedly watching such horror films remain unknown.

In an era where television and other electronic media rapidly transmit real and fictitious events into our homes, the effects of exposure to such stressors deserve evaluation. Witnessing a stressful event may have serious physiological consequences for the health of the observer. With sufficient exposure to psychological stress is it possible that an observer actually becomes a victim by proxy?

A Working Model of Neutrophil Behaviour in Response to Stress: the Key Players

Neutrophils are responsible for most of the ROS production seen in the blood samples (McLaren *et al.* 2003, Mian *et al.* 2003) A model of the interactions between neutrophils and other components of the stress response is outlined in Figure 3 and discussed below.

Plasma Factors

Stress causes the release of stress hormones including cortisol and adrenaline. A host of stress-related endocrine and non-endocrine plasma borne factors could potentially modify the sensitivity of circulating neutrophils to PMA and control their level of activation. For example, neutrophil behaviour, including ROS, is modified by both cortisol (e.g. Kurogi & Iida, 2002) and catecholamines (e.g. Bergmann & Sautner, 2002; Benschop 1999).

Cytokines

Non-endocrine plasma-borne factors could also potentially control the response of neutrophils in response to stress. In particular the cytokines IL- 1 & IL- 6, which are known to be released from activated endothelial cells, are known to affect neutrophil accumulation and activation(e.g. Joseph *et al.*, 1992). Also, IL- 8 is an important chemo-attractant for neutrophils and can also play a role in the production of ROS (McPhail & Harvath, 1993), and thus may play an important role in the recruitment and activation of neutrophils during stress.

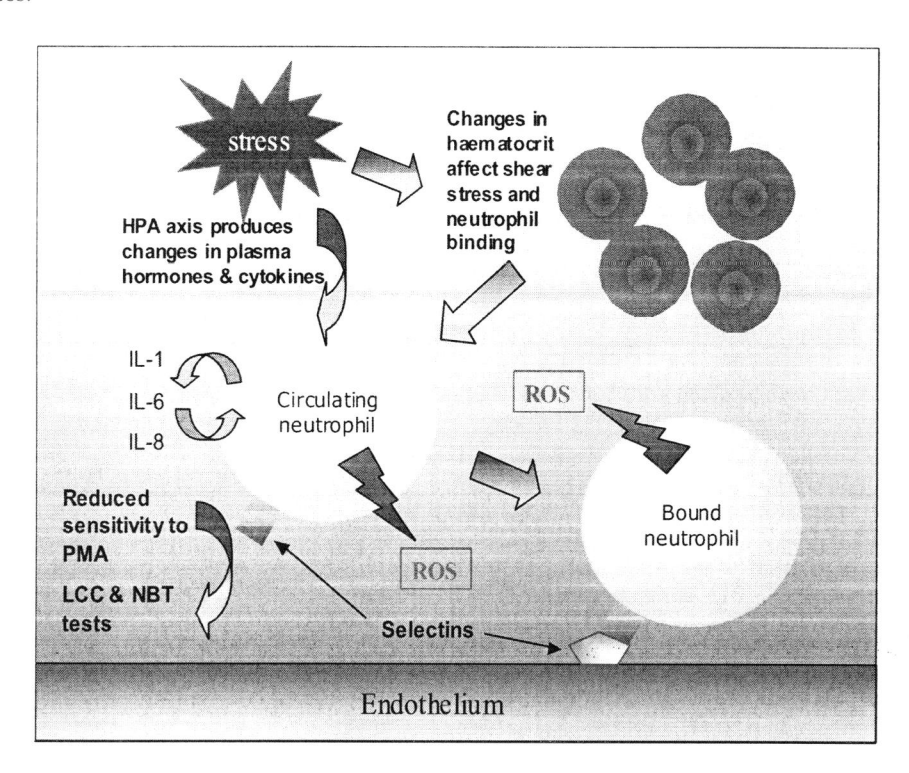

Figure 3.

Glutamine

Other factors that are important for neutrophil function, such as glutamine (Furukawa et al., 1997; 2000; Pithon-Curi et al., 2002) and glucose (Furukawa et al., 2000), could also affect the response of neutrophils to stress. In the case of glutamine, there is evidence to support the notion that glutamine depletion is related to immunosuppression in athletes (Castell & Newsholme 2001; Castell 2002).

Neutrophil-Endothelial Cell Interactions

The adhesion of neutrophils to the endothelium is another important component of neutrophil activation during stress (Jean et al., 1998; Figure 3) and modification of the receptors on either the endothelial cells or neutrophils can dramatically alter the number of adherent (and thus the number of free flowing) neutrophils and the distribution of leukocyte subsets (Ley, 1996; Maes 1999). Endothelial and neutrophil derived adhesion molecules serve important roles in properly orienting neutrophils temporally and spatially for activation along the endothelium (Park & Lucchesi, 1999;). Important regulators in this process are

TNFa, and ICAM-1. TNFa upregulates ICAM-1, which leads to increased neutrophil-endothelium interaction (Menger et al., 1999). The selectin family of adhesion molecules, which includes E- and L- selectin, mediate the first contact of neutrophils with the endothelium. (Ley, 1996). E- selectin is expressed on the surface of endothelial cells and L-selectin is expressed on the surface of neutrophils. L- selectin can also influence the production of reactive oxygen species (Nagahata et al., 2000). Furthermore, changes in shear stress, such as those brought about by stress related increases in red blood cell numbers, can modify neutrophil adhesion behaviour (Sheikh et al., 2003).

In summary stress-induced changes in leukocyte activation reflect changes occurring in the local environment.

THE COST OF IMMUNOSUPPRESSION: RESOURCE LIMITATION OR SELF PROTECTION?

The adaptive significance of immunosuppression is hypothesised to be related to either resource limitation or for self-protection through the avoidance of immunopathology (Råberg et al. 1998). The resource limitation hypothesis predicts that immunosuppression occurs so that energy and nutrients can be temporarily shifted away from the immune system and diverted into cells and tissues that are directly required to cope with the stressor. In this model there is a resource-based trade-off between the immune system and the costly behaviours associated with coping with the stressor. The extent of immunosuppression is thus predicted to be related to the intensity of the stressor and the condition of the animal.

The self-protection hypothesis predicts that the immune system is suppressed in order to protect the organism from 'hyperstimulation' of the immune system (Råberg et al. 1998). Some components of the immune system are activated by stress: for example some leukocytes (particularly neutrophils) can become activated and release oxygen free radicals (Mian et al. 2003; Montes et al. 2003; Montes et al. in press). Oxygen free radicals are potentially damaging to the host organism, costly to produce, and damage the activated leukocyte in the process of their release (Halliwell & Gutteridge 2000. Although the two hypotheses to explain immunosuppression are not mutually exclusive, they do make different predictions regarding the nature of stress-induced immunosupression.

There is considerable evidence that investment in the immune system is, in non-stress situations, dependent upon an animal's condition and nutritional status. For example, male Belding's ground squirrels (*Spermophilus beldingi*) that received a food supplement had a leukocyte count three times greater then control males (Bachman 2003). Furthermore, glutamine, an important fuel for immune cells (Castell 2002; Castell & Newsholme 2001), is known to enhance PMA- induced oxygen free radical production in neutrophils (Pithon-Curi et al. 2002). Low plasma glutamine is associated with a decrease in the functional ability of immune cells (Castell & Newsholme 2001) and in humans glutamine levels in the blood are decreased after prolonged, exhaustive exercise (Castell 2002).

To test the predictions of the two hypotheses. We subjected wild small mammals (woodmice Apodemus sylvaticus and bank voles Clethrionomys glareolus) to one of two treatments: handling (stressor) and non-handling(McLaren et al. submitted). We then measured the ability of animals' circulating leukocytes to produce oxygen free radicals in response to PMA challenge: the leukocyte coping capacity (LCC). Handling suppressed the LCC response, both in magnitude and variability. Heavier non-handled animals had a greater peak LCC, but this was not the case in handled animals, contrary to the predictions of the resource hypothesis. The self-protection hypothesis also failed to predict the observed variation we found in LCC in handled animals.

During an immune response, leukocytes are activated to produce oxygen free radicals during a stressful event, and this most likely occurs to prepare the body for physical damage and perhaps infiltration by bacteria (Mian 2003). In evolutionary terms it is tempting to speculate that stress would generally be linked to a fight or aggression that may lead to physical injury, thus the release of oxygen free radicals may be a 'pre-emptive strike' anticipating injuries and associated bacterial infection.

Once sufficient oxygen free radicals have been released it is possible that other mechanisms ensure that further production is suppressed to protect the body from physical damage. This model needs further investigation, in particular studies relating plasma glutamine levels to body weight in mammals and *in vitro* studies examining patterns of stress-related oxygen free radical production in relation to glutamine availability (Castell & Newsholme 2001; Pithon-Curi *et al.* 2002).

It is clear that the self-protection and resource hypotheses are not mutually exclusive, and both may play a part in the immunosuppression we observed in handled mice and voles. More generally, we hypothesize that the level and nature of stress-induced immunosuppression will vary between different components of the immune system depending upon: (1) the potential for the component of the immune response to cause harm to host tissues; (2) the energetic cost of the immune component; (3) the intensity, frequency and duration of the stressor; and (4) the condition of the animal. This hypothesis predicts that immune responses that are unlikely to damage the host may be more likely to be suppressed to save resources, whereas potentially damaging responses are suppressed to protect the host.

A WORKING MODEL OF NEUTROPHIL BEHAVIOUR IN RESPONSE TO STRESS

This diagram represents our working model of the interaction between stress and neutrophil behaviour. Stress brings about a shift in the behaviour of neutrophils, inducing the release of reactive oxygen species (ROS), and initiating a sequence of events that leads to neutrophils binding to the blood vessel endothelium, and (not shown) rolling along the endothelium and migrating into the tissues. Cytokines (including IL-1, IL-6, and IL-8) and stress hormones are likely to play a role in initiating and maintaining this behaviour, as is shear stress. This shift in responsiveness is limited to a subpopulation of neutrophils: those remaining in the circulation have a reduced sensitivity to PMA (see text for details), and this can be used as a measure of stress.

A New Look at Stress-Induced Production of Oxygen Free Radicals: Therapeutic Possibilities

Phagocytic leukocytes play a pivotal role in the innate immune response against bacteria, fungi, foreign particles and stress induced immuno-supression (Ellard *et al.* 2001, Mian *et a.l* 2003, McLaren *et al.* 2003). On the surface of phagocytic leukocytes lies NADPH oxidase, multisubunit enzyme that can assemble which when assembled can 'shoot' highly reactive oxygen species (ROS) through the membrane. NADPH oxidases are tightly controlled and thus generally do not blast highly reactive superoxide anions into healthy tissues. It has recently been shown that once 'superoxide shooting' commences, the leukocyte initiates a highly coordinated sequence of events which include fusion and release of several types of granules and activation of antimicrobial enzymes (Bokoch 2002).

The role of ROS is not thus just that of a reactive oxygen free radical, but may be a signal for subsequent alteration of electrons, movement of ions and ultimately release of granular contents (Bokoch 2002). Thus an alteration of stress-induced ROS (Figure 4 from Bokoch 2002) may signal a sequence of more sinister alterations of immune function.

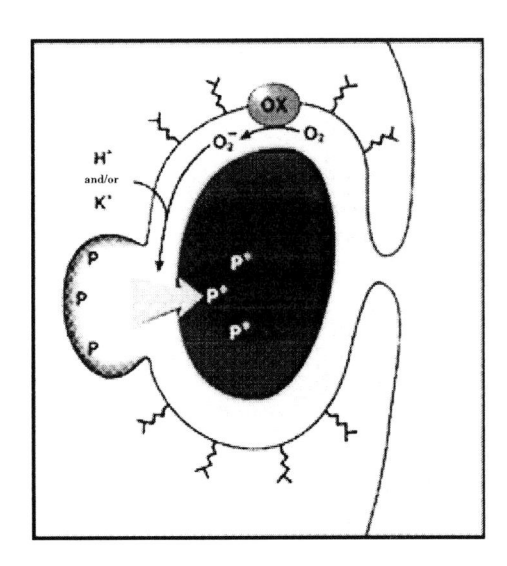

Figure 4. Figure reprinted from Bokoch (2002), with permission from GM Bokoch and the Nature Publishing Group.

The single electron reduction of molecular oxygen to form superoxide anion by the phagocyte NADPH oxidase (OX), stimulated by bacterial uptake (and possibly by substances e.g. adhesion molecules or cytokines released by stress), results in the transfer of electrons into the enclosed phagocytic vesicle. Dismutation of the superoxide generates OH^-, and the accumulating negative charge must be compensated by the influx of H^+ and/or K^+. The hypertonicity resulting from K^+ transport promotes the release of inactive cationic granule proteases (P) bound to an anionic sulfated proteoglycan matrix (cross-hatching). The released and active proteases (P^*) encounter the bacterium under optimal pH conditions within the phagocytic vesicle and degrade it. Cytoskeletal elements associated with the phagocytic vesicle (wavy lines) indirectly affect the killing process by modulating vesicular volume. pH and movement of ions may well be affected by gas signalling molecules. We speculate that this process may be intiated by stress. Pharmacological intervention with any of the processes discussed may modulate the production of ROS.

ROS Production in Disease States

Understanding the relationships between stress and ROS production is also important for disease studies. ROS have been implicated in a wide variety of autoimmune diseases such as rheumatoid arthritis (Halliwel *et al.*, 1992) inflammatory bowel disease (Kruidenhier & Verspaget 2002) and systemic lupus erythematosus (SLE) (Ames *et al.*, 1999) and psoriasis (Pereira *et al.*, 1999). Stress related psoriasis has been documented (Alabadie *et al.*, 1994). There is evidence that the occurrence of psoriasis is related to increased ROS production and decreased antioxidant capacity (Baz *et al.*, 2003). In an interesting experiment Kabat-Zinn *et al.*, (1998) demonstrated that stress reduction by meditation (in conjunction with ultraviolet light therapy) increased the rate at which psoriasis cleared in patients. ROS have been linked to such a variety of diseases because they of their potential for causing wide-ranging tissue damage. ROS can damage DNA and membranes and the oxidation products can induce protein damage, apoptosis, and the release of pro-inflammatory cytokines (Briganti & Picardo 2003), leading to serious tissue damage if antioxidant capacity is insufficient.

In patients with SLE the severity of the disease is known to be related to daily psychological stress (Pawlak *et al.*, 2003), and given that oxidative stress is a known factor in this disease (Ames *et al.*, 1999), the relationships between psychological stress, ROS production and disease onset and severity would be worth exploring further.

CONCLUDING COMMENTS

All mammals are subjected to psychological stress at some point in their lives. Whether man or mouse the nature, duration and intensity of the stress can result in a common endpoint : immunosupression and the release of reactive oxygen species from circulating leukocytes. Even vicarious, fictitious stress is sufficient to orchestrate what appears to be a basic instinctive response – the preparation for ensuing bacterial invasions. If the stress is of sufficient magnitude we appear to be hard wired to produce a defined physiological response. We prepare ourselves for action or injury. In anticipation, leukocytes prepare for battle and release their arsenal of weapons. The response is regulated. If however the stress continues, then this can have devastating consequences on the host (Irie 2003). Long term immunosupression can result in an increased vulnerability to opportunistic infections. Perhaps the ancient Egyptians were aware of the power of stress when they wrote curses on the tombs of pharaohs to deter thieves

> 'Moreover, as for him who shall destroy this inscription: He shall not reach his home. He shall not embrace his children. He shall not see success." (Budge 2001)

Such words would doubtless terrify a superstitious, and already anxious, tomb-raider. The resulting psychological stress, together with scattered invisible moulds scattered on the bodies of the mummies, which could remain dormant for thousands of years, could be a fatal combination. Believing in the curse could indeed have been a self-fulfilling prophesy. Unwittingly or otherwise than ancient Egyptians may have designed the first effective psycho-immunodeterrents.

REFERENCES

Alabadie, M. S., Kent, G. G. & Gawkrodger, D. J. 1994 The Relationship between stress and the onset and exacerbation of psoriasis and other skin conditions. *British Journal of Dermatology* 130, 199-203.

Atanackovic D. Brunner-Weinzierl MC. Kroger H. Serke S. Deter HC 2002. Acute psychological stress simultaneously alters hormone levels, recruitment of lymphocyte subsets, and production of reactive oxygen species. *Immunological Investigations.* 31(2): 73-91.

Atankovic, D. Schulze, J., Kröger, H., Brunner-Weinzierl, M.C. & Deter H.C. 2003 Acute psychological stress induces a prolonged suppression of the production of reactive oxygen species by phagocytes. *Journal of Neuroimmunology* 142, 159-165.

Ames, P. R. J., Alves, J., Murat, I., Isenberg, D. A. & Nourooz-Zadeh, J. 1999 Oxidative stress in systemic lupus erythematosus and allied conditions with vascular involvement. *Rheumatology* 38, 529-534.

Baz, K., Cimen, M. Y. B., Kokturk, A., Yazici, A. C., Eskandari, G., Ikizoglu, G., Api, H. & Atik, U. 2003 Oxidant/antioxidant status in patients with psoriasis. *Yonsei Medical Journal* 44, 987-990.

Benschop RJ. Rodriguez-Feuerhahn M. Schedlowski M. 1996 Catecholamine-induced leukocytosis: early observations, current research, and future directions. *Brain, Behavior, & Immunity.* 10(2):77-91

Bergmann, M. & Sautner, T. 2002 Immunomodulatory effects of vasoactive catecholamines. *Wien Klin Wochenschr* 114, 752-761.

Bokoch, G.M. 2002 Microbial killing: hold the bleach and pass the salt. *Nature Immunology* 3, 340-342.

Boxer, L.A. & Smolen, J.E. 1998 Neutrophil granule contents and their release in health and disease. *Haematology/Oncology Clinics of North America* 2, 101-134.

Briganti, S. & Picardo, M. 2003 Antioxidant activity, lipid peroxidation and skin diseases. What's new. *Journal of the European Academy of Dermatology and Venereology* 17, 663-669.

Budge EAA (2001)The Egyptian book of the dead p1-21 Publisher. Barnes & Noble London

Castell, L.M. 2002 Can glutamine modify the apparent immunodepression observed after prolonged, exhaustive exercise? *Nutrition* 18, 371-375.

Castell, L.M. & Newsholme, E.A. 2001 The relation between glutamine and the immunodepression observed in exercise. *Amino Acids* 20, 49-61.

Cavallone, E., Di Giancamillo, M., Secchiero, B., Belloli, A., Pravettoni, D. & Rimoldi, E. M. 2002 Variations of serum cortisol in Argentine horses subjected to ship transport and adaptation stress. *Journal of Equine Veterinary Science* 22, 541-545.

Delano, F.A., Forrest, M.J. & Schmidt-Schonbeim, G.W. 1997 Attenuation of oxygen free radical formation and tissue injury during experimental inflammation by P-selectin blockade. *Microcirculation* 4, 349-357.

Dhabhar, F.S., Miller, A.H., McEwen, B.S. & Spencer, R.L. 1995 Effect of stress on immune cell distribution - dynamics and hormonal mechanisms. *Journal of Immunology* 154, 5511-5527.

Ellard, D. R., Castle, P. C. & Mian, R. 2001 The effect of a short-term mental stressor on neutrophil activation. *International Journal of Psychophysiology* 41, 93-100.

Furukawa, S., Saito, H., Fukatsu, K., Hashiguchi, Y., Inaba, T., Lin, M., Inoue, T., Han, I., Matsuda, T. & Muto, T. 1997 Glutamine-enhanced bacterial killing by neutrophils from postoperative patients. *Nutrition* 13, 863-869.

Furukawa, S., Saito, H., Matsuda, T., Inoue, T., Fukatsu, K., Han, I., Ikeda, S., Hidemura, A. & Muto, T. 2000 Relative effects of glucose and glutamine on reactive oxygen intermediate production by neutrophils. *Shock* 13, 274-278.

Goebel, M.U.& Mills, P.J. 2000 Acute psychological stress and exercise and changes in peripheral leukocyte adhesion molecule expression and density. *Psychosomatic Medicine* **62**, 664-70.

Hou FY. Coe CL. Erickson C.1996 Psychological disturbance differentially alters CD4+ and CD8+ leukocytes in the blood and intrathecal compartments. *Journal of Neuroimmunology.* 68(1-2):*13-8.*

Irie M. Asami S. Nagata S. Miyata M. Kasai H 2001. Relationships between perceived workload, stress and oxidative DNA damage. *International Archives of Occupational & Environmental Health.* 74(2):*153-7*

Irie M. Asami S. Ikeda M. Kasai H. 2003 Depressive state relates to female oxidative DNA damage via neutrophil activation. *Biochemical & Biophysical Research Communications.* 311(4):*1014-8.*

Jean, W.C., Spellman, S.R., Nussbaum, E.S. & Low, W.C. 1998 Reperfusion injury after focal cerebral ischemia: the role of inflammation and the therapeutic horizon. *Neurosurgery* 43, 1382-1396.

Johansen C. Olsen JH.1997 Psychological stress, cancer incidence and mortality from non-malignant diseases. *British Journal of Cancer.* 75(1):*144-8.*

Johansen C. Olsen JH 1998. Psychological stress, occurrence of cancer and cause-specific mortality*Ugeskrift for Laeger.* 160(18):*2699-703.*

Halliwell, B. 1996 Antioxidants in human health and disease. *Annual Review of Nutrition* 16, 33-50.

Kabat-Zinn, J., Wheeler, E., Light, T., Skillings, A., Scharf, M. J., Cropley, T. G., Hosmer, D. & Bernhard, J. D. 1998 Influence of a mindfulness meditation-based stress reduction intervention on rates of skin clearing in patients with moderate to severe psoriasis undergoing phototherapy (UVB) and photochemotherapy (PUVA). *Psychosomatic Medicine* 60, 625-632.

Kanaley, J. A., Weltman, J. Y., Pieper, K. S., Weltman, A. & Hartman, M. L. 2001 Cortisol and growth hormone responses to exercise at different times of day. *Journal of Clinical Endocrinology and Metabolism* 86, 2881-2889.

Kiecolt-Glaser JK. Glaser R. 1999 Psychoneuroimmunology and cancer: fact or fiction?. *European Journal of Cancer.* 35(11):*1603-7.*

Kruidenhier, L. & Verspaget, H.W. 2002 Review article:oxidative stress as a pathogenic factor in inflammatory bowel disease – radicals or ridiculous. *Alimantary Parmacology and Theraputics* 16, 1997-2015.

Kurogi, J. & Iida, T. 2002 Inhibitory effect of cortisol on the defense activities of tilapia neutrophils in vitro. *Fish Pathology* 37, 13-16.

Laugero, K. D. & Moberg, G. P. 2000 Summation of behavioral and immunological stress: metabolic consequences to the growing mouse. *American Journal of Physiology* 279, E44-E49

Ley, K.1996 Molecular mechanisms of leukocyte recruitment in the Inflammatory process. *Cardiovascular Research* 32, 733-742.

Li J. Johansen C. Olsen J.2003 Cancer survival in parents who lost a child: a nationwide study in Denmark. [Clinical Trial. Journal Article. Randomized Controlled Trial] *British Journal of Cancer.* 88(11):*1698-701*

Lutz W. Tarkowski M. Dudek B. 2001.Psychoneuroimmunology. A new approach to the function of immunological system *Medycyna Pracy.* 52(3):*203-9.*

Madden K.S. & Livnat S. 1991 Catecholamine action and immunologic reactivity. In: R. Ader *et al. Psychoneuroimmunology* (2nd edn), Academic Press.

Macdonald D W & Newman C (2002) Population dynamics of badgers (Meles meles) in Oxfordshire U.K.: numbers density and cohort life histories and a possible role of climate change in population growth. *Journal of Zoology* 256, 121-138.

Maes, M., Van Der Planken, M., Van Gastel, A., Bruyland, K., Van Hunsel, F., *et al.*, (1998). Influence of academic examination stress on haematological measurements in subjectively healthy volunteers. *Psychiatry Research* 80, 201-12.

Maes M. Van Bockstaele DR. Gastel A. Song C. Schotte C. Neels H. DeMeester I. Scharpe S. Janca A.1999 The effects of psychological stress on leukocyte subset distribution in humans: evidence of immune activation. *Neuropsychobiology.* 39(1):*1-9.*

McLaren G.W., Macdonald, D. W., Georgiou, C., Mathews, F., Newman, C. & Mian, R. 2003 Leukocyte coping capacity: a novel technique for measuring the stress response in vertebrates. *Experimental Physiology* 88, 541-546.

McLaren, G.W., Mathews, F., Fell, R., Gelling, M. & Macdonald, D.W. In press Body weight responses as a measure of stress: a practical test. *Animal Welfare*

McPhail, L.C. & Harvath, L. 1993 Signal transduction in neutrophil oxidative matabolism and chemotaxis. In: *The Neutrophil*, ed Abramson JS & Wheeler JG, pp 63 – 107. Oxford University Press.

Menger MD, Richter S, Yamauchi J & Vollmar B (1999) Role of microcirculation in hepatic ischemia reperfusion injury. *Hepato-Gastroenterology* 46, 1452-1457

Mian, R. & Marshall, J. M. 1993 Effect of acute systemic hypoxia on vascular permeability and leukocyte adherence in the anaesthetised rat. *Cardiovascular Research* 27, 1531-1537.

Mian, R., Shelton-Rayner, G., Harkin, B. & Williams, P. 2003. Observing a fictitious stressful event: haematological changes, including circulating leucocyte activation. *Stress* 6, 41-47.

Moberg, G. P. 2000 Biological response to stress: implications for animal welfare. In: *The Biology of Animal Stress Basic Principles and Implications for Animal Welfare* ed G P Moberg & J A Mench pp 1-21. Wallingford: CABI Publishing

Montes, I., McLaren G.W, Macdonald D.W & Mian R In Press The Effect of transport stress on leukocyte activation in wild badgers. *Animal Welfare.*

Montes, I., McLaren G.W, Macdonald D.W & Mian R (2003). The effects of acute stress on leukocyte activation. *Journal of Physiology* 54P, 88P.

Nagahata, H., Higuchi, H., Yamashiki, N. & Yamaguchi, M. 2000 Analysis of the functional characteristics of L- selectin and its expression on normal and CD18-deficient bovine neutrophils. *Immunology and Cell Biology* 78, 264-271

Neveu J (2003) Brain-immune Cross-talk .Stress 6 (1) 3-4

Park JL & Lucchesi BR (1999) Mechanisms of myocardial reperfusion injury. *Annals of Thoracic Surgery* 68,1905-1912.

Pawlak, C. R., Witte, T., Heiken, H., Hundt, M., Schubert, J., Wiese, B., Bischoff-Renken, A., Gerber, K., Licht, B., Goebel, M., Heijnen, C. J., Schmidt, R. E. & Schedlowski, M. 2003 Flares in patients with systemic lupus erythematosus are associated with daily psychological stress. *Psychotherapy and Psychosomatics* 72, 159-165.

Pereira, P. R., Rebelo, I., Santos-Silva, A., Figueiredo, A., Ferra, M. I. A., Quintanilha, A. & Teixeira, F. 1999 Leukocyte activation and oxidative stress in psoriasis. *British Journal of Pharmacology* 127, 83P.

Pithon-Curi, T. C., Trezena, A. G., Tavares-Lima, W. & Curi, R. 2002 Evidence that glutamine is involved in neutrophil function. *Cell Biochemistry and Function* 20, 81-86

Rodriguez-Galen, M.C., Correa S.G., Cejas H. and Sotomayer, C.E. (2001) Imapired activity of phagocytic cells in Candia albicans infection after exposure to chronic varied stress, Neuroimmunomodulation 9 (4)), 193-202.

Rushen, J. 2000 Some issues in the interpretation of the behavioural responses to stress. In: *The Biology of Animal Stress: Basic Principles and Implications for Animal Welfare*, ed Moberg G P & Mench J A, pp. 23 – 42. CABI Publishing, Wallingford.

Sheikh, S., G. Rainger, E. Gale, Z., Rahman, M. & Nash, G.B 2003 Exposure to fluid shear stress modulates the ability of endothelial cells to recruit neutrophils in response to tumor necrosis factor-: a basis for local variations in vascular sensitivity to inflammation. *Blood* 102, 2828-2834.

Takase, S., Schmidt-Schonbein G. & Bergen, J.J., 1999 Leukocyte activation in patients with venous insufficiency. *Journal of Vascular Surgery* 30, 148-156.

Trouba, K. J., Hamadeh, H. K., Amin, R. P. & Germolec, D. R. 2002 Oxidative stress and its role in skin disease. *Antioxidants & Redox Signaling* 4, 665-673.

Viegas J 1999 ABC News: The curse of the pharoahs. *http://www.toxicmold.org/documents/0407.pdf*

Weiss, S.J. 1989 Tissue destruction by neutrophils. *New England Journal of Medecine* 320, 356-76.

In: Stress and Health: New Research
Editor: Kimberly V. Oxington, pp. 81-102
ISBN 1-59454-244-9
©2005 Nova Science Publishers, Inc.

Chapter IV

GROWTH IN EARLY LIFE IS ASSOCIATED WITH STRESS SYMPTOMS IN ADULTS

Yin Bun Cheung[*]

National Cancer Centre, Singapore
Lecturer, London School of Hygiene and Tropical Medicine, United Kingdom

ABSTRACT

Experimental studies of animals showed a relation between low birthweight and impaired coping and learning in stressful environments. In humans, concentrations of stress hormones in adults are related to birth weight. Furthermore, growth stunted children had higher levels of salivary cortisol concentrations and higher heart rates than non-stunted children. Studies have demonstrated that fetal and postnatal growth retardation has a negative impact on some aspects of psychological health in children and adolescents, but it is not known whether the impact is transient or not. In this chapter I report the findings from a cohort study of over 11,000 persons followed from birth to age 42. Parametric models were used to standardise birthweight for gestational age and weight at about age 7 for the age at measurement (in months). The resultant birthweight Z score and weight gain from birth to age 7 were the main independent variables, representing fetal and childhood growth respectively. Other variables included maternal smoking during pregnancy and father's social class when the participants were born. At ages 23, 33 and 42, the participants self-administered the Malaise Inventory. The psychological scale and somatic scale of the Malaise Inventory were the outcome measures. Multiple regression techniques were used to adjust for potential confounding by perinatal and childhood factors. The generalised estimation equations approach was used to adjust for correlation between repeated psychological assessments. Regression models with and without adjustment for social and health status in adulthood were compared to assess the extent to which the association was mediated by these mechanisms. It was found that slow growth

---

[*] Dr Yin Bun Cheung, MRC Tropical Epidemiology Group, Room 305a, London School of Hygiene and Tropical Medicine, Keppel Street, London WC1E 7HT, Tel: +44 (0) 20 7927 2101, Fax: +44 (0)20 7636 8739, E-mail: yinbun.cheung@lshtm.ac.uk.

had a long-term association with stress symptoms as measured by the psychological scale of the Malaise Inventory. A small part of the association was mediated by educational achievement in adults. The relative importance of growth and other factors was assessed by population attributable-risk fraction, adjusted for covariates. The fractions of incidence of high level of psychological distress attributable to below average birthweight, below average childhood weight gain, maternal smoking and father's social class status were, respectively, 3.0%, 3.0%, 5.9% and 6.8%.

INTRODUCTION

It has been hypothesised that fetal growth retardation or its determinants may have a long-term impact on the hypothalamic-pituitary-adrenal axis (HPAA) and sympathetic nervous system (SNS) (Barker, 1998; Clark, 1998). In a series of rat experiments, birthweight was reduced by fetal exposure to glucocorticoid in the maternal circulation. As adults the glucocorticoid exposed offspring rats showed impaired coping and learning in stressful environments (Welberg, Seckl & Holmes, 2000; Welberg, Seckl & Holmes, 2001). In humans, levels of stress hormones in children and adults were found negatively related to birthweight (Clark, Hindmarsh, Shiell, Law, Honour & Barker, 1996; Phillips, Walker, Reynolds, Flanagan, Wood, Osmond, Barker & Whorwood, 2000), giving support to the hypothesis about HPAA. It has also been found that low birthweight was associated with high resting pulse rate in adulthood (Phillips & Barker, 1997). This is consistent with the hypothesis that fetal growth retardation is linked to elevated SNS activities, although resting pulse rate is by no means a perfect indicator of SNS activity.

Postnatal growth retardation may also play a role in stress symptoms. Rats recovered from malnutrition show persistently increased emotionality and response to aversive situations (Levitsky & Barnes, 1970; Levitsky & Strupp, 1995; Smart, Whatson & Dobbing, 1975). In humans, growth retardation and under-nutrition in childhood also may affect children's psychological and behavioural characteristics (Barrett & Radke-Yarrow, 1985). Growth stunted children had higher level of salivary cortisol concentrations and higher heart rates than non-stunted children (Fernald & Grantham-McGregor, 1998). However, studies of children with protein-calories malnutrition found that their heighten cortisol concentrations return to normal level after the acute malnutrition stage, indicating that the impact of malnutrition in childhood may be transient (Castellanos & Arroyave 1961 and Alleyne & Young 1967, cited in Fernald & Grantham-McGregor, 1998).

Direct evidence about growth and stress symptoms or responses is limited. A study compared 21 neonates who had suffered from intrauterine stress conditions (i.e., intrauterine growth retardation, maternal hypertension or maternal smoking) with 30 normal controls. The two groups of neonates showed similar responses to stress tests designed to assess sympathetic and parasympathetic nervous activities (van Reempts, Wouters, Cock & van Acker, 1997). The authors reasoned that the sympathetic and parasympathetic effects of the stimuli might cancel each other, but due to ethical reasons they could not design an experiment to prevent this problem. Two recent studies demonstrated a relation between birth weight and stress in young adults. One was a study of Swedish conscripts. It showed an inverse relation between birthweight and susceptibility to stress at age 18 as assessed by psychologists of the army (Nilsson, Nyberg & Ostergren, 2001). Another was a study of British people born in 1970 (Cheung, 2002). It demonstrated that birth weight-for-gestational age was associated with the psychological score, but not somatic score, of the Malaise Inventory administered by the cohort members when they were 26 years old.

In addition to slow fetal and childhood growth, maternal smoking is another source of physiological insult that stresses the fetus. Maternal smoking is a risk factor of externalising behaviours in children and young adults (Batstra, Hadders-Algra & Neeleman, 2003; Fergusson, Woodward & Horwood, 1998) and schizophrenia in young adults (Jones, et al., 1998). It has been suggested that maternal smoking may alter the maturation of the autonomic nervous system and therefore responses to stress (van Reempts et al., 1997).

That parents' social class affects offspring's health and life chances has been one of the key issues in the studies about and debate on inequalities in Britain (Power, Manor & Fox, 1991; Townsend, Davidson & Whitehead, 1988). In addition, growth and maternal smoking are both associated with socio-economic status although the magnitude may be small (Cheung & Yip, 2001; Power & Matthews, 1997). For both reasons it is desirable to include parents' social class in the studies of the health effects of growth and perinatal factors.

Several investigators have suggested the relevancy of postnatal growth to hormones, metabolism and blood pressure (Cheung, Low, Osmond, Barker & Karlberg, 2000; Cianfarani, Germani & Branca, 1999). However, evidence on the association between growth in early childhood and stress-related outcomes in adults is scarce. Furthermore, the conventional focus of growth-related research is on the effects of "abnormal" versus "normal" growth status rather than the variation of growth rate across a broad spectrum. From the viewpoint of population health, a slightly below average growth rate may be more important than a grossly sub-normal one because the former is experienced by more people (van der Meulen, 2001). Barker (1998) repeatedly demonstrated that birth weight across a broad spectrum might have a continuous relation with certain health outcomes in adults, which was present even in newborns with birth weight above 2.5 kg, the cut-off defining low birthweight.

This study aims to test the hypothesis that birthweight and weight gain in childhood are associated with stress symptoms in adults. It also aims to examine whether maternal smoking during pregnancy and father's social class are related to the offsprings' stress levels, and to compare the fraction of population risk attributable to various factors. I draw on data from the UK National Child Development Study, which has followed a cohort of people from birth to age 42, to test the hypotheses.

PARTICIPANTS AND METHODS

The National Child Development Study

The National Child Development Study (NCDS) is a prospective study of about 17,000 people born in England, Wales and Scotland in the week 3 - 9 March 1958. It originated in the Perinatal Mortality Survey, which requested the National Health Service to identify all births in the target week and successfully obtained data on about 98% of the babies. The Survey then evolved into the NCDS, which assessed the cohort members when they were 7,

11, 16, 23, 33 and 42 years old by means of clinical examinations, face-to-face and self-administered interviews, survey of participants' parents, etc. The characteristics of the participants have been compared with those of other national samples of people in a similar age range. The NCDS participants were found representative of British nationals at similar ages. Details of the NCDS and the representativeness of the cohort have been reported elsewhere (Ferri, 1993; Power et al., 1991). The present study included singletons live-born between 35 and 43 weeks of gestation without congenital abnormality and who survived infancy. The total number of cohort members eligible for inclusion in the analysis was 14,108. The NCDS sample frame expanded to include immigrants to Britain born during the same week in 1958. The present analysis did not include these immigrants.

Variables Measured at Birth and Age 7

Data collected at birth included birthweight, gestational age (GA) in weeks determined by the last menstrual period method, birth order ("1st", "2nd to 3rd" and "4th or above"), mother's smoking habit during pregnancy ("non-smoking", "stop prior to 5th month", "<5", "5-14" or ">14" cigarette per day), father's social class defined according to the Registrar General's classification, mother's marital status ("married" or "unmarried"), and number of antenatal care visits ("<10", "10-14" or ">14"). At age 7 the cohort members' body weights were measured in a medical examination; housing tenure ("owner-occupier", "council renter", "private renter" or "others") was enumerated from a survey of the parents. The primary focus of this study was on intrauterine growth retardation as represented by birthweight standardised for GA and childhood growth as represented by weight gain from birth to age 7. Maternal smoking and father's social class were independent variables of secondary concern. Birth order, GA, mother's marital status, number of antenatal care visits, and housing tenure were included in the statistical modelling as potential confounders (Cheung, 2002; Petrou, Kupek, Vause & Maresh, 2001; Power et al., 1991).

Standardization of Growth Variables

To quantify intrauterine growth retardation, birthweight was standardised for GA separately for each sex, giving a birthweight standard deviation score or Z score. We used the parametric modelling approach described in detail by Royston and Wright (1998). Briefly, an exponential-normal distribution was used to model the relation between birthweight and GA. This distribution includes a parameter to capture the skewness of data. This distribution approaches the normal distribution as the skewness parameter approaches zero. Furthermore, fractional polynomials were used to model the level and variability of birthweight in relation to GA. The data collection at about age 7 took about 1 year to complete, so the age at body size measurement was variable. Weight at 7 was standardised for age in months, separately for each gender, using the same parametric modelling approach. Weight gain in childhood was measured as weight Z score at 7 years minus birth weight Z score. A higher value indicated a faster childhood growth.

Outcome Measures

At ages 23, 33 and 42, the cohort members self-administered the Malaise Inventory. The assessment at age 42 was computer-aided while the earlier two assessments were based on paper questionnaires. The Malaise Inventory was a questionnaire of 24 items developed by Rutter, Tizard and Whitmore (1970). It has been widely used to measure the level of stress experienced by carers of people with dependency needs (Grant, Nolan & Ellis, 1990). A series of two surveys demonstrated a moderate correlation between the Malaise Inventory and another stress symptoms scale and the taking of tranquillisers and sleeping tablets. (Hirst & Bradshaw, 1983). Whether the Inventory should be used as a single internally consistent measure of stress used to be a matter of debate (Bebbington & Quine 1987, cited in Grant et al., 1990). Recently a factor analysis demonstrated that the Inventory contains a psychological scale and a somatic scale; structural equation modelling also showed that the two factors were predictable by different stressors (Grant et al., 1990; Rodgers, Pickles, Power, Collishaw & Maughan, 1999). A study of the 1970 British birth cohort demonstrated a relation between birthweight and the psychological score but not the somatic score of the Malaise Inventory (Cheung, 2002). The present study employed the Malaise Inventory as a 15-item scale of psychological symptoms and an 8-item scale of somatic symptoms. There is a 9-item variant of the somatic symptom scale but it was not use in the present study as the validity of this variant had been questioned (Grant et al., 1990; Rodgers et al., 1999). Some sample questions of the psychological scale are: "Do you usually have great difficulty in falling or getting to sleep?", "Does very little thing get on your nerves and wear you out?" and "Are you easily upset or irritated?" Some sample questions of the somatic scale are: "Do you often have bad head-aches?" and "Do you suffer from an upset stomach?" Each question requires a yes or no answer. Each affirmative answer is counted as one symptom. A total of at least eight (psychological plus somatic) symptoms indicate a high risk of psychiatric morbidity (Power et al, 1991). This study proportionally assigned the cut-off of eight symptoms to the psychological and somatic scales to indicate a high level of distress in each – that is, at least five psychological symptoms and at least three somatic symptoms.

Intermediate Variables Measured at Ages 23, 33 and 42

In each of the three sweeps of follow-up in adulthood, the participants were asked about their educational qualifications, marital status and living arrangement, and whether they had "any long-standing illness, disability, or infirmity of any kind" (hereafter referred to as long-standing illness for brevity). Highest education qualification was categorised as "below O level", "O level", and "A level or above". (CSE and NVQ qualifications were converted to their O or A level equivalents in the categorisation.) Marital status was categorised as "married", "single", "cohabiting", or "previously married". Due to a relatively small number, the divorced, separated and widowed were combined to form the group of "previously married" people. Studies have demonstrated associations between growth and educational qualifications and marital status in adults (Philips, Handelsman, Eriksson, Forsen, Osmond & Barker, 2001; Richards, Hardy, Kuh & Wadsworth, 2002; van de Mheen, Stronks, Looman & Mackenbach, 1998). It is also known that these social situations affect psychological health

(Cheung, 1998; Power et al., 1991). The validity and reliability of self-reported long-term illness and disability was much discussed and established prior to the 1991 census in England and Wales (Thompson, 1995). It is now well-established that chronic illness in adults has early origins (Barker, 1998). Hence these three variables were included in the analysis as potential intermediate variables.

Statistical Analysis

The generalized estimating equations (GEE) multiple regression approach was used to analyse psychological and somatic scores, pooled across ages, in relation to birthweight Z score, weight gain, maternal smoking, father's social class and other variables (Zeger & Liang, 1986). An exchangeable correlation structure was used to adjust for the correlation between repeated measurements. A linear regression coefficient represents the difference in mean value of the psychological (or somatic) score associated with a unit increase in the explanatory variable. Furthermore, the odds of having a high level of psychological and somatic symptoms, as defined above, was analysed using GEE multiple logistic regression. An odds ratio (OR) represents the multiplicative change in the odds of reporting high level of distress associated with a unit increase in the explanatory variable. I first fitted a model with birthweight Z score and other variables measured at the time of birth (model I). A second model included weight gain and housing tenure at age 7 (model II). A comparison of the difference in regression coefficients reveals whether the influence of birthweight Z score was mediated by weight gain in childhood (Lucas, Fewtrell & Cole, 1999). A third model (model III) was fitted together with education, marital status and long-standing illness reported at the time of Malaise Inventory assessment. A comparison of the findings from models II and III would suggest whether the early exposures affect the adult outcomes via these potential intervening mechanisms.

For the purpose of examining non-linear relation between early growth and the outcomes, quadratic terms for birthweight Z score and weight gain were added into the models in supplementary analyses. For the purpose of examining interaction between birthweight and weight gain, a product term was included in the analysis. Furthermore, interaction terms between age at Malaise Inventory assessments and the growth variables were examined in supplementary analyses to check whether the associations were stable over the age range from 23 to 42.

The importance of an exposure in determining the health of a population depends on not only the level of excess risk associated with the exposure, but also the prevalence of the exposure. An exposure with low prevalence will have limited relevancy in population health even if it is highly associated with the outcome concerned. The population attributable-risk fraction (PAF) is a measure that quantifies the proportion of the incidence of a condition that is attributable to a risk factor, taking into account both the prevalence of the risk factor as well as the excess risk associated with the factor. The PAF can be estimated in a logistic regression framework, with adjustment for covariates (Bruzzi, Green, Byar, Brinton & Schairer, 1985; Greenland and Drescher, 1993). Conventionally a risk factor is often dichotomised in the calculation of PAF but this is not necessary. In the estimation of PAF, this study used birthweight and weight gain above zero Z score as the "no exposure" status while the values below zero were kept as continuous levels of exposure. Covariates were adjusted by using logistic regression.

All the analyses were performed using the statistical package Stata (StataCrop, 2001). The standardisation of weight and the estimation of PAF were performed using the Stata macros published by Wright and Royston (1997) and Brady (1998), respectively.

RESULTS

Descriptive Analysis

After excluding stillbirths, infant deaths, multiple births, births with congenital abnormalities and births with GA outside the range of 35 to 43 weeks or unknown GA, 14,108 cohort members were eligible for inclusion in this study. Birthweight data were available among 97 percents of the eligible subjects. About 20% of the subjects did not have their weight measured at age 7. Table 1 tabulates the growth data. Using all available data, the mean birthweight of men and women were 3.43 and 3.30 kg respectively. Their weights at 7 were 24.16 and 23.77 kg respectively. As expected, birthweight Z score had a mean value of 0.00 and a SD of 1.00 in both genders. The mean (SD) weight gain, defined as weight Z score at 7 minus birth weight Z score, was –0.01 (1.2) in both boys and girls. The sample of model 1 listed in table 1 refers to the subset of cohort members whose birthweight and values on perinatal factors were not missing and who had participated in at least one of the Malaise Inventory assessments at ages 23, 33 or 42. That of model 2 was further restricted to those whose weight and housing tenure at age 7 were known. The sample of model 3 was further restricted to those with non-missing data on education, marital status and long-standing illness at the time of Malaise Inventory assessments. Hence the sample size varied. The growth values of different samples were fairly similar, giving some assurance that there was no strong selection bias. Among men, mean birthweight and mean weight gain in the samples of models I to III were slightly higher (about 0.01 Z score) than the estimates based on all available data. Among women, mean birthweight was slightly higher (about 0.01 Z score) in the samples of models II and III than the estimates in all available data and model I.

Table 2 provides a descriptive summary of the subjects included in the main analysis, model II. That of subjects included in other models was similar and not listed here for brevity. Male and female cohort members had similar profiles. The mean GA was approximately 40 weeks. About 40% of the mothers smoked to some extent during the pregnancy. About 37% of the subjects were the first births and 48% the second or third. Traditionally in Britain the average number of antenatal visits was 13 (Petrous et al., 2001). In this study about 43% of the mothers had 10 to 14 visits, and the rest were roughly equally split between fewer or more visits. Fathers of the cohort members were mostly from the social class III (60%). Three percent of the mothers were not married. About 44% of the subjects lived as owner-occupiers at age 7.

Table 1. Mean value (sample size) of growth variables by gender

Sample	Variable	Men	Women
All available data	Birth weight (kg)	3.43 (7,009)	3.30 (6,653)
	Birth weight Z score	0.00 (7,009)	0.00 (6,653)
	Weight at 7 (kg)	24.16 (5,853)	23.77 (5,447)
	Weight gain (Δ Z score)	-0.01 (5,640)	-0.01 (5,287)
Model I (birth and outcome data)	Birth weight (kg)	3.44 (5,634)	3.30 (5,572)
	Birth weight Z score	0.01 (5,634)	0.00 (5,572)
	Weight at 7 (kg)	24.19 (4,777)	23.74 (4,665)
	Weight gain (Δ Z score)	0.00 (4,769)	-0.02 (4,652)
Model II (birth, age 7, and outcome data)	Birth weight (kg)	3.44 (4,768)	3.30 (4,648)
	Birth weight Z score	0.01 (4,768)	0.01 (4,648)
	Weight at 7 (kg)	24.19 (4,768)	23.75 (4,648)
	Weight gain (Δ Z score)	0.00 (4,768)	-0.01 (4,648)
Model III (birth, age 7, outcome and adult covariate data)	Birth weight (kg)	3.44 (4,755)	3.30 (4,638)
	Birth weight Z score	0.01 (4,755)	0.01 (4,638)
	Weight at 7 (kg)	24.18 (4,755)	23.75 (4,638)
	Weight gain (Δ Z score)	0.00 (4,755)	-0.01 (4,638)

Table 3 shows the mean (SD) number of psychological symptoms, as well as the prevalence of having a high level of psychological distress (≥ 5 symptoms), assessed by the psychological scale of the Malaise Inventory at ages 23, 33 and 42. Again, comparing the estimates from all available data and the three samples restricting to cohort members with certain non-missing data suggests no strong selection bias. Mean psychological score of men at age 23 in models II and III were slightly lower than that of the full sample and model I (1.3 vs 1.4). Mean psychological score of women at age 42 in models I to III was slightly lower than that of the full sample (2.8 vs 2.9). Women had visibly more symptoms and higher prevalence of at least 5 symptoms than men. Age 33 appeared to be a relatively stress free time, with a mean (SD) number of about 1.2 (1.9) and 1.9 (2.4) symptoms reported by men and women (all available data); the prevalence of high level of stress were about 6.4% and 12.4% for men and women at this age. The mean and prevalence were highest at age 42 in comparison with the younger ages: 2.1 symptoms and a prevalence of 15.5% in men and 2.9 symptoms and a prevalence of 23.1% in women (all available data).

Table 2. Descriptive data of variables other than growth measured at birth and age 7 in model II: mean (SD) or percentage

Variables	Unit / Category	Men (n = 4,768)	Women (n = 4,648)
Gestational age	Week	39.8 (1.5)	39.8 (1.5)
Maternal smoking	Non-smoking	60.5%	59.1%
	Stop during pregnancy	6.3%	8.4%
	<5 cigarettes/day	7.5%	7.5%
	5-14 cigarettes/day	21.3%	20.7%
	>15 cigarettes/day	4.5%	4.3%
Birth order	1st	36.5%	37.1%
	2nd or 3rd	48.2%	47.2%
	4th or above	15.3%	15.7%
No. of antenatal visits	<10	30.5%	30.3%
	10-14	42.0%	43.9%
	>14	27.5%	25.8%
Father's social class	I	4.6%	4.3%
	II	13.6%	13.4%
	III	59.9%	59.6%
	IV	11.2%	12.0%
	V	8.7%	8.3%
	Others	2.0%	2.4%
Mother's marital status	Married	97.4%	96.8%
	Unmarried	2.6%	3.2%
Housing tenure at age 7	Owner occupier	44.0%	43.7%
	Council renter	38.6%	39.5%
	Private renter	11.4%	11.2%
	Others	6.0%	5.7%

Regression Analysis

Table 4 shows the results of the GEE multiple linear regression analysis of psychological scores pooled over three ages. Model I included variables measured at birth and sex and age at follow-up as regressors. The total number of participants included was 11,206 and the total number of observations was 27,039, i.e. on average each participants contributed 2.4 observations. Birth weight had a significant negative association with the outcome. An increase of one Z score in birthweight was associated with a decrease of 0.05 in the mean psychological score (P<0.01). Maternal smoking at the levels of 5-14 and over 14 cigarettes per day was associated with an increase of 0.30 (P<0.01) and 0.41 (P<0.01) in the mean score. Father's social class and birth order had a dose-response relation with the outcome (each P<0.01). The lower the social class status and the higher the birth order, the higher the mean score. Children of unmarried mothers also had a higher level of symptoms when they grew up, the regression coefficient (coef.) being 0.42 (P<0.05). As in the above descriptive analysis, sex and age at follow-up were also related to the outcome. In contrast to a previous study that found a negative relation between GA and the psychological score (Cheung, 2002), this study could not replicate this finding. Furthermore, the number of antenatal visits was not associated with the outcome either.

Table 3. Levels of psychological symptoms as measured by the Malaise Inventory, by gender and age at follow-up

Sample	Age	Men N	Mean (SD)	% ≥ 5 symptoms	Women N	Mean (SD)	% ≥ 5 symptoms
All available data	23	5,041	1.4 (1.8)	6.6%	5,085	2.4 (2.5)	17.9%
	33	4,464	1.2 (1.9)	6.4%	4,596	1.9 (2.4)	12.4%
	42	4,526	2.1 (2.5)	15.5%	4,684	2.9 (2.8)	23.1%
Model I	23	4,765	1.4 (1.8)	6.6%	4,868	2.4 (2.5)	18.1%
	33	4,233	1.2 (1.9)	6.5%	4,405	1.9 (2.4)	12.5%
	42	4,287	2.1 (2.5)	15.3%	4,481	2.8 (2.8)	22.9%
Model II	23	4,079	1.3 (1.8)	6.4%	4,106	2.4 (2.4)	17.8%
	33	3,610	1.2 (1.9)	6.2%	3,685	1.9 (2.3)	12.5%
	42	3,661	2.1 (2.5)	15.4%	3,766	2.8 (2.8)	22.3%
Model III	23	4,079	1.3 (1.8)	6.4%	4,104	2.4 (2.4)	17.8%
	33	3,598	1.2 (1.9)	6.3%	3,677	1.8 (2.3)	12.6%
	42	3,660	2.1 (2.5)	15.4%	3,764	2.8 (2.8)	22.3%

Model II further included weight gain in childhood and housing tenure at age 7. The total number of participants included was 9,421 and the total number of observations was 22,916. Again, each participant on average contributed 2.4 observations. Birthweight and weight gain had a Pearson's correlation coefficient of –0.59, suggesting catch-up growth in infants born small (Karlberg & Albertsson-Wikland, 1995). Weight gain was negatively related to the mean psychological score (coef. = -0.06; P<0.01). Having adjusted for weight gain, the regression coefficient on birthweight changed from –0.05 to –0.09 (P<0.01). This suggests that the negative impact of a lighter birthweight could be partly compensated by a faster childhood weight gain. Housing tenure at age 7 was associated with the outcome. Children who lived as council renters (coef. = 0.31; P<0.01) or private renters (coef. = 0.32; P<0.01) had higher psychological scores. Having adjusted for housing tenure at age 7, the regression coefficients on father's social class moved closer to the null value but remain significant. The other regression coefficients remain quite similar to those in model 1.

Table 4. Mean psychological score: GEE multiple linear regression coefficients [a]

Group of variables	Variables	Unit / Category	Model I (n = 11,206)	Model II (n = 9,421)
Perinatal	Birth weight	Z score	-0.05**	-0.09**
	Gestational age	Week	0.00	0.01
	Maternal smoking	Non-smoking	0 [b]	0 [b]
		Stop in pregnancy	0.14	0.06
		<5 cigarettes/day	0.12	0.11
		5-14 cigarettes/day	0.30**	0.26**
		>14 cigarettes/day	0.41**	0.45**
	No. of antenatal visits	<10	0 [b]	0 [b]
		10-14	-0.07	-0.06
		>14	-0.03	-0.04
	Father's social class	I	0 [b]	0 [b]
		II	0.06	0.03
		III	0.35**	0.20*
		IV	0.48**	0.30**
		V	0.73**	0.44**
		Others	0.21	-0.08
	Birth order	1st	0 [b]	0 [b]
		2nd or 3rd	0.15**	0.13**
		4th or above	0.49**	0.37**
	Mother's marital status	Married	0 [b]	0 [b]
		Unmarried	0.42*	0.53**
Childhood	Weight gain	Δ Z score		-0.06**
	Housing tenure at age 7	Owner occupier		0 [b]
		Council renter		0.31**
		Private renter		0.32**
		Others		0.16
Demographic	Sex	Male	0 [b]	0 [b]
		Female	0.83**	0.82**
	Age at follow-up	23	0 [b]	0 [b]
		33	-0.35**	-0.34**
		41	0.60**	0.62**

**$p < 0.01$; * $p < 0.05$
a. Model I does not include childhood variables.
b. Reference category.

Table 5 gives the result of GEE multiple logistic regression analysis of the prevalence of having at least five psychological symptoms. The pattern of associations was basically similar to that of table 4. In particular, in model I birthweight had a significant relation with high psychological distress (OR = 0.95; $p < 0.05$). In model II, weight gain (OR = 0.92; $p < 0.01$) was negatively related to the odds and the odds ratio of birthweight strengthened to

0.91 (P<0.01). Maternal smoking, father's social class, parity, mother's marital status and housing tenure at 7 were also related to the outcome in a fashion similar to the linear regression analysis aforementioned.

Table 5. Odds of at least 5 psychological symptoms: odds ratio estimated by GEE multiple logistic regression [a]

Group of variables	Variables	Unit / Category	Model I (n = 11,206)	Model II (n = 9,421)
Perinatal	Birth weight	Z score	0.95*	0.91**
	Gestational age	Week	1.00	1.01
	Maternal smoking	Non-smoking	1 [b]	1 [b]
		Stop in pregnancy	1.09	1.03
		<5 cigarettes/day	1.12	1.09
		5-14 cigarettes/day	1.31**	1.25**
		>14 cigarettes/day	1.38**	1.41**
	No. of antenatal visits	<10	1 [b]	1 [b]
		10-14	0.97	0.97
		>14	1.01	1.01
	Father's social class	I	1 [b]	1 [b]
		II	1.09	0.99
		III	1.43**	1.15
		IV	1.66**	1.31
		V	2.01**	1.43*
		Others	1.36	1.03
	Birth order	1st	1 [b]	1 [b]
		2nd or 3rd	1.17**	1.16**
		4th or above	1.54**	1.38**
	Mother's marital status	Married	1 [b]	1 [b]
		Unmarried	1.38	1.52*
Childhood	Weight gain	Δ Z score		0.92**
	Housing tenure at age 7	Owner occupier		1 [b]
		Council renter		1.37**
		Private renter		1.36**
		Others		1.27*
Demographic	Sex	Male	1 [b]	1 [b]
		Female	2.07**	2.06**
	Age at follow-up	23	1 [b]	1 [b]
		33	0.75**	0.76**
		41	1.72**	1.74**

**P<0.01; * P<0.05
a. Model I does not include childhood variables.
b. Reference category.

Table 6 tabulates the relative frequency distribution of education, marital status and long-standing illness at age 42 by gender (using all available data). It also tabulates the mean birthweight and weight gain by gender and the social and health variables. In both genders approximately one-third of the cohort members were in each of the three education categories of below O level, O level, and A level or above. Slightly more than 70% of men and women were married. Twenty-eight percent of men and 29% of women reported long-standing illness. In men birthweight (P<0.01) and weight gain (P<0.05) were significantly related to education level, with the expected gradient of slower growth associated with lower educational achievement. Birthweight was also related to education in women (P<0.01), but weight gain was not. Without adjustment for any covariates these two growth variables were not related to marital status and long-standing illness. However, when a GEE multiple logistic regression analysis was used to adjust for covariates in model II, weight gain was related to long-standing illness (OR = 1.07; P< 0.01). Similar associations with the presence of long-standing illness at ages 23 and 33 were also found (details not shown). A previous study demonstrated an association between birthweight and subsequent marital status (Philips et al., 2001). In this cohort no such association was found even after covariates in model II were brought into account by way of multiple logistic regression (details not shown).

Table 6. Distribution of social and health status at age 42 by gender; mean (SD) of growth variables by social and health status at age 42 and gender

Gender	Variables	Category	%	Birth weight	Weight gain
Male	Education	Below O level	34.5%	-0.04 (1.00)	-0.05 (1.16)
		O level	34.9%	0.00 (1.00)	-0.02 (1.17)
		A level or above	30.6%	0.09 (0.97)	0.06 (1.12)
		ANOVA		P<0.01	P<0.05
	Marital status	Married	71.4%	0.04 (0.98)	0.00 (1.13)
		Single	9.7%	-0.08 (1.09)	0.09 (1.17)
		Previously married	9.1%	-0.03 (0.98)	-0.08 (1.26)
		Cohabitating	9.8%	-0.03 (0.98)	0.06 (1.16)
		ANOVA		P>0.05	P>0.05
	Long-standing illness	No	72.3%	0.02 (0.99)	-0.01 (1.16)
		Yes	27.7%	0.01 (0.99)	0.06 (1.13)
		ANOVA		P>0.05	P>0.05
Female	Education	Below O level	31.0%	-0.11 (1.04)	-0.06 (1.23)
		O level	39.5%	0.04 (1.00)	0.02 (1.21)
		A level or above	29.5%	0.11 (0.94)	0.01 (1.17)
		ANOVA		P<0.01	P>0.05
	Marital status	Married	72.4%	0.01 (1.01)	-0.01 (1.20)
		Single	7.1%	0.10 (0.98)	-0.01 (1.26)
		Previously married	11.8%	0.01 (0.98)	-0.03 (1.19)
		Cohabitating	8.7%	-0.02 (1.00)	0.00 (1.17)
		ANOVA		P>0.05	P>0.05
	Long-standing illness	No	71.0%	0.02 (1.00)	-0.01 (1.20)
		Yes	29.0%	0.01 (1.00)	0.00 (1.23)
		ANOVA		P>0.05	P>0.05

Table 7. Mean psychological score and odds of at least 5 psychological symptoms: GEE multiple linear and GEE multiple logistic regression (n = 9,393)

Group of variables	Variables	Unit / Category	Regression coefficient	Odds Ratio
Perinatal	Birth weight	Z score	-0.06*	0.93*
	Gestational age	Week	0.01	1.01
	Maternal smoking	Non-smoking	0 [a]	1 [a]
		Stop in pregnancy	0.06	1.02
		<5 cigarettes/day	0.07	1.04
		5-14 cigarettes/day	0.20**	1.17**
		>14 cigarettes/day	0.39**	1.32*
	No. of antenatal visits	<10	0 [a]	1 [a]
		10-14	-0.03	1.01
		>14	-0.01	1.04
	Father's social class	I	0 [a]	1 [a]
		II	-0.03	0.94
		III	0.04	0.97
		IV	0.10	1.06
		V	0.20	1.13
		Others	-0.17	0.92
	Birth order	1st	0 [a]	1 [a]
		2nd or 3rd	0.08	1.09
		4th or above	0.26**	1.23**
	Mother's marital status	Married	0	1 [a]
		Unmarried	0.42*	1.38
Childhood	Weight gain	Δ Z score	-0.05*	0.93**
	Housing tenure at age 7	Owner occupier	0 [a]	1 [a]
		Council renter	0.23**	1.25**
		Private renter	0.25**	1.27**
		Others	0.09	1.18
Adult	Education	Below O level	0 [a]	1 [a]
		O level	-0.42**	0.64**
		A level or above	-0.58**	0.54**
	Marital status	Married	0 [a]	1 [a]
		Single	0.05	1.08
		Previously married	0.65**	1.84**
		Cohabitating	0.19**	1.27**
	Long-standing illness	No	0 [a]	1 [a]
		Yes	0.78**	2.07**
Demographic	Sex	Male	0 [a]	1 [a]
		Female	0.84**	2.16**
	Age at follow-up	23	0 [a]	1 [a]
		33	-0.39**	0.69**
		41	0.41**	1.40**

**P<0.01; * P<0.05

Table 7 presents the results of the GEE multiple linear and logistic regression analyses that included perinatal, childhood, and adult covariates in the model (model III). The total number of participants and observations were 9,393 and 22,560, respectively. After inclusion of all the variables, birthweight and weight gain remained significantly associated with the mean score. The regression coefficient on birthweight changed from –0.09 in model II to –0.06 (P<0.05) here. That on weight gain changed only slightly from –0.06 in model II to –0.05 (P<0.05). Father's social class paled into insignificance, suggesting its relation with the outcome was intermediated by adult social or health status rather than direct. Maternal smoking and mother's marital status remained fairly strong in predicting psychological scores. More education was associated with lower distress (P<0.01). The previously married (coef. = 0.65; P<0.01) and those cohabiting (coef. = 0.19; P<0.01) had higher mean scores than the married. The presence of a long-standing illness was also associated with a higher mean psychological score (coef. = 0.78; P<0.01). Table 7 also shows the odds ratios about having at least 5 symptoms. The findings were similar to that of the linear regression analysis.

In models I to III and in both the linear regression and logistic regression analyses I explored whether there was interaction between the two growth variables and whether there were non-linear relation between the growth variables and the outcome. In no model were the interaction term and the second order polynomial terms for birthweight and weight gain significant (each P>0.10; details not shown). Furthermore, there was no significant interaction between age at assessment and the growth variables (each P>0.10; details not shown), suggesting that the potential impact of growth in early life was stable over the range of young to middle age.

No association between somatic symptoms and birthweight and weight gain was found (details not shown). All the linear regression coefficients were close to zero and all the odds ratios were close to one. This agrees with the previous study of the 1970 British birth cohort that growth in early life specifically relates to the psychological scores but not somatic scores (Cheung, 2002).

Population Attributable-Risk Fraction

Table 8 gives the fraction of population risk of having at least 5 symptoms attributable to slow growth, maternal smoking and father's social class. This calculation was based on the odds ratios estimated in model II. Model III was not used for this purpose because this would over-adjust as some of the variables might be intermediate factors. Birthweight and weight gain below average each accounted for 3.0% of the population risk; together they accounted for 6.0% of it. Although the odds ratio on smoking 5-14 cigarettes per day was smaller than that on smoking more than 14 cigarettes per day (1.25 vs 1.41, table 5), a higher fraction of population risk was attributable to the former than the latter (3.8% vs 0.7%) due to a much higher prevalence of smoking 5-14 cigarettes per day. All levels of maternal smoking together accounted for 5.9% of the population risk. The odds ratio on social class II versus social class I as reference was very close to 1. These two were combined as the reference category in the PAF calculation. Social classes III, IV and V individually accounted for 4.0%, 2.0% and 0.8% of the risk. Altogether social classes III to V accounted for 6.8% of the PAF.

Table 8. Fraction of population risk of having at least 5 symptoms attributable to growth and perinatal factors

Variables	Category	Fraction of population risk
Birth weight	≥ 0 Z score	Reference
	< 0 Z score	3.0%
Weight gain	≥ 0 Z score	Reference
	< 0 Z score	3.0%
Maternal smoking	Non-smoking	Reference
	Stop in pregnancy	0.4%
	<5 cigarettes/day	1.0%
	5-14 cigarettes/day	3.8%
	>14 cigarettes/day	0.7%
Father's social class	I or II	Reference
	III	4.0%
	IV	2.0%
	V	0.8%

DISCUSSION

A large amount of research since the 1960s demonstrated that fetal and childhood growth retardation and malnutritional are precursors of developmental deficits and behavioural problems. Birthweight is an important indicator of fetal growth and nutritional status (Beattie & Johnson, 1994); weight-for-age is one of the primary tools for assessing the nutritional and health status of children (WHO Working Group, 1986). Recent research in neuroendocrinology has provided new insights about how poor growth in early life may impair brain development. Levitsky and Strupp (1995) reviewed the recent literature and summarised that (a) the kind of long-term impairments may be more related to emotional responses to stressful events than to cognitive deficits, (b) the age range of vulnerability to these impairments may be much greater than expected, and (c) the minimal amount of malnutrition or hunger needed to produce these long-term effects is unknown.

The present study shows that birthweight standardised for GA as well as weight gain from birth to age 7 were associated with stress symptoms in adults, as measured by the psychological scale of the Malaise Inventory. Together with two other studies of the effects of fetal growth (Cheung, 2002; Nilsson et al, 2001), it establishes the plausibility of an association between fetal growth and stress in later life. As the review by Levitsky and Strupp (1995) suggests, concerns about poor growth should not be restricted to cognitive deficit alone. This study also shows that growth rate from birth to the age of 7 years was negatively associated with stress symptoms. It is of interest that the association between one unit change in birth weight Z score and the psychological score strengthened from –0.05 to –0.09 when adjusted for weight gain during childhood. A small size at birth is usually followed by some degree of postnatal catch-up (Karlberg & Albertsson-Wikland, 1995). The results indicate that the impact of fetal growth retardation may be partly compensated by a higher weight gain in postnatal life. Hence the coefficient was weaker when weight gain was not adjusted for. A study in Hong Kong found a relation between growth in the first two years of life and blood pressure in adults (Cheung et al., 2000). Since cardiovascular disease and stress share some common origins in the hypothalamic-pituitary-adrenal axis (HPAA) and sympathetic nervous system (SNS), this finding seems to corroborate the hypothesis studied here. Traditionally growth retardation is often dichotomised as normal versus abnormal, using, for example, –2 Z score or the 5th percentile of a normative data set, or birthweight of 2.5 kg as cut-offs. However, there is no evidence to presume that such severity is necessary to produce the long-term impact. From a population health point of view, a mild level of growth retardation may be more important as this is more prevalent and could affect more people. The analysis here utilised birthweight Z score and childhood weight gain as continuous rather than dichotomous variables. The association between growth and stress appeared to be linear; none of the quadratic terms for the growth variables were significant. It points to the lack of a clear threshold for growth retardation to affect stress symptoms. However, the study might not have enough power to detect non-linear associations. So we have to take the finding with a pinch of salt. The last two decades saw the rise of obesity as a modern epidemic (McCarthy, Ellis & Cole, 2003). The NCDS cohort spent their childhood in a relatively obesity free environment. So the linear relation found in the present study should not be extrapolated to modern cohorts to suggest that obese children would suffer less stress when they grow up.

Apart from HPAA and SNS activities, at least two more pathways of associations could be proposed to explain the association between growth in early life and psychological health in adulthood. Firstly, growth is related to life chances, such as education and, in one study (Phillips et al., 2001), marital status. Secondly, various chronic diseases are related to growth in early life (Barker, 1998). Social situations and health in adults therefore are possible intermediaries. In the analysis here, however, adjustment for these variables did not strongly modify the linear regression coefficients and odds ratios on birthweight Z score and weight gain. So they could not be major intermediate variables.

Maternal smoking and father's social class were also associated with the stress symptoms. The reduction of maternal smoking has been an obvious and uncontroversial target for public health programmes. The findings here provide one more reason for women not to smoke. Participants whose mothers quitted smoking prior to the fifth months of pregnancy did not have significantly more symptoms. So among women who do smoke, quitting is beneficial in this regard. The relation between parental social class and offspring's health has been one of the key issues in the debate on and studies of inequalities in Britain for decades. Cohort members from social classes I and II had significantly lower scores on the psychological scale. However, this advantage appeared to be largely an indirect effect exerted via parental influence on the participants' educational level. Once the educational qualifications of the participants were included in the multiple regression model, the effect of father's social class disappeared.

The population attributable-risk fraction (PAF) is a useful measure that takes into account strength of association as well as prevalence of the exposure. However, it relies on the strong assumption that the associations concerned are causal. To establish a causal relation beyond doubt is a very difficult task and the present study could not claim to have done so. The PAF's were estimated for the purpose of assessing the (relative) importance of the early exposures in a hypothetical situation that they were indeed the causal origins of high levels of stress in adults. The fractions of population-risk attributable to growth, maternal smoking and father's social class were not very large. A substantial fraction of the risk remained unexplained. Stress is a construct difficult to measure. Part of the unexplained variation is definitely due to measurement errors. Among the four variables discussed, slow fetal and childhood growth together accounted for 6% of the PAF. This is similar to the PAF maternal smoking (5.9%) and father's social class (6.8%) accounted for. The potential impact of slow growth was roughly equivalent to these two factors.

This study of the early origins of stress symptoms is unique in that sample size was very large, participants were followed up to 42 years of age, and data on both birthweight and childhood weight gain were available. One criticism about the studies of growth is that the findings could be confounded by social-economic status, congenital abnormalities, etc. (Chard, Yoong & Macintosh, 1993; Power et al., 1991). In the present study, multiple births and cohort members with congenital abnormalities were excluded to reduce the possible noises and confounding. The analyses adjusted for major covariates, such as parity and father's social class. That the growth variables did not relate to somatic symptoms is also against the scepticism about socio-economic confounding because the somatic symptoms are related to socio-economic situations (Cheung, 2002). Another common criticism concerns missing values and sample attrition. Losses to follow-up in such a longitudinal study over 40 years are inevitable. However, about 79% of the eligible cohort members were included in model I and about 67% in models II and III. These proportions are much larger than that of some other studies with shorter follow-up times. Comparison of the mean growth values and psychological scores of subjects included in the regression analysis and subjects with known growth or psychological score values but excluded due to incomplete data suggested that the excluded subjects might have slightly slower growth and slightly higher levels of psychological distress. This pattern of exclusion may lead to a dilution of associations (Cheung, 2001). Therefore, if there was a selection bias it was likely to be a bias towards the null value rather than a bias towards a spurious association.

The limitations of this study has suffered largely arose from the fact that the NCDS was not specifically designed for the present purpose. The definition of weight gain in early childhood as the difference in Z scores between birth and age 7 and the use of the Malaise Inventory as the outcome measure were based on data availability rather than theoretical considerations. Hence childhood growth and stress symptoms have not been conceptualised and measured in fine details in this study. Future studies should preferably take stages of human growth into account (Karlberg, 1989) and adopt a variety of measures to assess different aspects of stress (e.g. Compas, Connor, Osowiecki & Welch, 1997; Crawford & Henry, 2003).

The interpretation of growth pattern and its associations with health outcomes is not straightforward. Growth is usually considered an indicator of nutritional status. However, poor fetal nutrition does not necessarily imply a poor diet on the part of mothers. The fetus is at the end of a long nutritional supply line that extends from maternal intake, maternal metabolic and hormonal milieu, through the uterine blood supply and placental function, and finally to the fetus (Bloomfield & Harding, 1998). A disruption in any part of the supply line could incur a nutritional insult to the fetus and contribute to intrauterine growth retardation. While birthweight is largely unrelated to genetic factors, weight in childhood is (Brooks, Johnson, Steer, Pawson & Abdalla, 1995; Tanner, 1978). It is not impossible that both childhood growth and subsequent stress symptoms share the same genetic basis. To a considerable extent, the hypothesis about the relation between growth and stress has been shaped by animal studies in which dietary restriction were experimentally induced. Whether in humans the association represents the impact of diet or nutritional status remains uncertain. Further research will need to collect more detailed information about growth and its determinants, nutritional status, physiological and psychological measures of stress in order to better understand the complex web of associations. We should not presume that a better or heavier diet will help to stave off stress.

ACKNOWLEDGMENTS

I thank The UK Data Archive and the Centre for Longitudinal Studies, London, for providing the data of the National Child Development Study.

REFERENCES

Barker, D.J.P. (1998). *Mothers, babies and health in later life.* Edinburgh: Churchill Livingingstone.

Barrett, D.E. & Radke-Yarrow, M. (1985). Effects of nutritional supplementation on children's responses to novel, frustrating and competitive situations. *American Journal of Clinical Nutrition*, 42, 102-120.

Batstra, L., Hadders-Algra, M., Neeleman, J. (2003). Effect of antenatal exposure to maternal smoking on behavioural problems and academic achievement in childhood: prospective evidence from a Dutch birth cohort. Early Human Development, 75, 21-33.

Beattie, R.B. & Johnson, P. (1994). Practical assessment of neonatal nutrition status beyond birthweight: an imperative for the 1990s. *British Journal of Obstetrics & Gynecology*, 101, 842-846.

Bloomfield, F.H. & Harding, J.E. (1998). Experimental aspects of nutrition and fetal growth. *Fetal and Maternal Med Review*, 10, 91-107.

Brady, A.R. (1988). Adjusted population attributable fractions from logistic regression. *Stata Technical Bulletin Reprints*, 42, 137-143.

Brooks, A.A., Johnson, M.R., Steer, P.J., Pawson, M.E. & Abdalla, H.I. (1995). Birth weight: nature or nurture ? *Early Human Development*, 42, 29-35.

Bruzzi, P., Green, S.B., Byar, P., Brinton, L.A. & Schairer C. (1985). Estimating the population attributable risk for multiple risk factors using case-control data. *American Journal of Epidemiology*, 123, 904-914.

Chard, T., Yoong, A. & Macintosh, M. (1993): The myth of fetal growth retardation at term. *British Journal of Obstetrics & Gynecology*, 100, 1076-1081.

Cheung, Y.B. & Yip, P.S.F. (2001) Social patterns of birth weight in Hong Kong, 1984-1997. *Social Science & Medicine*, 52, 1135-1141.

Cheung, Y.B. (1998). Can marital selection explain the differences in health between married and divorced people? *Public Health*, 112, 113-117.

Cheung, Y.B. (2001). Adjustment for selection bias in cohort studies. An application of a probit model with selectivity to life course epidemiology. *Journal of Clinical Epidemiology*, 54, 1238-1243.

Cheung, Y.B. (2002). Early origins and adult correlates of psychosomatic distress. *Social Science & Medicine*, 55, 937-948.

Cheung, Y.B., Low, L.C.K., Osmond, C., Barker, D.J.P. & Karlberg, J.P.E. (2000). Fetal growth and early postnatal growth are related to blood pressure in adults. *Hypertension*, 36, 795-800.

Cianfarani, S., Germani, D. & Branca, F. (1999). Low birthweight and adult insulin resistance: the "catch-up growth" hypothesis. *Archives of Diseases in Childhood: Fetal & Neonatal Edition*, 81, F71-F73.

Clark, P.M. (1998). Programming of the hypothalamo-pituitary-adrenal axis and the fetal origins of adult disease hypothesis. *European Journal of Pediatrics*, 157, S7-S10.

Clark, P.M., Hindmarsh, P.C., Shiell, A.W., Law, C.M., Honour, J.W. & Barker DJ. (1996). Size at birth and adrenocortical function in childhood. Clinical Endocrinology (Oxf), 45, 721-726.

Compas, B.E., Connor, J., Osowiecki, D. & Welch, A. (1997). Effortful and involuntary responses to stress: Implications for coping with chronic stress. In B.H. Gottlieb (Eds.), *Coping with chronic stress* (pp. 105-130). NY: Plenum.

Crawford, J.R. & Henry, J.D. (2003). The Depression Anxiety Stress Scales (DASS): Normative data and latent structure in a large non-clinical sample. *British Journal of Clinical Psychology*, 42, 111-131.

Fergusson, D.M., Woodward, L.J., Horwood, L.J. (1998). Maternal smoking during pregnancy and psychiatric adjustment in late adolescence. *Archive of General Psychiatry*, 55, 721-727.

Fernald, L.C. & Grantham-McGregor, S.M. (1998). Stress response in school-age children who have been growth retarded since early childhood. *American Journal of Clinical Nutrition*, 68, 394-405.

Ferri, E. (1993). *Life at 33: The fifth follow-up of the National Child Development Study*. London: National Children's Bureau.

Grant, G., Nolan, M. & Ellis, N. (1990). A reappraisal of the Malaise Inventory. *Social Psychiatry and Psychiatric Epidemiology*, 25, 170-178.

Greenland, S. & Drescher, K. (1993). Maximum likelihood estimation of the attributable fraction from logistic models. *Biometrics*, 49, 865-872.

Hirst, M.A. & Bradshaw, J.R. (1983). Evaluating the Malaise Inventory: A comparison of measures of stress. *Journal of Psychosomatic Research*, 27, 193-199.

Jones, P.B., Rantakallio, P., Hartikainen, A.L., Isohanni, M., Sipila, P. (1998). Schizophrenia as a long-term outcome of pregnancy, delivery, and perinatal complications: A 28-year follow-up of the 1966 North Finland general population birth cohort. *American Journal of Psychiatry* 155, 355-364.

Karlberg, J. (1989). A biologically-oriented mathematical model (ICP) for human growth. *Acta Paediatrica Scandinavia*, 350, S70-S94.

Karlberg, J. & Albertsson-Wikland, K. (1995). Growth in full-term small-for-gestational-age infants: from birth to final height. *Pediatric Research*, 38, 733-739.

Levitsky, D.A. & Barnes, R.H. (1970). Effect of early malnutrition on the reaction of adult rats to aversive stimuli. *Nature*, 225, 468-469.

Levitsky, D.A. & Strupp, B.J. (1995). Malnutrition and the brain: changing concepts, changing concerns. *Journal of Nutrition*, 125, 2212S-2220S.

Lucas, A., Fewtrell, M.S. & Cole, T.J. (1999). Fetal origin of adult disease: the hypothesis revisited. *British Medical Journal*, 319, 245-249.

McCarthy, H.D., Ellis, S.M. & Cole, T.J. (2003). Central overweight and obesity in British youth aged 11-16 years: cross-sectional surveys of waist circumference. *British Medical Journal*, 326, 624.

Nilsson, P.M., Nyberg, P. & Ostergren, P.O. (2001). Increased susceptibility to stress at a psychological assessment of stress tolerance is associated with impaired fetal growth. *International Journal of Epidemiology*, 30, 75-80.

Petrou, S., Kupek, E., Vause, S. & Maresh, M. (2001). Clinical, provider and socio-demographic determinants of the number of antenatal visits in England and Wales. *Social Science & Medicine*, 52, 1123-1134.

Phillips, D.I. & Barker, D.J. (1997). Association between low birthweight and high resting pulse in adult life: is the sympathetic nervous system involved in programming the insulin resistance syndrome? Diabetics Medicine, 14, 673-677.

Phillips, D.I., Walker, B.R., Reynolds, R.M., Flanagan, D.E., Wood, P.J., Osmond, C., Barker, D.J.P. & Whorwood, C.B. (2000). Low birthweight predicts elevated plasma cortisol concentrations in adults from 3 populations. *Hypertension*, 35, 1301-1306.

Phillips, D.I.W., Handelsman, D.J., Eriksson, J.G., Forsen, T., Osmond, C. & Barker, D.J.P. (2001). Prenatal growth and subsequent marital status: longitudinal study. *British Medical Journal*, 322, 771.

Power, C. & Matthews, S. (1997). Origins of health inequalities in a national population sample.*Lancet*, 1997, 350, 1584-1589.

Power, C., Manor, O. & Fox, J. (1991). *Health and class: The early years*. London: Chapman & Hall.

Richards, M., Hardy, R., Kuh, D. & Wadsworth, M.E.J. (2002). Birthweight, postnatal growth and cognitive function in a national UK birth cohort. *International Journal of Epidemiology*, 31, 342-348.

Rodgers, B., Pickles, A., Power, C., Collishaw, S. & Maughan, B. (1999). Validity of the Malaise Inventory in general population samples. *Social Psychiatry and Psychiatry Epidemiology*, 34, 333-341.

Royston, P. & Wright, E.M. (1998). A method for estimating age-specific reference intervals ('normal ranges') based on fractional polynomials and exponential transformation. *Journal of the Royal Statistical Society, Series A*, 161, 79-101.

Rutter, M., Tizard, J. & Whitmore, K. (1970) *Education, health and behaviour*. London: Longmans.

Smart, J.L., Whatson, T.S. & Dobbing, J. (1975). Thresholds of response to electric shock in previously undernourished rats. *British Journal of Nutrition*, 34, 511-516.

StataCorp. (2001). *Stata Statistical Software: Release 6.0.* College Station, TX: Stata Corporation.

Tanner, J.M. (1978). *Foetus into man: Physical growth from conception to maturity.* London: Open Books.

Thompson, E.J. (1995) The 1991 census of population in England & Wales. *Journal of the Royal Statistical Society, Series A*, 158, 203-240.

Townsend, P., Davidson, N. & Whitehead, M. (1988). *Inequalities in health.* Harmondsworth: Penguin.

van de Mheen, H., Stronks, K., Looman, C.W.N., Mackenbach, J.P. (1998). Role of childhood health in the explanation of socioeconomic inequalities in early adult health. *Journal of Epidemiology and Community Health*, 52, 15-19.

van der Meulen, J.H.P. (2001). Early growth and cognitive development. *International Journal of Epidemiology*, 30, 72-74.

van Reempts, P.J., Woutersn A., de Cock, W., & van Acker, K.J. (1997). Stress responses to tilting and odor stimulus in preterm neonates after intrauterine conditions associated with chornic stress. *Physiology & Behavior*, 61, 419-424.

Welberg, L.A., Seckl, J.R. & Holmes, M.C. (2000). Inhibition of 11beta-hydroxysteroid dehydrogenase, the foeto-placental barrier to maternal glucocorticoids, permanently programs amygdala GR mRNA expression and anxiety-like behaviour in the offspring. *European Journal of Neuroscience*, 12, 1047-1054.

Welberg, L.A., Seckl, J.R. & Holmes, M.C. (2001). Prenatal glucocorticoid programming of brain corticosteriod receptors and corticotrophin-releasing hormone: possible implications for behaviour. *Neuroscience*, 104, 71-79.

WHO Working Group. (1986). Use and interpretation of anthropometric indicators of nutritional status. *Bulletin of the World Health Organization*, 64, 929-941.

Wright, E. & Royston, P. (1997) Age-specific reference intervals ("normal ranges"). *Stata Technical Bulletin Reprints*, 6, 91-104.

Zeger, S.L. & Liang, K.Y. (1986). Longitudinal data analysis for discrete and continuous outcomes. *Biometrics*, 42, 121-130.

In: Stress and Health: New Research
Editor: Kimberly V. Oxington, pp. 103-123
ISBN 1-59454-244-9
©2005 Nova Science Publishers, Inc.

Chapter V

EVALUATING PARENTAL STRESS EXPERIENCES FOLLOWING PRETERM BIRTH

Rosalind Lau and Carol Morse
Royal Women's Hospital
Victoria University
Australia

ABSTRACT

A controlled prospective longitudinal study was carried out to evaluate stress experiences of parents whose preterm infants were admitted to a special care nursery in a tertiary level maternity hospital. The control group consisted of parents of fullterm infants matched on maternal age, parity and socioeconomic status. Sixty mothers and 59 fathers of preterm infants and 60 mothers and fathers of fullterm infants were followed from birth to 16 weeks after discharge home. A battery of self-reports was utilised that have been well validated. These instruments were used to collect information on feelings, moods, marital/partner relationships, availability and satisfaction with perceived social support and salivary markers of stress (cortisol and tribulin) were collected. Data were collected on five occasions with parents of preterm infants and on three occasions with parents of healthy term infants. Findings revealed that parents of preterm infants reported higher subjective stress levels than parents of term infants within the first week of their infant's birth but returned lower objective markers of stress. Mothers of preterm infants were more anxious and stressed when compared to fathers of preterm infants. The stress levels for parents of preterm infants reduced over time and appeared to illustrate positive effect from the support of health care professionals. There was no direct correlation between self-reported stress and the biochemical markers of stress. Issues for future research are discussed.

INTRODUCTION

Parenthood is one of the most frequently experienced life transitions in our society and for most people, this event is part of a normal life course. However, even this normative event is not easy for any new parent and is a challenge that is influenced by multiple factors, such as parental age, length of relationship, previous experience with children, role adjustment, availability of social support, the value and expectation parents place on the infant, and individual coping patterns [1]. This challenge is compounded by the birth of a preterm infant. Previous research has shown that parents of preterm infants experience a range of mixed emotions [2]. The most commonly reported responses are anxiety, helplessness, fear, uncertainty, and worry about the outcome of their infant. Other common responses reported by mothers are sadness, guilt, shame, a sense of failure and depression. These findings indicate that not only is the birth traumatic for the parents but the appearance and behaviours of the preterm infant may trigger mixed emotions, that can, not infrequently includes produce feelings of rejection of the child. The subsequent hospitalisation of the infant further contributes to the parental stress.

Previous studies of parents of preterm infants have tended to focus on the mothers in particular and on the neonatal intensive care unit (NICU). Given that special care nurseries have assumed a wider responsibility for monitoring infants of increasing immaturity and poorer health status than previously, it is important that parental responses to this hospitalisation is examined. This was the first study in the world that examined the stress experiences of mothers and fathers with preterm infants in the tertiary-based special care nursery (SCN) environment. In this study, to identify the stress levels of these parents both self-report questionnaires and objective biochemical markers of stress were measured. The study design utilised a controlled comparison that compared the stress levels of parents of preterm infants in the special care nursery with parents of healthy term infants in the postnatal ward in a tertiary maternity setting.

CONCEPTUAL FRAMEWORK

The conceptual framework for this study was based on the transactional model of stress and coping proposed by Richard Lazarus and his colleagues [3,4].

The transactional model of Lazarus and colleagues views stress and coping as productions of cognition, as products of the way an individual appraises his or her relationship with the environment in a continuing changing transaction. Further, that it is these interactions between an individual and the environment that result in stress experiences and not simply whether or not a serious or significant event occurs. The second component of the transactional model includes a consideration of the coping skills and strategies an individual has at their disposal through which to respond to the stressful event (stressor). This model has been widely used because of its emphasis on the individual and his or her ability to cope with demands. It is not stress per se that is important in adaptation but it is the way we both perceive and cope with the event(s) and situation(s).

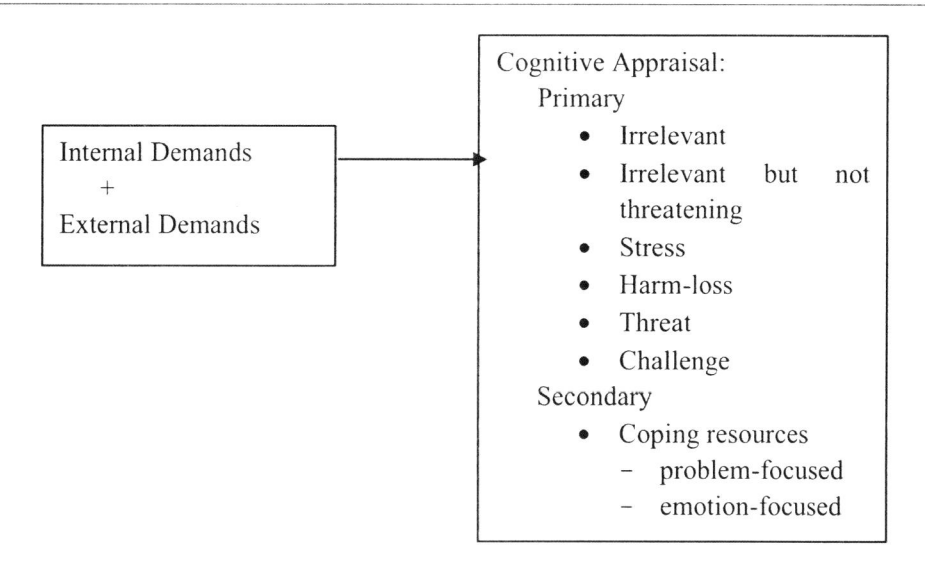

```
┌──────────────────┐          ┌─────────────────────────────────┐
│ Internal Demands │          │ Cognitive Appraisal:            │
│        +         │─────────▶│ Primary                         │
│ External Demands │          │   • Irrelevant                  │
└──────────────────┘          │   • Irrelevant but not          │
                              │     threatening                 │
                              │   • Stress                      │
                              │   • Harm-loss                   │
                              │   • Threat                      │
                              │   • Challenge                   │
                              │ Secondary                       │
                              │   • Coping resources            │
                              │       - problem-focused         │
                              │       - emotion-focused         │
                              └─────────────────────────────────┘
```

Adapted from Lazarus and colleagues transactional model of stress and coping (1978, 1984).

Figure 1 Transactional model of stress and coping

The transactional view of stress and coping has an important central feature. It emphases the process, on what is happening between the individual and the environment in any given stressful encounter and how changes, which occur over time or across encounters, are interpreted and reacted to. Thus, the process contains two elements which can be applied to the present focus of study. The first element focuses on the actual interchange between the individual and the environment e.g. with the birth of a preterm infant, the focus is on the specific stressful encounter faced by the parents brought about by the premature rather than the expected full term birth. The second element focuses on the flow and transformation of the interchange. It emphases flux and change over time in diverse encounters [5]. That is, a stressful encounter is not a momentary static stimulus in the environment to which the individual gives a single response. Rather, it is a continuous flow of events over seconds or minutes, days or weeks e.g. the coping process of responding to the concerns and distress common to parents following giving birth to a preterm infant. The process tends to occur over an extended time and encompasses many encounters that continuously trigger a range of psychological and emotional changes. Initially, the parents may experience a range of negative feelings (shock, loss, guilt and sadness). Eventually, they may accept the loss of an expected full term infant and, through successful adaptation, and resolution of feelings and negative reactions, hopefully come to accept the premature birth.

Transaction has two meanings: (1) transaction means not only does the environment affect the individual but the individual affects the environment, both influencing the other mutually in the course of an encounter; and (2) the transaction brought about by the interaction between the individual and the environment forms a series of new relationships. According to Lazarus and Launier [3], the individual and the environment are seen to be in a dynamic relationship of reciprocal interaction, each affecting and in turn being affected by the other.

Cognitive Appraisal

According to Morse [6], the key factor in Lazarus theory of stress transaction is the cognitive system. Cognition refers to attitudes, attributes, beliefs, inferences and thoughts that operate at conscious, unconscious and preconscious levels [7]. The cognitive system produces interpretations of events that are designed to make meaningful sense of myriad incoming sensations from both external social sources and the internal physiological environment. According to Lazarus [8], the individual's cognitive system appraises incoming stimuli in two ways. Primary appraisal refers to the interpretation of stimuli into inferences of irrelevance, challenge or threat-harm. Secondary appraisal refers to the evaluation of one's coping resources that are presently or potentially available for dealing with the demand that has arisen. Accordingly, it is the quality of these appraisals that determines whether these transactions are stressful or not, and not only because of some intrinsic entity in the stimuli themselves. In Lazarus's stress model [8], secondary appraisal refers to the second phase in the stress transaction, that involves one's subjective evaluations about the possible responses available through applying acquired skills and knowledge that can be brought to bear on the stress experience.

This secondary appraisal is concerned with judgements about readily available or potential *coping* strategies. These include personal resources (attitudes, beliefs, abilities, self-concept), styles (strategies, defences) and efforts (internal and external actions) [9]. Coping, then, is primarily a psychological construct concerning inner struggles with perceived demands, conflicts and the emotional distress generated by these. It is a continuous process characterised by attempts to master and gain control over an external social world event; to maintain emotional and physiological equilibrium (internal reactions) in order to execute effective motivated actions and decision-making; to retain/regain flexibility of action; and to increase one's tolerance for negative realities in order to hold on to a positive self-image [4].

Coping

Lazarus's definition of coping refers to the process of managing demands both external and internal that are appraised as taxing or exceeding the resources of an individual [10]. This definition has three important characteristics. Firstly, it is process-oriented. Coping refers to what an individual actually thinks or does in relation to a perceived challenge or stressor and the changes in these thoughts and actions as the situation unfolds. Secondly, the definition is contextual which emphasises that the transaction and process for any two events are not the same. Individuals use different coping strategies at varying phases of implementing efforts to solve a given problem. Thus, coping is not determined solely by personal disposition but also by the individual's appraisal of the demands of a particular situation. Thirdly, coping is exercised without reference to its outcome.

Coping refers to the efforts to manage a challenging event moment by moment, not necessarily to the success of these efforts. People are often confronted with situations that cannot be mastered or controlled. In such cases, effective coping involves coming to terms with undesirable outcomes rather than mastering them. Originally, Lazarus [8] referred to this category as 'palliative coping'. Coping consists of efforts to manage, reduce, tolerate or minimise the demands created by the stressful transactions. Clearly, the relationship between coping and a stressful event represents a dynamic process and coping can be seen to be a set of reciprocal transactions by which the event and the individual influence each other.

Lazarus and Folkman [4] identified two forms of coping: (1) problem-focused coping which is the management of the problem that is causing the distress and (2) emotion-focused coping, the management of the emotions or distress that arise from the stressful transactions. *Problem-focused* coping is directed at defining the problem, generating alternative solutions and weighing up the options for action in terms of their costs and benefits. Problem-focused coping embraces an array of problem-oriented actions, which include strategies that are directed at the environment and those that are directed at the self which include cognitive problem identification and solving and decision making. Each of these may include interpersonal conflict resolution, information gathering, and advice seeking. *Emotion-focused* coping, previously referred to as *palliative coping*, consists of the mobilisation of cognitive processes directed primarily at reducing the emotional distress occasioned by the challenge or stressor and includes strategies that utilise a range of intrapsychic defensive processes (such as denial, repression and distancing, suppression or intellectualisation).

Emotion-focused coping is used to minimise anxiety, maintain hope and optimism, to reduce the reality of the event and to acknowledge that the event is harmful. Other strategies include reappraisal by changing the way an encounter is construed without changing the objective of the situation e.g. threat is diminished by changing the meaning of the situation, "I decided that there are more important things to worry about" (denial or suppression), "or looking at the brighter side of things" (rationalisation or intellectualisation). Problem- and emotion-focused forms of coping can be mutually facilitative. Coping has been named a "shifting" process in which a person must, at certain times, rely on one form of coping, say emotion-solving strategy and at other times, on a problem-solving strategy, as the demands of the situation change.

There are numerous studies on the experiences of parents of preterm infants. These studies tended to focus predominately on mothers with preterm infants in the neonatal intensive care nursery only. The studies of today tend to include the fathers. In the past decade special care nursery in a tertiary-based centre has become more technically orientated making it possible to provide more care to smaller and sicker infants that would normally been cared for in a NICU. Thus resulted in the SCN having the potential to alienate the parents from their infants. This indicates that there is a real need to study the experiences of parents (both mothers and fathers) of preterm infants admitted to a special care nursery. For a more comprehensive monitoring of stress experiences, it is regarded that psychosocial indicator alone is insufficient and therefore biochemical markers of stress were measured simultaneously.

METHODS

This study was carried out at in Melbourne, Australia, from December 1997 to June 2000 at one of the large public tertiary teaching hospitals. The research design utilised a controlled prospective longitudinal study. The Control group (n-120) was composed of both parents of healthy term infants who were matched by maternal age (within 5 years), and by parity and socioeconomic status (such as occupation). The gestational age was recorded from the baby's history which was determined by the attending neonatologist. The Experimental group (n=119) was both parents of preterm infants. Approval for the study was obtained from the Human Research Ethics Committees of the hospital and the University. Informed written consents were obtained from both parents in both groups.

Inclusion Criteria for Parents of Preterm and Term Infants

a) Both parents consenting to be involved
b) Primigravida and multigravida mothers and their partners
c) Parents aged between 20-40 years
d) Parents who were able to read and write English
e) Parents giving birth to a singleton
f) Parents with no known psychiatric history as recorded in the maternal history
g) Parents of infants with no congenital anomalies
h) Parents with no previous experience in a NICU/SCN

Sample Size

For the estimation of sample size for two groups, with α set at .05, power 80%, and 2 Tailed, the State-Anxiety Scale [11], and Stress/Arousal Checklist (SACL) [12] were used. The State-Anxiety Inventory scores which were used to calculate the sample size was based on an earlier study of maternal stress within the first postnatal week in NICU following hospitalisation of their preterm infant [13]. With a mean of 37.6 and a standard deviation of 7.1 for mothers of preterm infants and mean of 31.8 with a standard deviation of 10.6 for mothers of term infants (control group), it was estimated that 50 in each group would give a power of 89% [14].

Using the Stress/Arousal Checklist (SACL), the sample size was calculated based on the original sample of Women's Clinic Patients [12] with a mean of 38 and a standard deviation of 13. Accepting that parents of term infants would experience the same degree of stress (M 38, sd 13) and allowing for a minimum of half a standard deviation increase for parents of preterm infants admitted to a SCN (M 45, sd 13), the sample size would be 50 in each group to yield a power of 85% [14]. Based on previous study of first time parents [15] and allowing for an estimated attrition of up to 20% (N=10), 60 couples were recruited to each group. A total of 120 mothers entered the study but only 119 fathers (1 father of preterm infant consented to the study but did not return the questionnaire). Results of the total number of 239 are reported.

MEASURES

A series of validated psychological measures were used to assess feelings, moods, marital/partner relationship quality and social support.

Subjective Measures

Current levels of anxiety and anger feelings were assessed using the *State Personality Inventory*, two 10-item, four-point Likert scales of statements reflecting these feelings [11]. In responding to the state-anxiety and anger items, subjects report how they feel "right now" by rating the intensity of their anxiety or anger feelings on a four-point scale: where 1 = not at all; 2 = somewhat; 3 = moderately so; and 4 = very much so. For the trait-anxiety and –anger scales, subjects report how they "generally" feel by rating themselves on the Likert type four-point frequency scale where 1 = almost never; 2 = sometimes; 3 = often; 4 = almost always. Internal consistency of the scales is high with alpha = 0. 84 – 0.92 for state-anxiety; 0.90 – 0.92 for state-anger; 0.80 – 0.85 for trait-anxiety and 0.82 – 0.85 for trait –anger [16].

Stress/Arousal Checklist is an 18-item scale of stress adjectives (10 positive and 8 negative) and 12 items (7 positive and 5 negative) reflecting states of arousal [12]. The alpha coefficient was 0.89 for stress and 0.84 for arousal. There are two forms of scoring, short and long scoring. For the short scoring, the response scale is dichotomised and the two halves are scored either '0' and '1' according to whether the adjective is positive or negative. The long scoring is computed by scoring the individual response categories on a '1' to '4' Likert type scale.

Short-Form Dyadic Adjustment Scale is a 7-item, Likert-scale that assesses the couple's relationship quality. Internal consistency on an Australasian sample is high with alpha = 0.90 [17]. The one global item "overall happiness" showed 65% of cases to be classified correctly which indicated that the one global item was regarded as sufficient for a brief, rapid screening [18].

Beck Depression Inventory-Short Form is a 13-item self-report measure of symptoms and cognition only of depressed mood [19]. The shorter 13-item form was developed for use as a rapid screening instrument in clinical settings of general practice [20]. The short form correlates at 0.96 with the original 21-term inventory and 0.61 with the clinician's ratings of depression [20].

Short Form Social Support Questionnaire [21] is a six item questionnaire that assesses (a) the number of available others the individual feels he or she can turn to in times of need and (b) the individual's degree of satisfaction with the perceived support. The satisfaction with perceived support is measured on a 6-point Likert scale from 1=very dissatisfied to 6=very satisfied. The internal reliabilities range from 0.90 to 0.93 for both number and satisfaction level respectively.

Objective Measures

The human response to highly stressful conditions involves increased sympathetic–adreno medullary activity, increased hypothalamic-pituitary-adrenal cortisol activity and also enhanced turnover of the brain monoamine [22]. Thus, there is strong evidence that a relationship exists between perceived stress and raised levels of biochemical markers of cortisol and monoamine oxidase (MAO) inhibitory activities (tribulin) [23,24]. Therefore, ways to monitor biochemical indices of stress effects may be done by measuring the levels of cortisol and MAO inhibitory secretions in relation to stressful events.

Cortisol is secreted in an unbound state, however it binds to plasma proteins mainly to globulin and to a lesser extend to albumin [25]. It is the non-protein bound cortisol which is present in saliva and is regarded as the best indicator of psychological stress. The acinar cell lining the salivary glands prevents proteins and protein-bound molecules from entering the saliva and therefore the cortisol is of the unbound free hormone fraction that provides acceptable reliability [26]. Cortisol is known to have a very strong diurnal cycle where levels are highest in the morning and decrease throughout the day to reach a nadir around 8-9 pm [27,28]. The normal values at 8 am are 16 ± 8.2 nmol\L (range 6.4 to 32.2 nmol\L) for men and 9.8 ± 3.1 nmol\L (range 4.8 to 18.2 nmol\L) for women; the value at 8 pm for men and women are 3.9 ± 0.2 nmol\L (range 2.2 to 4.2 nmol\L) [29,30].

Earlier studies [31,32] measuring cortisol secretion have relied on serum and urine cortisol measurements, but recent advances in salivary cortisol assays have demonstrated a salivary sample to be a simple, non-invasive procedure that is readily accessible. Monoamine oxidase is present in the outer mitochondrial and nuclear membranes of the brain at synaptic endings [33]. MAO, a flavoenzyme is responsible for the metabolism of both endogenous and exogenous biogenic amines [34]. The presence of endogenous urinary monoamine oxidase inhibitory activity, [35] *tribulin*, [36] appears to be increased in a variety of conditions associated with anxiety or stress [37,38]. It has been reported that tribulin peaks to just over 50% immediately following a stressor [39]. Both cortisol and tribulin have been shown to exhibit a marked circadian pattern of activation with high level in the morning and low levels in the evening and night. Thus, the salivary samples for this study were collected between 4-8pm taking into consideration the usual circadian patterns of activation of both cortisol and tribulin. As well, the routine of the hospital (such as visiting times) inhibited the parents from completing the questionnaires.

A convenient and hygienic sampling device called the 'Salivette' (Sarstedt Inc., Rommelsdorf, Germany) was used. The salivette consists of a small cotton roll, which fits inside a standard centrifugate tube. It facilitates pipetting of the sample. The cortisol assays were determined using a radioimmunoassays commercial kit (Coat-A Count^R, Diagnostic Products Corporation, CA, USA) and the tribulin assays were determined by measuring its inhibition of MAO.

PROCEDURES

Psychological measures and biochemical assays were collected from each mother and father in both the target and control groups. Parents of preterm infants were invited to participate in the study within 24 hours after their infant's admission to the SCN. Data were collected separately from the mothers and fathers of both the preterm and term infants. Salivary samples were collected using a small dental roll from each parent of preterm and term infants on the days they completed the questionnaires with instructions to collect these between 4-8pm. Each parent was instructed to orally rinse with plain water, to place the roll in the mouth and suck on it for the duration of the time it took to complete the questionnaire (approximately 20 minutes in total). For Times 4 and 5, the questionnaires and the container with the cotton roll with an explanatory note were mailed to the parents with an addressed envelope for immediate return included. The salivary samples were then stored at the university at –80°C until analysed. Studies have shown that salivary cortisol concentrations do not appear to be affected by the storage temperature nor by the immediate or delayed centrifugation of samples [23,40].

For the parents of preterm infants, measures were collected separately on the following occasions:

T1 - within 24 hours after the parent's first visit to SCN
T2 – a week after their infants was admitted to SCN
T3 – at the time of their infant discharge from the SCN
T4 - 1 week after discharge home
T5 – 16 weeks after discharge home

Measures at Times 1, 4 and 5 only were collected from the Control group, as the mother and the healthy term infant are normally discharged home on day 2-5, therefore, the three measuring occasions were feasible and desirable and Times 2 and 3 were omitted.

Table 1 shows the times of the different measurements collected from the parents of preterm infants.

Table: 1. Timing of measures for parents of preterm infants

Measures	T1	T2	T3	T4	T5
State Anxiety & Anger	√	√	√	√	√
Trait Anxiety & Anger	√				√
Stress/Arousal	√	√	√	√	√
SDAS	√				√
BDI-SF	√				√
SSQ	√				√
Salivary Sample	pm	pm	pm	pm	pm

Table 2 shows the times of the different measurements collected from the parents of term infants.

Table 2: Timing of measures for parents of term infants

Measures	T1	T4	T5
State Anxiety & Anger	√	√	√
Trait Anxiety & Anger	√		√
Stress/Arousal	√	√	√
SDAS	√		√
BDI-SF	√		√
SSQ	√		√
Salivary Sample	pm	pm	pm

DESCRIPTIVE FINDINGS

The data were analysed using the Statistical Packages for the Social Sciences (SPSS, Version 9) [41].

Descriptive analyses were carried out on all variables. In the mothers' group, to reduce extreme skewness and kurtosis, the state-anger scores at Times 1, 4, and 5 were logarithmically transformed using Log^{10} because they were substantially positively skewed. Cortisol and tribulin values at Times 1, 4, and 5 which were moderately positively skewed were logarithmically transformed using the square root conversion. In the fathers' group, to reduce the extreme skewness and kurtosis, the state-anger and cortisol values at Times 1, 4, and 5 which were substantially positively skewed were also logarithmically transformed using Log^{10}.

The sample consisted of two groups of parents, 119 parents (60 mothers and 59 fathers) of infants born between 30-35 weeks gestation and 120 parents (60 mothers and 60 fathers) of infants born at full term, i.e. between 38-42 weeks gestation. One father of a preterm infant consented to be involved in the study but did not return the questionnaires. Two sets of parents of preterm infants were withdrawn from the study after they had completed the questionnaires at Time 1 because both infants were transferred to the neonatal intensive care nursery (NICU). One of these infants developed respiratory distress and required respiratory support and the other infant developed non-perforated necrotising enterocolitis and required respiratory support. However, the answers of these parents were included in the Time 1 analysis. Further losses of participants occurred over time. There were no demographic differences between those who continued with the study and those who did not.

Demographic profiles of all the parents recruited to the study are shown in Table 3.

Preterm Group

The average maternal age was 30 years (range 21-40 years), 57% (34) had undergone college and higher education and 42% (25) were in professional occupations. The average paternal age was 33 years (range 22-55 years), 53% (31) had received college and higher education and 53% (31) were in professional occupations. Just over 82% (98) of the parents were caucasian and the remainder 18% (21) were of Asian background with one couple of Aboriginal origin. In this group, 87% (52) babies were born by vaginal delivery and 13% (8) by elective caesarean section. Seventy three percent (44) of mothers were having their first baby (primigravida) and 27% (16) were having subsequent babies (multigravida).

Term Group

In the term group, the average maternal age was 30 years (range 23-40 years), 63% (38) had received college and higher education and 50% (30) were in professional occupations. The average paternal age was 32 years (range 22-43 years), 54% (32) had undergone college and higher education and 57% (34) were in professional occupation. Just over 85% (102) of the parents were caucasian and the remainder 15% (18) were of Asian background. In this group, 92% (55) babies were born by vaginal delivery and 8% (5) by elective caesarean section. There were 77% (46) primigravida and 23% (14) multigravida.

Table 3: Demographic profiles of the parents

	Preterm Mothers N=60	Term Mothers N=60	Preterm Fathers N=59	Term Fathers N=60
Age (yrs): M (sd)	30 (5)	30 (4)	33 (6)	32 (5)
Ethnicity: N (%)				
Australian	36 (60)	38 (63)	37 (63)	42 (70)
British	6 (10)	3 (5)	4 (7)	0 (0)
European	8 (13)	10 (17)	7 (12)	10 (17)
Asian	9 (15)	9 (15)	10 (16)	8 (13)
Others	1 (2)	0 (0)	1 (2)	0 (0)
Education: N (%)				
Primary	1 (2)	0 (0)	0 (0)	0 (0)
Secondary	25 (42)	16 (27)	18 (30)	11 (18)
Trade/Apprenticeship	0 (0)	6 (10)	9 (15)	17 (28)
Certificate/Diploma	10 (17)	8 (13)	10 (17)	10 (17)
Bachelor Degree/Higher	24 (40)	30 (50)	21 (36)	22 (37)
Missing	0 (0)	0 (0)	1 (2)	0 (0)
Occupation: N (%)				
Professional	25 (42)	30 (50)	31 (53)	34 (57)
Tradesperson/Related Workers	5 (8)	9 (15)	18 (53)	23 (38)
Clerical/Related Workers	16 (27)	15 (25)	2 (3)	2 (3)
Labourers	4 (7)	0 (0)	1 (2)	0 (0)
Home duties	10 (17)	5 (8)	0 (0)	0 (0)
Other	0 (0)	1 (2)	7 (12)	1 (2)
Parity: N (%)				
Primiparous	44 (73)	46 (77)		
Multiparous	16 (27)	14 (23)		
Mode of delivery : N (%)				
Vaginal	52 (87)	55 (92)		
Caesarean section	8 (13)	5 (8)		

There were no significant differences in the demographic profiles of the mothers in both groups in terms of age (p.729), education level (p.161), occupation (p.111), parity (p.676) and mode of delivery (p.382). In the fathers, there were no significant differences in age (p.097), and educational level (p.489), but a significant difference in occupation (p.021) indicating more fathers in the term group were in professional and trades occupations.

The characteristics of the preterm and term infants are shown in Table 4. The mean gestational age of the preterm babies was 33 weeks (range 30-35 weeks) and the mean birth weight was 2066g (range 1064-3128g). The mean gestational age of the term babies was 40 weeks (range 38-41 weeks) and the mean birth weight was 3444g (range 2475-4260g). As expected, there were significant differences between the infant groups in gestational age ($p<.001$), birth weight ($p<.001$), and number of days of hospitalisation ($p<.001$) with the preterm infants more underage and under-developed or lower birth weight and remaining in hospital for longer.

Table 4: Demographic characteristics of the infants

	Preterm M (sd) N=60	Term N=60	p
Gestation (wk)	33 (1)	40 (1)	<.001
Birth weight (gm)	2066 (397)	3444 (391)	<.001
Hospitalisation (day)	26 (10)	4 (1)	<.001
Sex: N%			
Male	32 (53)	31 (52)	NS
Female	28 (47)	29 (48)	NS

Univariate Analysis

Univariate analysis examined separately each variable. Table 5 shows the results of the self-reports of anxiety, anger, arousal, stress, cortisol and tribulin (biochemical markers of stress); maternal depression; marital/partner relationship; and social support measures at each time period for parents of preterm and term infants.

In the mothers, at Time 1, there were significant differences between the groups in state-anxiety ($p<.001$), state-anger (p.008), self-reported stress ($p<.001$), indicating that the mothers of preterm infants were the more stressed and distressed. The group differences in trait-anxiety were significant (p.027) indicating that mothers of preterm infants were more prone to anxiety compared to mothers of term infants.

At time 1, between the fathers' groups, there were significant group differences in state-anxiety ($p<.001$), self-reported stress (p.003), arousal (p.008), relationship quality (p.003), and satisfaction with perceived support (p.041). The result indicated that the fathers of preterm infants reported more stress, inversely related to arousal levels, while their relationship and perceived/received social support was also less positive. At Time 1, fathers of term infants reported a better relationship quality with their partners and also were more satisfied with perceived support than fathers of preterm infants.

Table 5: Univariate analysis of profiles of measures for parents of preterm and term infants

		Mothers				Fathers			
		Preterm		Term		Preterm		Term	
Variables	Time	N		N		N		N	
State-anxiety	1	60	21.4 (6.7)**	60	16.8 (4.7)	59	20.1 (5.9)**	60	16.4 (4.6)
	4	60	17.4 (4.9)	60	16.8 (4.9)	59	16.7 (5.1)	60	17.0 (5.0)
	5	60	14.5 (4.6)	60	16.3 (4.9)	59	16.2 (4.4)	60	16.5 (4.5)
State-anger (transformed Log 10)	1	60	1.1(9.2E-02)**	60	1.0 (5.7E-02)	59	1.1 (0.1)	60	1.1 (8.2E-02)
	4	60	1.1 (7.7E-02)	60	1.0 (8.1E-02)	59	1.1 (9.7E-02)	60	1.1 (8.0E-02)
	5	60	1.0 (9.3E-02)	60	1.1(7.8E-02)	59	1.1 (0.1)	60	1.1 (9.9E-02)
Stress	1	60	40.2 (12.3)**	60	31.5 (8.6)	59	36.2 (10.7)**	60	30.6 (9.1)
	4	60	33.8 (9.0)	60	31.3 (9.1)	59	31.4 (10.6)	60	30.0 (8.1)
	5	60	29.7 (10.0)	60	29.9 (10.7)	59	30.6 (9.0)	60	31.5 (9.4)
Arousal	1	60	33.8 (9.0)	60	31.3 (9.1)	59	30.8 (6.6)**	60	34.0 (6.5)
	4	60	28.7 (6.5)	60	29.7 (6.7)	59	32.6 (5.8)	60	34.0 (6.0)
	5	60	32.5 (6.1)	60	31.8 (6.8)	59	34.8 (6.5)	60	32.5 (6.8)
Cortisol (transformed square root)	1	47	2.2 (0.9)	47	2.5 (1.2)	48	4.8 (3.8)	48	5.2 (4.4)
	4	46	2.3 (1.2)	46	2.3 (1.1)	47	5.0 (6.0)	47	5.0 (5.4)
	5	47	1.9 (0.8)	46	1.9 (0.8)	45	3.8 (3.4)	46	5.4 (6.5)
Tribulin (transformed square root)	1	47	2.6 (1.1)	47	2.8 (1.4)	48	8.5 (5.9)	48	8.7 (7.4)
	4	46	3.0 (1.4)	46	3.1(1.3)	47	9.2 (6.9)	47	9.2 (5.5)
	5	47	3.1 (1.1)	46	2.8 (1.3)	45	10.2 (6.3)	46	10.5(6.3)
Trait-anxiety	1	60	18.3 (4.8)*	60	16.6 (3.3)	59	17.1 (5.1)	60	16.7 (4.2)
	5	60	17.4 (4.6)	60	16.8 (4.6)	59	16.4 (4.2)	60	17.0 (4.5)
Trait-anger	1	60	18.3 (4.1)	60	17.1 (3.3)	59	17.1 (4.1)	60	17.6 (3.6)
	5	60	17.5 (3.8)	60	17.4 (3.7)	59	16.7 (3.5)	60	17.1 (4.4)
Relationship quality	1	60	5.8 (1.3)	60	6.2 (0.9)	59	5.6 (1.2)**	60	6.1 (0.7)
	5	60	5.2 (1.2)	60	5.2 (1.3)	59	5.2 (1.5)	60	5.5 (1.1)
Depression	1	23	2.6 (1.3)	23	1.9 (1.3)				
	4	23	3.0 (0.7)	23	2.8 (1.3)				
Social support: Number	1	60	21.0 (11.2)	60	23.8 (12.9)	59	18.6 (13.7)	60	20.0 (10.9)
	5	60	20.5 (9.8)	60	21.2 (11.0)	59	16.4 (11.3)	60	14.9 (9.4)
Satisfaction	1	60	33.6 (4.5)	60	34.3 (2.3)	59	31.4 (7.4)*	60	33.5 (2.6)
	5	60	32.6 (4.0)	60	32.7 (4.6)	59	31.6 (4.2)	60	32.1 (2.7)

**p<0.01 *p<0.05

MANOVA Analysis

The cross-sectional results of MANOVA comparing the mothers of preterm and term infants are shown in Table 6.

Table 6: Mothers of preterm and term infants: MANOVA comparing combined measures of self-reports and biochemical markers of stress as a function of gestation type (N=94, 92, 93)

	N	Preterm M (sd)	N	Term M (sd)	P
Time 1	47		47		
State-anxiety		21.1 (6.5)**		16.5 (4.1)	<.001
State-anger (Log 10 transformed)		1.1 (9.4E-02)**		1.0 (5.7E-02)	.010
Stress		39.9 (12.1)**		31.2 (7.5)	<.001
Arousal		33.9 (8.7)		30.5 (8.5)	.063
Trait-anxiety		18.3 (4.8)*		16.4 (3.1)	.021
Trait-anger		18.4 (4.4)		17.2 (3.1)	.131
Cortisol (Square root transformed)		2.2 (0.9)		2.5 (1.2)	.326
Tribulin (Square root transformed)		2.6 (1.1)		2.8 (1.4)	.522
Relationship quality		6.0 (1.2)*		6.0 (1.1)	.047
Social support number		20.3 (11.3)		22.7 (12.0)	.322
Satisfaction		33.6 (3.6)		34.2 (2.1)	.347
Time 4	46		46		
State-anxiety		17.0 (4.6)		16.5 (4.8)	.578
State-anger (Log 10 transformed)		1.1 (6.7-02)		1.1 (7.0E-02)	.199
Stress		34.1 (8.8)		30.7 (8.6)	.065
Arousal		29.0 (7.0)		29.7 (5.8)	.591
Cortisol (Square root transformed)		2.0 (1.2)		2.3 (1.1)	.902
Tribulin (Square root transformed)		3.0 (1.4)		3.1 (1.3)	.647
Time 5	47		46		
State-anxiety		14.3 (4.1)		15.5 (4.5)	.184
State-anger (Log transformed)		1.0 (5.7E-02)		1.0 (6.6E-02)	.269
Stress		29.9 (8.7)		29.8 (9.9)	.795
Arousal		32.3 (6.7)		31.8 (6.1)	.748
Trait-anxiety		17.5 (4.4)		16.7 (4.5)	.414
Trait-anger		17.6 (4.0)		17.2 (3.7)	.655
Cortisol (Square root transformed)		1.9 (0.8)		1.9 (0.8)	.951
Tribulin (Square root transformed)		3.1 (1.1)		2.9 (1.4)	.284
Relationship quality		5.3 (1.1)		5.3 (1.1)	.907
Social support number		20.6 (10.0)		20.8 (10.3)	.938
Satisfaction		32.9 (3.6)		32.4 (5.1)	.520

**$p<0.01 *p<0.05

At Time 1 there were statistically significant differences between the mothers of preterm and term infants in anxiety (p<.001), anger (p.010), self-reported stress (p<.001), trait-anxiety (p.021), and relationship quality (p.047), indicating that mothers of preterm infants were more stressed with more negative moods and at the same time they reported a less satisfactory relationship with their partners at Time 1.

Table 7: Fathers of preterm and term infants: MANOVA comparing combined measures of self-reports and biochemical markers of stress as a function of gestation type (N=96, 94, 91)

	N	Preterm M (sd)	N	Term M (sd)	P
Time 1	48		48		
State-anxiety		19.3 (4.9)*		16.8 (4.8)	.013
State-anger (Log 10 transformed)		1.1 (9.5E-02)		1.1 (8.9E-02)	.484
Stress		34.7 (9.4)*		31.0 (9.3)	.050
Arousal		31.2 (6.4)*		34.3 (6.2)	.018
Trait-anxiety		17.7 (5.3)		16.7 (4.4)	.326
Trait-anger		16.9 (4.1)		17.3 (3.3)	.570
Cortisol (Square root transformed)		4.8 (3.8)		5.2 (4.4)	.624
Tribulin (Square root transformed)		8.5 (5.9)		8.7 (7.4)	.896
Relationship quality		5.6 (1.2)*		6.2 (0.6)	.004
Social support					
Number		19.1 (14.2)		19.7 (10.8)	.822
Satisfaction		31.3 (7.8)		33.5 (2.7)	.069
Time 4	47		47		
State-anxiety		16.3 (4.7)		17.1 (5.1)	.473
State-anger (Log 10 transformed)		1.1 (8.2E-02)		1.1 (8.0E-02)	.808
Stress		30.9 (9.6)		30.6 (8.1)	.686
Arousal		32.9 (5.9)		34.3 (5.9)	.239
Cortisol		5.0 (6.0)		5.0 (5.4)	.969
Tribulin		9.2 (7.0)		9.2 (5.5)	.994
Time 5	45		46		
State-anxiety		16.4 (4.3)		16.6 (4.1)	.799
State-anger (Log 10 transformed)		1.1 (9.9E-02)		1.1 (8.8E-02)	.688
Stress		30.2 (8.7)		31.7 (9.0)	.401
Arousal		34.8 (6.7)		33.2 (6.4)	.254
Trait-anxiety		16.1 (4.2)		16.9 (4.7)	.429
Trait-anger		16.4 (3.4)		16.5 (3.8)	.955
Cortisol		3.8 (6.3)		5.4 (6.5)	.145
Tribulin		10.3 (6.3)		10.5 (6.3)	.848
Relationship quality		5.2 (1.4)*		5.8 (0.9)	.030
Social support					
Number		15.6 (11.1)		15.3 (9.9)	.871
Satisfaction		31.6 (4.4)		32.4 (2.7)	.330

**p<0.01 *p<0.05

Utilising MANOVA, longitudinal analysis at Time 4 was carried out controlling for stress levels at Time 1 in mothers of the two groups. Results showed a significant difference only in self-reported stress (p.009). The same procedure was performed at Time 5 controlling for stress at Time 1 that showed a significant difference in trait-anxiety (p.007) between both groups.

Findings of the fathers' cross-sectional reports at each time phase using MANOVA at Time 1 (Table 7), revealed significant differences between the two groups of fathers in anxiety (p.013), self-reported stress (p.050), arousal (p.018), and quality of relationship (p.004). These results reflected those revealed in the mothers, indicating that fathers of preterm infants had more negative moods and the fathers of term infants reported a more satisfactory relationship. There was also a significant difference in relationship quality (p.030) at Time 5 indicating a more satisfactory relationship with their partners compared to fathers of preterm infants.

Utilising MANOVA for the two groups of fathers, longitudinal analysis at Time 4 controlling for stress levels at Time 1, showed significant differences in anxiety (p<.001), anger (p.005), stress (p<.001), and arousal (p.002), indicating that fathers of preterm infants were more anxious. Interestingly, fathers of term infants were more angry and had higher arousal levels. The same procedure was performed at Time 5 and again there were significant differences in anxiety (p.017) stress (p.008), and arousal (p<.001), trait-anxiety (p<.001), relationship quality (p.002), and satisfaction with perceived support (p.023). The results indicated that fathers of term infants had more negative feelings, but were less aroused and reported less satisfactory relationships with their partners.

DISCUSSION

The results reported in this study indicated that mothers of preterm infants were significantly stressed at Time 1 but less stressed at Time 5. Mothers of preterm infants were also more prone to depression at Time 1 compared to mothers of term infants. Even though mothers of preterm infants self-reported feeling were stressed at Time 1 their cortisol levels were lower than in the mothers of term infants indicating that they were in fact not more stressful than mothers of term infants. However, there were no differences in the tribulin levels for mothers of both groups and values were within the norms [29,30].

The fathers of preterm infants also reported more negative moods of anxiety and self-reported stress (SACL) at Time 1 than did the fathers of term infants. Even though fathers of preterm infants reported greater stress levels at Time 1, their arousal levels were lower than in the fathers of term infants indicating that self-reported stress and arousal were inversely related and that fathers of preterm infants were stressed but had low energy level.

Comparing the experiences of mothers and fathers of preterm infants, the mothers were more anxious and stressed at Times 1 and 4 compared to the fathers. The fathers reported higher arousal levels than mothers at Times 4 and 5. The fathers also reported higher cortisol and tribulin levels than the mothers at all three time periods.

Mothers of term infants were slightly stressed at Times 1 and 4 but the fathers were more stressed at Time 5. However, it is interesting to note that fathers had higher arousal levels than the mothers at each of the three time periods. This group of parents had a more satisfactory relationship at the birth of their infant but scores reduced over time suggesting the perceived quality of the relationship had deteriorated by 16 weeks after the infants were discharged from the hospital.

LIMITATIONS/WEAKNESSES OF THE STUDY

Method and Attrition

Recruitment and retention of an adequate number of subjects are crucial to the success of any study and the most serious problem of a longitudinal design is attrition of subjects or loss of subjects at different points of the study. In this study, parents of preterm infants at Time 3 had the lowest number of subjects and this is mainly due to the timing of the early discharge of the infants from the hospital. As the infants who were recruited into this study were not all booked for delivery at the tertiary level maternity hospital where they were located, once their conditions were stable, they were transferred back to the referral hospital which could have been up to 200 kilometres from Melbourne in regional or rural settings. So there were difficulties following up these infants. There was some attrition at other times in the study also even though several telephone calls were made when the parents had not returned the questionnaires.

Obtaining salivary specimens at one point in time and not repeatedly over time on a specific day only provides spot measurements. Obtaining measurements over time per day were not practical in this study, and therefore one needs to balance what is ideal and what is practical. Another limitation of the present study occurred when some parents collected their salivary specimens in the morning when the levels were high due to the usual circadian rhythms instead of in the late afternoon after 4 pm as instructed, when it was hypothesised that higher than normal levels would occur in those parents who were stressed. As well, many samples were not sufficient in quantity for analysis of both cortisol and tribulin. This emanated from inadequate attention being paid by the participants to the instructions to produce sufficient saliva through sucking on the cotton roll for at least 10 minutes during the time taken to complete the questionnaire in order to obtain a fully stimulated saliva flow. This was clearly not done by some of the parents.

Measures

In hindsight, the self-report questionnaires could have included a measure of locus of control and the multidimensional health locus of control instrument (MHLC) [42] would have been the measure of choice. Locus of control is a personality trait that is related to general psychological wellbeing and independent of the impact of life events [43]. An external locus of control (E-LOC) refers to beliefs that outcomes to demands are unrelated to one's behaviours, while an internal locus of control (I-LOC) refers to beliefs that the control of life experiences depends on one's own efforts to effect change. Since high internal people believe that they can determine their own fate and effect control, it is reasonable to say that these people would seek to be in control of their situation and therefore would be less anxious when facing a potentially stressful situation like having a baby and one that is premature requiring hospitalisation. An internally controlled individual is likely to engage in coping strategies that will moderate the impact of potentially stressful experiences. Thus, it is reasonable to expect an internally controlled person experiencing the birth of a preterm infant would be less affected on measures of negative moods (anxiety, and/or depression). Alternatively, people who seek/desire control in situations that are uncontrollable (e.g. following admission of their preterm infant to a special care nursery) would be more likely to experience stress. It is obvious that locus of control does play some role in affecting the ways in which people cope with their experience. In this study, the parents of the preterm infants felt assured that their infants were in SCN, being cared for by the medical and nursing staff (Powerful Others) at Time 1, yet their negative moods were significantly higher than the parents of term infants.

The sympathetic adreno-medullary system is very responsive to a variety of conditions that involve change, resulting in an increased production of catecholamines. Also, unpredictable and/or uncontrollable events have been shown to result in increased catecholamines (adrenaline and noradrenaline) production [44]. If control is achieved, adrenaline levels decrease near to normal but noradrenaline remains slightly elevated as long as attention demands prevail. Any state of under-stimulation or over-stimulation will be characterised by raised catecholamines output that corresponds closely to the subject's reports of feelings of discomfort or unpleasantness. Therefore, in hindsight it would have been valuable to measure catecholamines as well as cortisol and to have mapped the changes over time. Alternate advice was received during the planning stage of this study that tribulin was a suitable alternative biochemical marker [45] as an indicator of hypothalamic-pituitary-adrenal cortical activity of monoamine oxidase inhibitors, a key marker of anxiety. Given the results of the study, this might appear to have been a less suitable decision. In reality, tribulin levels rise in situations of acute stress in general and do not differentiate particularly how the individual is responding to the situation over time. In a harm/loss situation, it is expected there would be high levels of cortisol, adrenaline and noradrenaline output especially in the presence of felt helplessness. Alternately, in a challenge situation, noradrenaline levels will be moderately high but cortisol and adrenaline levels will be very high [46,47].

Future Research

From the literature review, this is the first study of its kind where the parents' experiences were examined when their preterm infants were admitted to a special care nursery. It was also one of a few studies where the collection of subjective and objective data of stress reactions were obtained simultaneously. Most of the parents in this study were caucasian, from middle class socioeconomic backgrounds, well-educated and with supportive networks. Further investigations are needed to assess the possible effects of ethnicity, lower social class, and poor supportive networks on parent's experiences when a preterm infants is born and subsequently admitted to a SCN. Future research should replicate this study in different SCN settings and in particular, these should preferably include objective measurements of both catecholamines and subjective reports of Locus of Control and stressful life event. This information would be most useful if it is supported by a concurrent qualitative data. Infants admitted to a SCN tend to be less smaller and sicker than infants admitted to a NICU. Therefore, it would be logical to expect lesser stress responses in parents in the former category. Hence, it would be interesting to compare the experiences of the parents whose preterm infants were admitted to a SCN with the parents whose preterm infants were admitted to a NICU.

REFERENCES

[1] Kenner, C. 1995. Transition to parenthood. In Gunderson, L.P. and Kenner, C. (eds.), *Care of the 24-25 week gestational age infant: A small baby protocol.* 2nd edition. Petaluma, CA: NICU INK

[2] Lau, R. and Morse, C. 1998. Experiences of parents with premature infants hospitalised in neonatal intensive care units: A literature review. *Journal of Neonatal Nursing*, 4 (6): 23-29

[3] Lazarus, R. and Launier, R. 1978. Stress-related transactions between person and environment. In Pervin, L. and Lewis, M. (eds.), *Perspectives in interactional Psychology.* New York: Plenum Press

[4] Lazarus, R. and Folkman, S. 1984. *Stress, appraisal, and coping.* New York: Springer

[5] Lazarus, R. 1981. The stress and coping paradigm. In Esidorfer, C., Cohen, D., Kleiman, A., et al. (eds.), *Models for clinical psychopathology.* Lancaster, England: MTP Press

[6] Morse, C.A. 1989. *Premenstrual syndrome: An integrated cognitive-hormonal analysis and treatment.* Doctoral dissertation, The University of Melbourne

[7] Dixon, N.F. 1981. *Preconscious processing.* New York: John Wiley and Son

[8] Lazarus, R. 1966. *Psychological stress and coping process.* New York: McGraw-Hill

[9] Menaghan, E.G. 1983. Individual coping efforts: Moderators of the relationship between life stress and mental outcomes. In Kaplan, H.B. (ed.), *Psychosocial stress: Trends in theory and research.* New York: Academic Press

[10] Lazarus, R. 1993. Coping theory and research: Past, present and future. *Psychosomatic Medicine,* 55:234-237

[11] Spielberger, C.D., Gorsuch, R.L. and Lushene, R.D. 1970. *STAI: Manual for the State-Trait Anxiety Inventory.* Palo Alto: Consulting Psychologists Press

[12] Gotts, G. and Cox, T. 1988. Stress and Arousal Checklist: Administration, scoring and interpretation. Australia: Swinburn Press

[13] Gennaro, S. 1988. Postpartal anxiety and depression in mothers of term and preterm infants. *Nursing Research,* 37(2):82-85

[14] *Sample power.* 1.0. 1997. SPSS Inc. USA

[15] Morse, C.A., Buist, A. and Durkin, S. 2000. First-time parenthood: Influences on pre- and postnatal adjustment in fathers and mothers. *Journal of Psychosomatic Obstretrics and Gynecology,* 21:109-120.

[16] Spielberger, C.D., Jacob, G., Crane, R., et al. 1979. *Preliminary manual for the state-trait personality inventory (STPI).* University of South Florida: Tampa.

[17] Sharpley, C.F. and Cross, D.G. 1982. A psychometric evaluation of the Spanier dyadic adjustment scale. *Journal of Marriage and the Family*, 44:739-741

[18] Sharpley, C.F., and Rogers, H.J. 1984. Preliminary validation of the abbreviated Spanier dyadic adjustment scale: Some psychometric data regarding a screening test of marital adjustment. *Educational and Psychological Measurement*, 1045-1049

[19] Beck, A.T., Ward, C.H., Mendelson, M., et al. 1961. An inventory for measuring depression. *Archives of General Psychiatry*, 4:561-571

[20] Beck, A.T. and Beck, R.W. 1972. Screening depressed patients in family practice: A rapid technique. *Postgraduate Medicine*, 52(6):81-85

[21] Sarason, I.G., Sarason, B.R., Shearin, E.N., et al. 1987. A brief measure of social support: Practical and theoretical implications. *Journal of Social and Personal Relationships*, 4:497-510

[22] Dantzer, R. 1989. Neuroendocrine correlates of control and coping. In Steptoe, A. and Appels, A. (eds.), *Stress, personal control and health*. New York: John Wiley and Sons

[23] Kahn, J.P, Rubinow, D.R. and Davis, C.L. 1988. Salivary cortisol: A practical method for evaluation of adrenal function. *Biological Psychiatry*, 23:335-349

[24] Doyle, A., Hucklebridge, F., Evans, P., et al. 1996. Salivary monoamine oxidase A and B inhibitory activities correlate with stress. *Life Sciences*, 59(16):1357-1362

[25] Greenspan, F.S. 1991. *Basic and clinical endocrinology*. 3rd edition. San Mateo, California: Appleton and Lange

[26] Kirschbaum, C. and Hellhammer, D.H. 1994. Salivary cortisol in psycho-neuroendocrine research: Recent developments and applications. *Psychoneuroendocrinology*, 19(4):313-333

[27] Kirschbaum, C. and Hellhammer, D.H. 1989. Salivary cortisol in psychobiological research : An overview. *Neuropsychobiology,* 22:150-169

[28] Ockenfels, M.C, Porter, L., Smyth, J., et al. 1995. Effect of chronic stress associated with unemployment and salivary cortisol: Overall cortisol levels, diurnal rhythm, and acute stress reactivity. *Psychosomatic Medicine,* 57(5):460-467

[29] Orth, D.N., Kovacs, W.J. and Debold, C.R. 1992. Adrenal the adrenal cortex. In Wilson, J.D. and Foster, D.W. (eds), *Williams Textbook of endocrinology*, London: W.B. Saunder

[30] Laudat, M.H., Cerdas, S., Fournier, C., et al. 1988. Salivary cortisol measurement: A practical approach to assess pituitary-adrenal function. *Journal of Clinical Endocrinology and Metabolism,* 66(2):343-348

[31] Roth-Isigkeit, A.K., Dibbelt, L. and Schmucker, P. 2000. Blood levels of corticosteroid-binding globulin, total cortisol and unbound cortisol in patients undergoing coronary artery bypass grafting surgery with cardiopulmonary bypass. *Steroids*, 65(9):513-520

[32] Kelly, K.S., Hayslip, B.Jr., Carter, A.P., et al. 1999. Comparisons of urinary verus serum cortisol in older persons. *Experimental Aging Research*, 25(2):161-167

[33] Muller, E.E. and Nistico, E. 1989. *Brain messengers and the pituitary*. New York: Academic Press

[34] Finch, C.C., Ho, S.L., Williams, A.C., et al. 1995. Platelet MAO activities and MAO protein concentrations in Parkinson's disease and controls. In Yu, P.M., Lipton, K.F.

and Boulton, A.A. (eds.), *Current neurochemical and pharmacological aspects of biogenic amines*. New York: Elsevier
[35] Glover, V., Raveley, M.A. and Sandler, M. 1980. A monoamine oxidase inhibitor in human urine. *Biochemistry Pharmacology*, 29:467-470
[36] Sandler, M. 1982. The emergency of tribulin. *Trends Pharmacology Science*, 471-472
[37] Clow, A., Glover, V., Sandler, M., et al. 1988. Increased urinary tribulin output in generalised anxiety disorder. *Psychopharmacology*, 95:378-380
[38] Clow, A., Glover, V., Weg, M.W., et al. 1988. Urinary catecholamine metabolite and tribulin output during lactate infusion. *British Journal of Psychiatry*, 52(1):122-126
[39] Hucklebridge, F., Sen, S., Evans, P.E., et al. 1998. The relationship between circadian patterns of salivary cortisol and endogenous inhibitor of monoamine oxidase A. *Life Science*, 62(25):2321-2328
[40] Leonard, J.P., MacKenzie, F.J., Patel, H.A., et al. 1991. Hypothalamic noradrenergic pathways exert an influence on norendocrine and clinical status experimental autoimmune encephalomyelitis. *Brain Behaviour Immunology*, 5:328-338
[41] *SPSS for Windows* [computer program]. SPSS 1. 10.0.7. 2000
[42] Wallston, K.A. and Wallston, B.S. 1978. Development of the multi-dimensional health locus of control (MHLC) scales. *Health Education Monographs*, 6(2):161-170
[43] Rotter, J.B. 1966. Generalized expectancies for internal versus external control of reinforcement. *Psychological Monographs 80* (Whole No.609)
[44] Frankenhaeuser, M. 1975. Sympathetic-adrenomedullary activity, behaviour and the psychosocial environment. In Venables, P.H. and Christie, M.J. (eds.), *Research in Psychophysiology*. New York: John Wiley
[45] Norman, T. 1997. Department of Psychiatry, Austin Repatriation Medical Centre, Melbourne, Victoria, Australia
[46] Frankenhaeuser, M., Nordheden, B., Myrsten, A., et al. 1971. Psychophysiological reactivity to understimulation and overstimulation. *Acta Psychologica*, 35:298-308
[47] Lundberg, U. and Frankenhaeuser, M. 1980. Pituitary-adrenal and sympathetic-adrenal correlates of distress and effort. *Journal of Psychosomatic Research*, 24:125-130

In: Stress and Health: New Research
Editor: Kimberly V. Oxington, pp. 125-141
ISBN 1-59454-244-9
©2005 Nova Science Publishers, Inc.

Chapter VI

CORTISOL RESPONSES TO EXPERIMENTAL STRESS IN PATIENTS WITH WHIPLASH ASSOCIATED DISORDER

Mariëtte Blokhorst[a], Pinel Schrijver[a], Stefan Meeldijk[a], Rob Hermans[b], Richel Lousberg[a,c] and Gerrit Zilvold[a].

[a] Roessingh, Research & Development, Enschede, the Netherlands
[b] Dept. Pharmacol.Toxicol., Cardiovasc. Res. Inst. Maastricht, Univ Maastricht, the Netherlands
[c] Dept. of Psychiatry, Academic Hospital Maastricht, the Netherlands

ABSTRACT

An experiment was carried out to explore cortisol levels and cortisol response as a result from a mental stress task, in patients with a Whiplash Associated Disorder (WAD) compared to healthy subjects and subjects in a relax-control condition. In addition, it was investigated whether the amount and appraisal of severity of daily hassles predicted cortisol response. It was expected that WAD patients had higher cortisol levels in time and that they showed a stronger increase in cortisol levels after performing a mental stresstask, compared to healthy subjects and subjects in a relax-control condition. Both the frequencies and appraisal of daily problems were assumed to be significant predictors of cortisol responsivity.

As was expected, results revealed that WAD patients had significant higher cortisol levels in time. Although the differences were not significant, there seems to be a trend towards an increase in cortisol concentrations after performing a mental stress task in the experimental WAD group, compared to the healthy control group and relax control groups.

Cortisol responsivity in the experimental groups is predicted by the amount of daily hassles and especially by the appraisals of severity of daily problems. The frequency and intensity ratings of daily hassles are significant higher in WAD patients compared to healthy persons.

It is concluded that chronic WAD patients have higher cortisol levels compared to healthy subjects. Because both the amount and appraisal of severity of daily problems are significant predictors of cortisol responsivity due to an acute mental stressor, it is plausible that a subgroup of WAD patients is more vulnerable to subsequent stressors after the whiplash injury. For this reason, 'stressmanagement' should be an important topic in rehabilitation programmes for chronic WAD patients. Study of HPA-axis in WAD patients offer new, interesting perspectives in the WAD phenomenon.

Key words: Whiplash Associated Disorder, Pain, Cortisol; Stress, Daily Hassles.

INTRODUCTION

There is consistent evidence that patients with a Whiplash Associated Disorder (WAD) experience a great deal of emotional distress following the onset of physical symptoms (Radanov, Di Stefano, Schnidrig, Ballinari, P., 1991; Merksey, 1993; Barnsley, Lord, Bogduk, 1994; Radanov, Di Stefano, Schnidrig, Sturzenegger, 1994; Drottning, Staff, Levin, Malt, 1995; Radanov, Begre, Sturzenegger, Augustiny, 1996; Mayou, 1997; Blokhorst, Lousberg, Vingerhoets, Winter, Zilvold, 2002; Sterling, Kenardy, Jull, Vicenzino, 2003). A WAD is a hyper-extension / flexion trauma of the neck, resulting after an injury (often an automobile accident) and is accompanied by pain in the neck, headache, fatigue, dizziness, attentional problems and emotional distress (Spitzer, et al., 1995). Most authors agree that the distress WAD sufferers report is a consequence of the physical injury itself and its profound effects on daily life (Radanov, Di Stefano, Schnidrig, Sturzenegger, 1994; Mayou, 1997; Blokhorst, Lousberg, Vingerhoets, Winter, Zilvold, 2002). Recent results revealed that both the amount of problems related to personal functioning, as well as WAD patient's excessively negative interpretations of stressors contribute to the level of distress (Blokhorst, Lousberg, Vingerhoets, Winter, Zilvold, 2002).

It seems reasonable to assume that the emotional distress WAD patients exhibit, leads to activation of the Hypothalamic-Pituitary-adrenocortical (HPA) axis and release of the stresshormones ACTH and cortisol. Whereas research in chronic painsyndromes like Fibromyalgia and Rheumatoid Arthritis has provided evidence of HPA-axis disturbances (Catley, Kaell, Kirschbaum, Stone, 2000), HPA-axis research in WAD patients has not yet been conducted. A valid method to examine the functioning of the HPA-axis is to investigate the changes in cortisol levels in response to an experimental psychological challenge or a stresstask (Cohen, Kessler, Underwood, 1995). The purpose of the present study was to examine changes in salivary cortisol levels, after performing a mental stresstask, in both WAD patients and healthy controls, and to compare these changes to a relax-control condition. The concentration of salivary free cortisol has proved to be a reliable method for assessing cortisol responses in man (Cohen, Kessler, Underwood, 1995; Hawk & Baum, 2001). It was hypothesised that WAD patients will show an increase in complaints (pain, fatigue, tension) and cortisol levels after performing a mental stresstask, compared to healthy control subjects and subjects in a relax-control condition.

Another important issue investigated in this study is whether the amount of daily hassles predicts cortisol response induced by a mental stresstask, in WAD patients and healthy control subjects. 'Daily hassles' means the chronic everyday problems (or chronic life stress) patients may perceive in several domains of their life (for example the problems in family life, living conditions, working conditions of physical appearance and general performance) (Blokhorst, Lousberg, Vingerhoets, Winter, Zilvold, 2002). Various studies suggest a possible link between chronic life stress and the stresshormone system. For instance, Brosschot et al. (1994) showed that high numbers of daily hassles are associated with a more pronounced decrease in immune cell traffic, induced by an acute stressor in healthy human subjects. This suggests that a high degree of life stress "sensitizes" the individual to subsequent stress. Daily hassles may lead to sustained physiological activation, which in turn changes the magnitude or duration of physiological responses. Pike et al. (1997) demonstrated that cortisol levels of persons undergoing chronic life stress, remained increased above base line during recovery, after they had undergone a psychological challenge, indicating sustained activation. In contrast, persons with a low level of stress returned to base line cortisol levels during recovery. Smyth et al. (1998) reported that the number of daily hassles were significantly related to cortisol levels in normal healthy subjects.

Based on these previous results, it was hypothesised that the amount of daily hassles predicts significantly the cortisol response induced by a mental stresstask.

Because HPA-axis activation is also associated with an inability to cope with stressfull events and helplessness (Cohen, Kessler, Underwood, 1995; Peters, Godaert, Ballieux, van Vliet, Willemsen, Sweep, Heijnen, 1998; Smyth, Ockenfels, Porter, Kirschbaum, Hellhammer, Stone, 1998), it was further hypothesised that (besides the self-reported frequencies of daily hassles) the seriousness or intensity ratings of these problems significantly predicts cortisol response.

METHODS

Participants

Twenty-eight WAD patients (16 females), referred to a rehabilitation centre for treatment because of chronic whiplash related complaints, participated in this research project. The patients in this study had a mean age of 32 years (± 7 years). The injury occurred more than six months before testing, which means that all patients were in the chronic phase (mean interval= 38 months; ± 24 months). All patients encountered the whiplash injury in a car-accident (rear-end collision); none was to blame for the accident. All patients were still in litigation. Patients, who reported that they lost consciousness after the whiplash injury, had recent narcoses or pre-morbid head injury, were excluded, to eliminate the possibility of significant head trauma. Psychiatric comorbity and premorbid migraine were also exclusion criteria. Fifty-seven percent of the patients had a low/middle educational level and the other 43 percent of patients had a middle/high educational level. Thirty-nine percent of the patients were able to work, whereas 57% had a workman's compensation. Following the Quebec Task Force's clinical-anatomic axis that corresponds to the severity of the whiplash injury, this study concerns only patients with chronic complaints after a W.A.D. Grade I and II. This means neck complaints of pain, stiffness, or tenderness eventually accompanied by musculo-skeletal sign(s) (Spitzer et al., 1995).

Twenty-eight healthy control subjects (16 females), farmost working in the rehabilitation centre, were selected and matched for educational level and age. These variables are related to performance on the mental stress task (Elsmore, 1994) used in this experiment and should therefore be controlled for (see procedure). The distribution of the variable 'sex' is shown in Table 3: both experimental groups have more females compared to both control groups.

None of the participants reported to be under treatment with medication. At the moment of testing, none of the subjects had used medication of influence on the central nervous system. All subjects gave their written informed consent. A medical ethical committee approved the study.

Measures

Salivary Cortisol

Saliva samples were collected. At the beginning of the session, each subject was given a 20-ml polyethylene vial with a mark on the side at the 5-ml level. Subjects collected saliva in their mouths and deposited it into the vials up the 5-ml marks on the side. Samples were stored at
–60° C until cortisol determination. For the determination of cortisol in salivary samples an HPLC method was used based on previously described methods (Gotelli, Wall, Kabra, Marton, 1981; Nozaki, Ohata, Ohba, 1991; Mason, Ward, Reilly, 1992; Hermans, van Essen, Struijker-Boudier, Johnson, Theeuwes, Smits, 2002). Briefly, 30 pmol of 4-androsten-11, 17-diol-3-one-17- carboxylic acid (Steraloids, New Port, USA) was added to the saliva samples to serve as internal standard. Following acidification of the saliva with HCl, steroids were extracted and derivatized with sulfuric acid essentially as described (Gotelli, Wall, Kabra, Marton, 1981; Nozaki, Ohata, Ohba, 1991; Mason, Ward, Reilly, 1992). Subsequently, the obtained fluorescent products were extracted with a 4/1 v/v mixture of diethylether (Merck Darmstadt, Germany) and methylene chloride (Biosolve, valkenswaard the Netherlands) in order to remove the sulphuric acid. Fluorescent products were analysed on HPLC within 18 hours. The HPLC consisted of a Nucleosil C18 column (150x3.2 mm, Supelco-Sigma, St Louis, USA) as stationary phase and a 1/640/360 v/v/v mixture of trifluoroacetic acid (Sigma st. Louis, USA), methanol (Biosolve, Valkenswaard, the Netherlands) and water as mobile phase. Cortisol and internal standard were detected by their fluorescence at excitation and emission wavelengths of 367 and 532 nm respectively. Cortisol concentrations were derived by calculating peak area ratios and comparing them with calibration curves. For every subject all samples were analyzed within one assay. The HPLC method had a detection limit of about 0.3 pmol and an intra-assay variation of 13 %.

Daily Hassles

The Daily Problems Checklist (DPC) is a 114-item self-report questionnaire that assesses both the frequency and perceived severity or impact of daily hassles during the preceding two months (Vingerhoets & van Tilburg, 1994). This questionnaire is partly based on the Daily Hassles Scale of Lazarus and co-workers (Kanner, Coyne, Schaefer, et al., 1981; DeLongis, Coyne, Dakof, et al., 1982; Brosschot, Benschop, Godaert, Olff, de Smet, Heijnen, Ballieux, 1994). The scale has a test-retest reliability of $R=0.87$. Both questionnaires are claimed to be valid (including validity in predicting psychological and physical complaints) (Van de

Willige, Schreurs, Tellegen, Zwart, 1985; Vingerhoets, Jeninga & Menges, 1989; Vingerhoets & van Tilburg, 1994) and are among the tests most widely used for stress research in Dutch-speaking countries.

Respondents were asked to check the items, describing events and/ situations that they experienced in the past two months (frequency of daily hassles). Next, they are asked to rate the level of severity of the stressor, indicating the impact of the stressor on the subjects' daily life (intensity of daily hassles). The questionnaire discriminates between person-dependent and person-*in*dependent stressors. Person-dependent stressors represent events and conditions that are likely caused by the individuals themselves and that depend on the functioning and mental status of a person. An example is "you could not realise your ambitions", or "you had problems with friends". The person-*in*dependent stressors represent situations beyond human control (e.g. "things you wanted to buy were suddenly more expensive" or "someone of the family was the victim of a crime").

SCL-90

In order to investigate the level of distress in our population, the Dutch version of the SCL-90 was applied (Arrindel & Ettema, 1986). The SCL-90 is a self-report symptom checklist composed of 90 items, each describing a physical or psychological symptom (Derogatis, 1983; Arrindel & Ettema, 1986). The instructions require patients to respond on a 5-point scale (ranging from 'not at all' to 'extremely') to indicate how much an item has bothered them over the past week. The Global Severity Index (GSI) is a measure of general distress which is obtained from the eight subscale scores plus other items of the questionnaire not included in these scores. The SCL-90 has proven to be a useful device for describing the distress of chronic pain patients in general, including the psychological and physical symptoms after a whiplash injury (Bernstein, Matthew & Hinkley, 1994; Wallis, Lord, Barnsley & Bogduk, 1996). Psychometric properties (such as test-retest reliability, internal consistency and validity coefficients) are satisfactory (Derogatis et al., 1983; Arrindel & Ettema, 1986).

State-Dependent Measures: Headache, Neck Pain, Fatigue, Tension

Subjective 'state' dependent feelings were measured by means of the Visual Analogue Scale (VAS). Patients were asked to rate the level of headache, neck pain, fatigue and tension several times during the experiment (see procedure). A 10-cm line was provided with written anchors at the two extremes: e.g. 'no pain' and 'unbearable pain'.

Laboratory Task

The 'Synwork' task, a divided attentional task, was used as a mental stress task (Elsmore, 1994; Cremer, 1998). This task consists of four subtasks: a memorytask, an arithmetic task, a visual monitoring task and an auditive monitoring task. The subject has to alternate his attention on those four tasks. Every seven minutes, the task becomes more complex by increasing the speed of stimulus presentation and/or raising the number of target items (e.g. in the working memory task and the auditive monitoring task). The other two tasks are self-paced: a new stimulus is presented just after a response is given. The test consists of six sessions of seven minutes. Subjects get 10 points for every right reaction and they lose 10 points when they neglect certain stimuli (e.g. stimuli of the visual monotoring task). They are instructed to collect as much points as possible. Their score is visible in the middle of the screen. Before the test starts, subjects perform a practice-session (lasting 10 minutes), in which initially every subtask is executed separately before all subtasks are presented together. Subjects may choose which task they want to perform and in which order they execute the tasks, so in fact they may develop their own strategy.

Synwork is known as a dynamic and complex task, which simulates the many-sidedness of worksituations (Elsmore, 1994). The task is also used in mental capacity assessment (Cremer, 1998).

In order to investigate the self-perceived effort to perform this task, subjects were asked to rate the level of effort by means of a Visual Analogue Scale (VAS-scale), ranging from zero (no effort) through 10 (extreme effort) after they had executed the task.

Experimental Stress Procedure

All subjects were instructed not to use any coffee/tea, not to smoke and not to take medication of influence on the central nervous system. They had a light breakfast at least two hours before the experiment started. All subjects arrived one hour before baseline measurement. After arriving, subjects filled in a state-check list. In all groups, half of the subjects started at 8.30 AM with pre-measurement and at 9.30 AM with base line measurement (T-0), while the other half started with pre-measurement at 10.30 AM and at 11.30 AM with base line measurement (T-0). The first saliva sample was collected as soon as subjects came in (Pre-1). Thirty minutes later, another saliva sample was collected and subjects rated their state-related feelings (Fatigue, Neckpain, Headache, Tension) (Pre-2).

Next, all subjects underwent a noise-tolerance test for twenty minutes: subjects were offered five different noise-intensities (ranging from 57dB - 95dB) by means of an audiometer. The results of this test will be published elsewhere (Blokhorst, Meeldijk, van Luijtelaar, van Toor, Lousberg, & Ganzevles, 2005).

The base line sample (T-0) was collected just before the intervention took place (mental stress condition or relax condition). Subjects also rated their complaints (fatigue, neck pain, headache and tension). After this, half of the WAD-patients and half of the healthy subjects performed the mental stress task (WAD-experimental group and Healthy-experimental group) which lasted for about 60 minutes. Subjects were instructed as follows:

> "You have to perform an attentional task on this computer. This task measures your ability to execute several tasks at the same time. The task consists of four parts. Task one is a letter-recognition task: you have to recognize a letter out of several other letters. Task two is an arithmetic task: you have to add two numbers. In task three you have to prevent a vertical dash from being longer than one second at both ends of a horizontal line. In task four you have to push your left-mouse button on a reactangle on your screen, when you hear a high sound."

Next, subjects were able to practice all four tasks separate and later on together (practice session lasted about ten minutes).

After the practice-session, the test began and subjects got the following instruction:

"As you have seen, you get ten points for every right reaction. Your score is visible in the middle of the screen. However, when you forget to react to the visual-monotoring task (the "dash-task"), your score will decrease. The better you are able to react to all the different tasks, the higher your score will be. The test consists of six sessions of seven minutes. Try to increase your score with every new session!"

The two control groups (WAD-control and Healthy-control) had to rest and were allowed to relax. After completion of synwork, saliva samples were collected in the four groups (T+60 min) and VAS-scales were rated concerning state-related feelings and subjective feeling of effort relating to the stresstask in the two experimental groups. Next, all subjects again received the same noise-tolerance test. After this test, saliva samples were collected (T+90 min) and after thirty minutes rest again (T+120 min).

Statistical Procedure

Statistical analyses were performed with the Statistical Package for Social Sciences (Norusis, 1999). The mental stresstask performance and subjective feelings of mental effort were calculated for the two experimental groups and expressed in means and standard deviations.

In order to investigate differences on state-related variables (in time) between the four groups, non-parametric tests were performed.

Differences between the frequency and intensity of daily hassles (DPC-variables), were investigated by means of MANOVA between the WAD-patients and healthy subjects. A *t*-test was performed regarding the data of the Synwork task.

Normality tests revealed that the cortisol data were not distributed normally. As was indicated by Hair (1998), the cortisol data were log-transformed. This transformation resulted in normally distributed data. ANOVA for repeated measures was performed in order to measure cortisol changes from Pre-1 to Base line (T-0). Next, ANOVA for repeated measures were applied on the four different moments (T-0, T+60, T+90, T+120), in order to investigate the differences in cortisol response between the four groups. Starttime and sex were entered as covariates in the analyses, because these factors influence acute cortisol stress responsivity that would have otherwise complicated the analyses (Cohen, Kessler & Underwood, 1995; Kirschbaum, Wust, Hellhammer, 1992).

Cortisol responsivity was calculated as changes in cortisol from baseline to the three post stress-task measures (T+60, T+90, T+120) and expressed as percentages relative to baseline levels (Negrão, Deuster, Gold, Singh, Chrousos, 2000). In order to investigate the relationship between daily hassles/ severity appraisals on the one hand and the cortisol responsivity after a mental stresstask (independent variables) on the other hand, separate regression analyses were performed within the two experimental groups, with respect to the three different post-task cortisol responsivity measures.

RESULTS

Frequency of Daily Hassles and Self-Perceived Stress-Load

The data of the DPC-variables were normally distributed. Mean and standard deviations are listed in Table 1. MANOVA revealed significant differences between WAD patients and healthy subjects on the person-dependent frequency and intensity variables (e.g. one-tailed) (see Table 1). The person-*in*dependent variables showed no significant differences between the WAD-patients and healthy subjects.

Table 1: Mean and SD of Daily Problem Checklist in WAD patients and Healthy subjects

DPC			P*
Person-dependent FREQ	7.0 ± 4.0	5.1 ± 3.4	0.03
Person-dependent INT	1.5 ± 0.5	0.9 ± 0.6	0.001
Person-independent FREQ	4.1 ± 2.7	4.1 ± 2.5	0.45
Person-independent INT	1.4 ± 0.7	1.1 ± 0.6	0.09

*P-values are one-tailed and refer to MANOVA-analysis

Mental Stress Performance

An independent *t*-test was conducted to explore whether performance on the mental stress task (Synwork) was different between the WAD-experimental group and the Healthy-experimental group. The results revealed no significant differences, indicating that both groups performed equally well on this test ($P=0.3$).

Subjective feelings of mental effort were recorded just after the mental stress task. A Mann-Whitney U test revealed no significant difference between the two experimental groups on the mental-effort VAS-scale ($P= 0.40$); WAD-group: $M=62$ mm ± 23; Healthy-group: $M=54$ mm ± 22.

'State' Characteristics of the WAD and Control Group during the Laboratory Session

The question 'How tense are you at this moment?' was used in order to check whether the abstination of cigarettes, coffee and tea had possibly caused an abnormal high level of tension. The responses ranged from 'not at all' through 'extremely tensed' (five-point scale). The results revealed that none of the subjects were 'fairly tensed' or 'extremely tensed'. Twenty-one percent of the WAD patients and 7% of the healthy subjects said to be a little tense and the other 79% of the WAD patients and 93% of the healthy subjects were not tense (at all). This indicated that the influence of the abstination of cigarettes and coffee/tea on the subjective feeling of tension was not relevant.

Table 2: State-measures in mm of the four groups, before and after a mental stress task (experimental groups) or rest (control-groups) (N=56)

	Headache			Neck Pain			Fatigue			Tension		
	Before	After	P*	Before	After	P	Before	After	P	Before	After	P
WAD exp.	20±23	31±28	.005	34±19	50±25	.002	29±24	43±25	.003	10±11	17±21	.015
Healthy exp.	1±3	1±2	.32	1±3	3±4	.14	4±6	5±6	.48	2±5	2±5	.59
WAD cont.	32±22	36±21	.24	40±24	37±21	.92	36±22	39±29	.47	22±23	16±20	.08
Healthy cont.	2±4	2±3	1.0	1±5	1±3	.32	5±8	5±8	.57	2±5	2±4	.68

*All P-values (two-tailed) refer to Wilcoxan Signed Ranks Tests

Mann-Whitney U tests showed that the 'state'-levels just before the mental stresstask (base-line) (headache, neck pain, fatigue, tension) were not significantly different between the two WAD-groups (all P-values ≥ 0.1). However, WAD patients had significantly more complaints on all moments compared to healthy-subjects (all P-values ≤ 0.001). Performance of the mental stress task did not induce more complaints in both healthy groups (all P-values ≥ 0.14). In addition, the subjects of both control groups did not perceive more complaints (see Table 2).

In contrast, the level of state-variables in the experimental WAD-group increased significantly, just after the mental stress task was performed (see Table 2). Wilcoxon Signed Ranks Tests revealed that at T+90, neck pain and tension remained on the same level, while headache and fatigue increased further in the experimental WAD group (all P-values ≤ 0.02). At T+120 all levels remained the same compared to T+90, except for the variable fatigue, which significantly decreased, after a relax period of thirty minutes.

The level of headache and fatigue in the WAD control-condition did not change during the experiment (all P-values ≥ 0.09). The level of neck pain increased at T+90 ($P= 0.01$). The level of tension decreased after a relax-period ($P=0.05$) and remained on the same level after this.

The data of the Global Severity Index (GSI) were not normally distributed (transformations of the data did not succeed in a normal distribution). A Kruskall-Wallis Test showed that the difference on the GSI-index between the WAD-groups and the healthy-groups is significant ($P\leq 0.001$): the GSI-index of WAD patients is much higher than the index of healthy subjects, indicating more distress in the patient groups (WAD-group: $M= 156 \pm 45$; Healthy-group: $M= 114 \pm 33$).

Cortisol Response in Experimental- and Control Groups

Cortisol data were incomplete for four WAD patients and two healthy controls due to technical difficulties in assay or not having enough saliva. Repeated measures of variance of the three pre-treatment cortisol samples showed no significant main effect for Time (pre-1, pre 2, T-0), Group (WAD / healthy), Condition (experimental / control), nor significant interaction effects. Starttime and sex were covariates: Starttime was significant ($P<0.002$) and sex was not.

The raw average salivary cortisol values recorded during the laboratory session for both WAD and healthy groups from base line to the end of the experiment are shown in Table 3.

Repeated measures of variance were conducted with the four cortisol samples as dependent variables ('Time': T-0, T+60, T +90, T+120) and Group (=Patient/ Healthy), Condition (= Mental stresstask/ Rest) as independent variables. Starttime (Early/ Late in the morning) and sex (male/female) were entered as a covariates in the analysis. Results showed a main effect for Group ($F (1, 49)= 9.2, P=0.004$); as can be seen from Table 3, the average cortisol level of WAD patients is higher than the average cortisol level of healthy subjects. Furthermore, a significant main effect of Time was present ($F (3, 47)= 5.5, P<0.003$). An interaction effect of Time by Group was also significant ($F (3, 47)=3.1, P<0.03$). Inspection of Table 3 demonstrated that the cortisol levels of WAD patients remained stable or increased in time, whereas the cortisol levels of healthy subjects decreased.

Table 3: First colum: distribution of the variable 'sex'. Colum 2-5: mean levels and standard deviations of raw cortisol concentrations in saliva (nmol/l) recorded in WAD and Healthy groups before (base line) and at three moments after a mental stress task (experimental groups) or before and after a break (control- groups) (N=56)

	Sex : Females	T-0 : Base line*	T+60 :	T+90 :	T+120 :
WAD-exp.	11	2.8 ± 1.7	5.4 ± 7.4	6 ± 8.7	3.1 ± 2.2
WAD-control	5	4.5 ± 5.9	3.5 ± 4.9	4.3 ± 7.5	5.3 ± 8.3
Healthy-exp.	12	1.8 ± 1.5	± 1.0	1.2 ± 1.0	0.9 ± 0.7
Healthy-control	4	4.3 ± 3.1	2.4 ± 1.4	1.7 ± 1.3	1.8 ± 2.0

* in every group half of the cortisol concentrations were measured at 9.30 AM and half at 11.30 AM.

Results showed that the factor 'sex' was significant in this analysis, indicating a different stressreponse for men and women (F (1,49)=4.1, P=0.05). Inspection of the means showed higher mean cortisol levels for men compared to women, during all measurements.

Relationship Between Daily Hassles / Severity Appraisal and Cortisol Responsivity

In order to investigate the relationship between daily hassles / severity appraisal and cortisol change as results of a mental stress task, separate regression analyses were performed within the two experimental groups with respect to the cortisol change at T+60, T+90 and T+120.

The basic model consisted of the new calculated dependent variable T+60-change, T+90-change or T+120-change and the basic predictor variables 'Group and Starttime'. This basic model did not predict cortisol change significantly at moments T+60, T+90 and T+120.

Furthermore, the variables 'duration of complaints', 'age' and the 'GSI-index' were not significant predictors.

With respect to the daily stressors, both the frequency and intensity measures of the *in*dependent stressors were not related to T+60, T+90 of T+120 cortisol change. In contrast, both the frequency and the intensity measures related to personal functioning were significant predictors for T+60 cortisol change (see Table 4).

Only the person-dependent intensity variable is still a significant predictor of T+90-change in the experimental groups (P=0.03). Because the person-dependent variables are significantly related to Group (Patient/Healthy), this last variable disappeared in the best predicting model for T+90-change (see Table 4). The best predicting model of T+120-change was the level of tension just before the mental stresstask (T-0), combined with the variables Group, Starttime and sex (R^2=0.55; P=0.003).

Table 4. Prediction of percentage cortisol change at several Post-task moments as result of a mental stress task: regression analyses in WAD and Healthy Intervention groups (N=25)

	B	SE B	ß	P
Model 1(dependent: cortisolchange at T+60)*				
Constant	-.74	.32		.03
Starttime	-.02	.24	-.01	.93
Person-dependent intensity	.83	.22	.73	.001
Person-dependent frequency	-.09	.04	-.52	.01
Model 2(dependent: cortisolchange at T+90)*				
Constant	-.93	.39		.03
Starttime	.14	.30	.09	.63
Person-dependent intensity	.60	.26	.47	.03
Model 3(dependent: cortisolchange at T+120)*				
Constant	-1.6	.45		.002
Starttime	0.84	.33	.41	.02
Patient/Healthy	0.83	.34	.41	.02
Male/Female	0.84	.43	.31	.06
Tension at baseline (T-0)	-0.07	.02	-.57	.004

*Note: R^2=0.44 for Model 1 (P=0.009); R^2= 0.21 for Model 2 (P<0.09); R^2=0.55 for Model 3 (P<0.003)

DISCUSSION

In line with the results of previous studies, the WAD patients in this study reported more general distress and daily hassles (related to personal functioning) and perceived them as more serious than healthy subjects (Wallis, Lord, Barnsley, Bogduk, 1996; Blokhorst, Lousberg, Vingerhoets, Winter, Zilvold, 2002).

The results showed no differences in performance on the mental stresstask between WAD patients and healthy subjects. Furthermore, both groups perceived the stresstask as equally strenuous. This implicates that the WAD patients in this study were not underperforming or aggravating (because in case of underperformance or aggravation, the performance and complaints of WAD patients should have been worse compared to healthy subjects) (Schmand, de Sterke & Lindeboom, 1999). Hence, the results can be interpreted as valid.

Confirming the expectations, the mental stresstask did not induce complaints of fatigue, pain or tension in healthy subjects. However, WAD patients did report significantly more headache, neck pain and were more fatigued and tensed after performing the mental stresstask. In contrast, the complaints of WAD patients in the relax-condition stayed roughly the same (e.g. headache, neck pain, fatigue) or decreased (e.g. tension).

Results demonstrated that WAD patients had significantly higher cortisol levels compared to healthy subjects during the experiment. Furthermore, cortisol levels of WAD patients showed a different time-course during the experiment: cortisol levels in WAD patients remained the same or increased, whereas the cortisol concentrations in healthy subjects decreased. Despite the fact that the interaction term between Group x Time x Condition was not significant, it can be seen from Table 3 that there is a trend towards an increase in cortisol concentrations in WAD patients, after performing a mental stress task. It is conceivable that an extension of this experiment with more subjects will reveal a significant change in cortisol concentration in the experimental WAD group compared to control groups.

In conclusion, WAD patients may perform as well as healthy subjects on a mental stress task, but in order to achieve this 'normal' result, it probably requires extra effort for them, whereas their processing resources are limited (Klein, 1997; Blokhorst, Meeldijk, van Luijtelaar, van Toor, Lousberg, Ganzevles, submitted). This enhanced effort results in more pain, fatigue, tension and a higher cortisol secretion.

The results of this study are in accordance with the results of previous studies which demonstrated elevated cortisol concentrations in other chronic pain syndromes like fibromyalgia and Rheumatoid Arthritis (Catley, Kaell, Kirschbaum, Stone, 2000; Crofford, Pillemer, Kalogeras, et al., 1994).

Analysis revealed a significant relationship of the factor 'sex' with cortisol levels, indicating higher cortisol levels for men. This result is in line with previous results (Kirschbaum, Wust, Hellhammer, 1992).

Because previous studies have demonstrated a high level of distress in WAD patients, which is related to the chronic daily stressors patients perceive (related to personal functioning), it was hypothesised that the amount of daily hassles predicts significantly the cortisol response induced by a mental stresstask in WAD patients and healthy persons (Radanov, Di Stefano, Schnidrig, Sturzenegger, 1994; Mayou, 1997; Blokhorst, Lousberg, Vingerhoets, Winter, Zilvold, 2002). It was further hypothesised that (besides the self-reported frequencies of daily hassles) the seriousness ratings of these problems by the subjects significantly predicts cortisol response. Results demonstrated that cortisol responsivity in the experimental groups is indeed predicted by both the amount of daily hassles and appraisal of severity of the daily problems. Especially this last factor has proven to be a significant predictor of cortisol responsivity 30- and 60 minutes after termination of the stressor. These results are in agreement with other results concerning the positive relationship between frequency and intensity ratings of daily hassles and cortisol secretion as a result of an acute psychological stressor (Brosschot, Benschop, Godaert, Olff, de Smet, Heijnen, Ballieux, 1994; Pike, Smith, Hauger, et al., 1997; Smyth, Ockenfels, Porter, Kirschbaum, Hellhammer, Stone, 1998).

The present findings have to be interpreted with care, because of the relatively small group of subjects. Definite conclusions cannot be drawn. Nevertheless, the present results offer new, interesting perspectives in the WAD phenomenon.

To substantiate our findings and in order to reveal the mechanisms behind the observed differences between healthy subjects and WAD patients, further research is necessary. Investigating cortisol levels and cortisol response at various time points post-injury, may give an indication about the time course of the changed HPA-axis sensitivity and may offer insight into the natural development of this syndrome, including different contributing factors, as is explained by the 'biopsychosocial model' (Ferrari & Schräder, 2001). Of particular interest is the investigation of the cortisol stress-reaction in the acute phase of the WAD syndrome.

Previous results have revealed that the initial emotional response to the injury and the existence of stressors independently of the injury are significant prognostic factors (Drottning, Staff, Levin, Malt, 1995; Smed, 1997; Blokhorst, Lousberg, Vingerhoets, Winter, Zilvold, 2002; Sterling, Kenardy, Jull, Vicenzino, 2003). Therefore, a cortisol stress-reaction in the acute phase will be expected in those subjects who exhibit this strong emotional distress in the acute phase. This kind of evidence would further objectivate a vulnerability to stress in some WAD patients.

In conclusion: although the number of subjects in the present study is relatively small and therefore no definite conclusions can be drawn, the results indicated significantly higher cortisol concentrations in WAD patients compared to healthy persons. Furthermore, the results demonstrated that the cortisol change as result of an acute mental stressor is related to the amount of daily hassles (related to personal functioning) and especially the appraisal of severity of daily problems. Likely, WAD patients have become more sensitive to subsequent stressors after the whiplash injury, because of chronic daily hassles and disfunctional coping strategies. For this reason 'stressmanagement' should be an important topic in rehabilitation programmes for chronic WAD patients.

It is concluded that study of HPA-axis in WAD patients offers new, interesting perspectives in the WAD phenomenon.

ACKNOWLEDGEMENTS

This research project was financially supported by the Nardy Roeloffzen Foundation and the Hubertus foundation. The authors are grateful to I. Blokhorst for her assistance and G. van Luijtelaar for his advice.

REFERENCES

Arrindel, W.A. & Ettema, J.H.M. (1986). *SCL-90: Handleiding bij een psychopathologie-indicator*. Swets & Zeitlinger, Lisse (The Netherlands).

Barnsley, L., Lord, S., & Bogduk, N. (1994). Clinical review: Whiplash Injury. *Pain*, 283-307.

Bernstein, I.H., Matthew, E.J. & Hinkley, B.S. (1994). On the utility of the SCL-90-R with Low-Back Pain Patients. *Spine*, 19, 42-48.

Blokhorst, M.G.B.G., Lousberg, R., Vingerhoets, A.J.J.M., Winter, F.A.M., Zilvold, G. (2002). Daily hassles and stress vulnerability in patients with a Whiplash Associated Disorder. *International Journal of Rehabilitation Research*, 25, 173-179.

Blokhorst, M.G.B.G., Meeldijk, S. van Luijtelaar, G., van Toor, T., Lousberg, R. & Ganzevles, P. (2005). Noise intolerance and state dependent factors in patients with Whiplash Associated Disorder, accepted for publication in *Journal of Whiplash and Related Disorders*; vol.4 (1).

Brosschot, J.F., Benschop, R.J., Godaert, G.L.R., Olff, M., De Smet, M., Heijnen, C.J. & Ballieux, R.E. (1994). Influence of Life Stress on Immunological Reactivity to Mild Psychological Stress, *Psychosomatic Medicine*, 56 (3), 216-224.

Catley, D, Kaell, A.T., Kirschbaum, C. & Stone, A.A. (2000). A naturalistic evaluation of cortisol secretion in persons with fibromyalgia and rheumatoid arthritis. *Arthritis Care Research*, 13 (1), 51-61.

Cohen, S., Kessler, R.C., Underwood, G..L. (1995). Strategies for measuring stress in studies of psychiatric and physical disorders. In: *Measuring Stress; a Guide for Health and Social Scientists* (Cohen S, Kessler RC, Underwood, G.L, eds.). Oxford: Oxford University Press, 3-26.

Cremer, R. (1998). *Mentaal Belastbaarheids Onderzoek*, internal report TNO, Amsterdam.

Crofford, L.J., Pillemer, S.R., Kalogeras, K.T., Cash, J.M., Michelson, D. Kling, M.A., Sternberg, E.M., Gold, P.W. Chrousos, G.P., Wilder, R.L. (1994). Hypothalamic-pituitary-adrenal axis pertubations in patients with fibromyalgia. *Arthritis Rheum*, 37, 1583-1592.

DeLongis, A., Coyne, J.C., Dakof, G. et al. (1982). Relationship of daily hassles, uplifts, and major life events to health status. *Health Psychol.*, 1, 119-136.

Derogatis, L.R. (1983). *SCL-90R. Annual II. Clinical Psychometric research*. Towson: Clinical Psychometric Research.

Drottning, M., Staff, P.H., Levin, L. & Malt, U.F.R. (1995). Acute emotional response to common whiplash injury predicts subsequent pain complaints. *Nord. J. Psychiatry*, 49, 293-299.

Elsmore, T.F. (1994). Synwork 1: A PC-based tool for assessment of performance in a simulated work environment. Behavior Research Methods, *Instruments & Computers*, 26 (4), 421-426.

Ferrari, R. & Schrader, H. (2001). The late whiplash syndrome: a biopsychosocial approach. *Journal of Neurosurg Psychiatry*, 70, 722-726.

Gotelli, G.G., Wall, J.H., Kabra, P.M., and Marton, L.J. (1981). Fluorometric liquid-chromatographic determination of serum cortisol. *Clin. Chem.*, 27, 441-443.

Hair, J.S., Anderson, R.E., Tatham, R.L., Black, W.C. (1998). Multivariate data analysis. London: Prentice Hall.

Hawk, L.W. & Baum, A. (2001). Endocrine assessment in behavioral medicine. In: *Assessment in Behavioral Medicine* (Vingerhoets, A., Ed.). East-Sussex: Brunner-Routledge, 413-440.

Hermans, J.J.R., Van Essen, H., Struijker-Boudier, H.A.J., Johnson, R.M., Theeuwes, F. & Smits, J.F.M. (2002). Pharmacokinetic advantage of intrapericardially applied substances in the rat. *Journal of Pharmacol. Exp. Ther.*, 301, 672-678.

Kanner, A., Coyne, J.C., Schaefer, C. et al. (1981). Comparison of two modes of stress measurements: Daily hassles and uplifts versus major life events. *J. Beh. Med.*, 4, 1-39.

Klein, M. (1997). Attentional performance in Young and Old patients with Cervical Acceleration Deceleration Injury. In: *Cognitive Aging, Attention, and Mild Traumatic Brain Injury (Thesis)*. Maastricht: Neuropsych Publishers. 155-170.

Kirschbaum, C., Wust, S. & Hellhammer, D. (1992). Consistent sex difference in cortisol responses to psychological stress. *Psychosomatic Medicine*, 54 (6), 648-657.

Mason, S.R., Ward, L.C., Reilly, P.E.B. (1992). Fluorimetric detection of serum corticosterone using high-performance liquid chromatography. *J. Chrom.*, 581, 267-271.

Mayou, R. (1997). The psychiatry of road traffic accidents. In: *The Aftermath of Road Accidents* (Mitchell, M., ed.). London/New York: Routledge, 33-48.

Merksey, H. (1993). Psychological consequences of whiplash. In: *Spine state of the art reviews; Cervical flexion-extension/Whiplash injuries* (Teasell, R.W. & Shapiro, A.P., eds.). Philadelphia: Hanley & Belfus, 471-480.

Negrão, A.B., Deuster, P.A., Gold, P.W., Singh, A., Chrousos, G.P. (2000). Individual reactivity and physiology of the stress response. *Biomed. & Pharmacother.*, 54, 122-128.

Norusis, M.J. (1999). *SPSS-user Guide: version 9.0.*, Chicago.

Nozaki, O., Ohata, T., Ohba, Y. 1991. Determination of serum cortisol by reversed-phase liquid chromatography using precolumn sulphuric acid-ethanol fluorescence derivatization and column switching. *J. Chrom.*, 570, 1-11.

Peters, M.L., Godaert, G.L.R., Ballieux, R.E., van Vliet, M., Willemsen, J.J., Sweep, F.C.G.J. & Heijnen, C.J. (1998). Cardiovascular and endocrine responses to experimental stress: effects on mental effort and controllability. *Psychoneuroendocrinology*, 23 (1), 1-17.

Pike, J.L., Smith, T.L., Hauger, R.L., Nicassio, P.M., Patterson, T.L., McClintick, J, Costlow, C. & Irwin, M.R. (1997). Chronic life stress alters sympathetic, neuroendocrine, and immune responsivity to an acute Psychological Stressor in Humans. *Psychosomatic Medicine*, 59, 447-457.

Radanov, B.P., Di Stefano, G., Schnidrig, A. & Ballinari, P. (1991). Role of psychosocial stress in recovery from common whiplash. *The Lancet*, 338, 712-715.

Radanov, B.P., Di Stefano, G., Schnidrig, A., Sturzenegger, M. (1994). Common whiplash: psychosomatic or somatopsychic? *J. Neurol. Neurosurg. Psychiat.*, 57, 486-490.

Radanov, B.P., Begre, S., Sturzenegger, M. & Augustiny, K.F. (1996). Course of psychological variables in whiplash injury – a 2-year follow-up with age, gender and education pair-mathced patients. *Pain*, 64, 429-434.

Schmand, B., de Sterke, S. & Lindeboom, J. (1999). *Amsterdamse Korte Termijn Geheugen Test*. Lisse: Swets & Zeitlinger Publishers.

Smed, A. (1997). Cognitive function and distress after common whiplash injury. *Acta Neurologica Scandinavica*, 95, 73-80.

Smyth, J., Ockenfels, M.C., Porter, L., Kirschbaum, C., Hellhammer, D.H., Stone, A.A. (1998). Stressors and mood measured on a momentary basis are associated with salivary cortisol secretion. *Psychoneuroendocrinology*, 23 (4), 353-370.

Spitzer, W.O., Skovron, M.L., Salmi, L.R., et al. (1995). Scientific monograph of the quebec task force on whiplash-associated disorders: redefining "whiplash" and its management. *Spine*, 20 (7), 7-73.

Sterling, M., Kenardy, J., Jull, G. & Vicenzino, B. (2003). The development of psychological changes following whiplash injury. *Pain*, 106(3), 481-489.

Van de Willige, G., Schreurs, P., Tellegen, B. & Zwart, F. (1985). Het meten van 'life-events': de vragenlijst recent meegemaakte gebeurtenissen (VRMG). *Nederlands Tijdschrift voor de Psychologie*, 40, 1-19.

Vingerhoets, A.J.J.M., Jeninga, A., & Menges, L.J. (1989). Het meten van chronische en alledaagse stressoren: eerste onderzoekservaringen met de Alledaagse Problemen Lijst (APL) II. *Gedrag en Gezondheid*, 17, 10-17.

Vingerhoets, A.J.J.M. & Van Tilburg, M.A.L. (1994). *Alledaagse Problemen Lijst (APL)*. Lisse: Swets en Zeitlinger.

Wallis, B.J., Lord, S.M., Barnsley, L., & Bogduk, N. (1996). Pain and Psychologic Symptoms of Australian Patients with Whiplash. *Spine*, 21, 804-810.

In: Stress and Health: New Research
Editor: Kimberly V. Oxington, pp. 143-172

ISBN 1-59454-244-9
©2005 Nova Science Publishers, Inc.

Chapter VII

CYTOKINES IN BEHAVIORAL MEDICINE RESEARCH: IMPORTANCE FOR PSYCHOLOGICAL STATES OF STRESS, DEPRESSION AND FATIGUE AND HEALTH OUTCOMES

Shamini Jain and Paul J. Mills[*]

Department of Psychiatry, Behavioral Medicine Program, University of California, San Diego, UCSD Medical Center, San Diego, CA. 92103

ABSTRACT

Cytokines are important immune transmitters that mediate effects of psychological states on disease processes and health outcomes. Cytokines have diverse effects not only on immune system function but also on the central nervous system and hypothalamic-pituitary axis activity, providing multiple routes for their actions. Alterations in cytokine levels have been identified in a number of disorders that are particularly important to stress and behavioral medicine research. The purpose of this chapter is to familiarize the behavioral medicine researcher with cytokines, providing descriptions of their classifications, functions, techniques of measurement and interactions with physiological systems relevant to stress and negative psychological states. We review the literature and present original data on associations of cytokines with stress, depression and fatigue. Included in the discussion is the relevance of cytokines to disease processes and mechanisms by which cytokines might help mediate health outcomes.

---

[*] Paul J. Mills, UCSD Medical Center, 200 West Arbor Drive, San Diego, CA. 92103-0804, (619)-543-2506; (619)-543-7517 (fax); pmills@ucsd.edu

INTRODUCTION

Behavioral Medicine has expanded greatly in research methodology and practice since its formal U.S. inception in the late 1970s. With advances in knowledge within the field, there has been an increased focus on refining study design, including selecting markers that are relevant to processes of disease and health outcomes. Psychoneuroimmunology (PNI), a discipline with high relevance to behavioral medicine and stress research, seeks to understand interactive communication among the immune, neuroendocrine, and nervous systems, especially as this communication relates to psychological states and disease processes. Developments within PNI parallel the overall growth of behavioral medicine research with seemingly exponential advances in discoveries and techniques that allow us to better understand how psychological states affect health. The search for mediators of such processes has brought considerable attention to the importance of cytokines as cellular messengers that not only mediate immune function, but also are implicated in psychological, neuroendocrine, and nervous system processes within the individual that affect health. Cytokines play an important role in physiological and psychological processes and appear increasingly important for understanding the pathological mechanisms of a variety of medical illnesses. In addition to playing a substantial role in primarily immune-related disorders such as cancer, rheumatoid arthritis and asthma, knowledge of cytokines is important for understanding other medical pathologies including cardiovascular disease, chronic pain, and sleep disorders. Furthermore, studies have examined the role of cytokines in psychological states such as depression, stress, and fatigue and their implications for contributing to disease outcomes associated with these states (Anisman & Merali, 2003; Kiecolt-Glaser, McGuire, Robles, & Glaser, 2002; Kronfol & Remick, 2000).

This chapter begins with a basic review of cytokines, describing their physiological structure and function as well as techniques of assessment. We then provide examples of how cytokines interact with the central nervous system and hypothalamic-pituitary-adrenal axis, particularly as these interactions relate to stress responses. Next, we discuss data relevant to cytokine associations with psychological and physiological states of stress, deperssion, and fatigue, as well as health outcomes. We conclude by discussing the potential for behavioral interventions to affect cytokine levels as part of an effort to ameliorate stress and its negative physiological concomitants.

BASIC CYTOKINE STRUCTURE AND FUNCTION

Cytokines are a diverse group of potent, low molecular weight proteins and glycoproteins that are secreted by white blood cells (most notably, T-helper cells and macrophages, although natural killer, T-cytotoxic, and mast cells are also significant sources of cytokines as well as other cells in the body, including in the brain). The functions of cytokines are diverse: they assist in development and proliferation of immune cell subsets, promotion of inflammatory as well as non-inflammatory processes, and alteration of neurochemical and neuroendocrine processes that affect overall physiology and behavior. Cytokines may be thought of as similar to neurotransmitters and hormones in that they are mediators of specific physiological responses, rely on receptor-ligand interactions, and have self (autocrine), local (paracrine) and distal (endocrine) effects (although the ability of cytokines to act in a long-range endocrine fashion is limited compared to hormones because of their relatively short half-life in the blood). Indeed, cytokines carry out their specific functions through various mechanisms of action: namely, pleiotropy, redundancy, synergy, antagonism, and cascade induction (Goldsby, Kindt, Osborne, & Kuby, 2003).

Pleiotropy refers to the ability of a single cytokine to influence different target cells in different ways. For example, among the varied pleiotropic actions of the cytokine interleukin 6 (IL-6) are inducing B-cell differentiation in antibody-secreting plasma cells, promoting T cell proliferation and differentiation, inducing neural differentiation and stimulating hepatocytes to produce and release acute-phase proteins (such as C-reactive protein and fibrinogen) that participate in inflammatory responses (Naka, Nishimoto, & Kishimoto, 2002). *Redundancy* refers to cytokines having the same function, e.g., IL-2, IL-4, and IL-5, all promote B cell differentiation. *Synergy* occurs when two or more cytokines co-create a shared effector response that is more than additive. For example, the combined actions of IL-4 and IL-5 promote a greatly increased ability to induce a B-cell to switch its antibody production from one class to another, beyond the sum of the individual effects IL-4 and IL-5 (Goldsby et al., 2003). Cytokines also may exhibit *antagonism* or inhibition of another cytokine's effects. An example is the ability of the cytokine interferon-gamma (IFN-γ) to inhibit the class switching induced by IL-4 as described above. IFN-γ also exemplifies the ability of cytokines to promote *cascade induction,* or the release of other cytokines in a hierarchical fashion. For example, IFN-γ stimulates macrophages to secrete another cytokine, IL-12, which in turn activates T-helper cells to release, in addition to more IFN-γ, other cytokines including tumor necrosis factor-alpha (TNF-α) and IL-2 (Goldsby et al., 2003). Examining these mechanisms of action allows one to appreciate the vast complexity and ability of cytokines to affect diverse cellular and physiological processes throughout the body.

CLASSIFICATION OF CYTOKINE FAMILIES

Because of their notable variability in structure and function, there have been many attempts to classify cytokines. Traditional classifications include the *hematopoietin, interferon, chemokine, and tumor necrosis factor* families. These families are differentiated both by structure, and, to a certain extent, function (Goldsby et al., 2003). Certain cytokines are often classified as *interleukins,* referring to the fact that they are secreted by some leukocytes (white blood cells) and affect other leukocytes. Because of the pleiotropy of many cytokines, classification systems are limited. However, a classification system that has proven useful for stress and behavioral medicine researchers is the classification of cytokines as either *pro-inflammatory* or *anti-inflammatory*. These are sometimes referred to as T_H1 vs. T_H2 secreted cytokines, referring to the specific subset of T-helper cells that secrete pro-inflammatory and anti-inflammatory cytokines, respectively.

Pro-inflammatory cytokines, which include IL-1, IL-2, IL-6, TNF-α, and IFN-γ, promote a variety of cell functions that stimulate and enhance inflammation. For example, IL-1, IL-6 and TNF-α promote differentiation of cytotoxic T cells, helping to prime these cells to respond to current and future immune insults. The release of these cytokines also stimulates production of antibodies on B cells, most notably IgG2a, which, through interactions with the complement system, promote phagocytosis (engulfing of microorganisms) by cells such as macrophages and neutrophils (which are themselves activated through cytokines TNF-α and IFN-γ). Inflammatory cytokines also increase inflammation by promoting increased vascular permeability and cellular adhesion, allowing cells to leave the blood vessels and migrate to tissues. For example, IL-1 activates the expression of the endothelial adhesion molecule intercellular adhesion molecule-1, (ICAM-1) which, when bound to the properly conformed integrin (e.g., LFA-1) on the surface of immune cells, promotes firm adhesion to endothelial cells for eventual extravasation (migration of cells from the circulation to tissue) (Figure 1). TNF-α promotes a similar process for neutrophils by stimulating the production of the adhesion molecule E-selectin on the endothelium, which binds to adhesion molecules on neutrophils. TNF-α, IL-6, and IL-1 also promote the activity of *chemokines*, small polypeptides that may directly assist in the adhesion process as well as subsequently guide cells to their proper destinations in the tissues via chemical diffusion gradients. Finally, some proinflammatory cytokines, including IL-6 and TNF-α, mediate further inflammatory processes by promoting liver production and release of acute phase proteins such C-reactive protein, an inflammatory mediator and important marker of cardiovascular risk (Shah & Newby, 2003). These inflammatory immune responses are often described as T_H1 *responses*, referring to the T-helper cell subset that generally produces the cytokines that initiate these inflammatory processes.

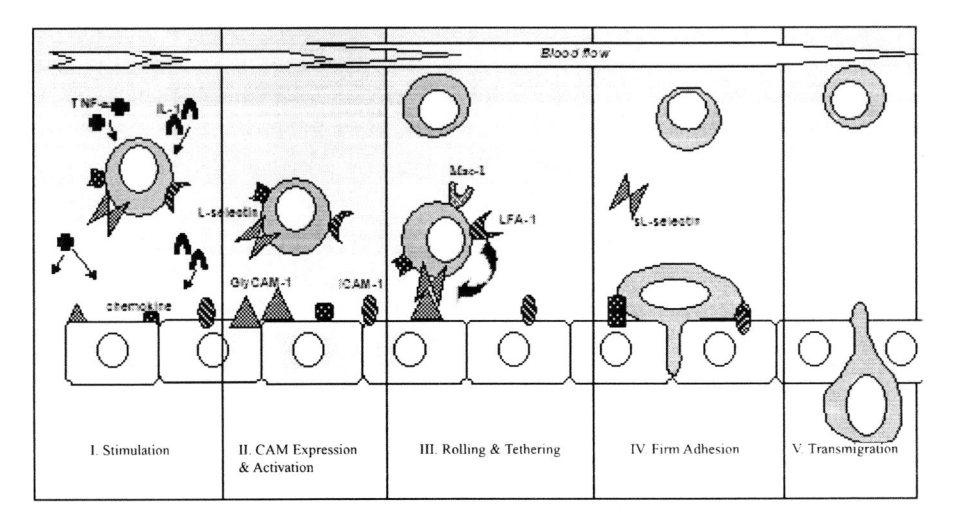

Figure 1: Schematic diagram of homing and adhesion of leukocytes through cytokine mechanisms. I & II. Stimulating factors including pro-inflammatory cytokines result in the activation of leukocytes and endothelial cells and lead to subsequent increased expression and activation of adhesion molecules on both endothelial and immune cells. III. Selectins (e.g., L-selectin) bind to ligands on the endothelium (e.g., GlyCam-1) causing leukocytes to be 'captured, roll and tether'. IV. Activation and binding of integrins (e.g., LFA-1) to ligands (e.g., ICAM-1) lead to attachment and further activation of leukocytes. V. Leukocytes transmigrate through the endothelial wall (adapted from Goebel & Mills, 2000).

Anti-inflammatory cytokines, which include IL-3, IL-4, IL-5, IL-10, and IL-13, may be thought of as immunosuppressors due to their ability to inhibit the T_H1-mediated inflammatory response (often via direct antagonism of the T_H1-secreted inflammatory cytokines). However, these cytokines themselves promote certain increases in the immune response, most notably increased overall production of antibodies and increased eosinophil and mast cell production. For example, IL-3, IL-4, and IL-10 increase production of mast cells, which when activated release histamine, promoting mucus secretion and vasodilation. In addition, as mentioned earlier, IL-4 promotes class switching in B cells to the immunoglobulin IgE, which when crosslinked promotes degranulation of mast cells thereby inducing these cells to release histamine as well as other cytokines. IL-4 also regulates the clonal expansion of these IgE expressing B cells. IL-3 and IL-5 enhance the maturation, activation, and accumulation of eosinophils, which, when activated, release products that mediate inflammation. Often called the *T_H2 response,* these cascades of cytokine-induced immune activation support allergic reactions (Goldsby et al., 2003). It is important to note that some cytokines support both pro- and anti-inflammatory effects depending on the situation (e.g., IL-6, IL-8), thus rendering the nomenclature of cytokines as either pro-inflammatory or anti-inflammatory less that perfect (Diehl & Rincon, 2002). For the most part, however, the classification of cytokines as either T_H1 and T_H2 has been useful within certain limitations in understanding the specific balance of cytokines in pro-inflammatory and anti-inflammatory processes relevant to disease states.

Disruption in the T_H1/T_H2 balance has been noted in several disorders. For example, a shift to greater T_H2 dominance has been found in insomnia unassociated with other medical conditions (Sakami et al., 2002), asthma (Meltzer, 2003), and other allergic conditions (Frieri, 2003). A decrease in cell-meditated T_H1 activation, as well as aberrant production of T_H2 cytokines, are often prevalent in cancer, impeding proper tumor detection and removal (Skinnider & Mak, 2002). A shift toward increased T_H1 dominance and decreased T_H2 dominance has been found in type 1 diabetes, multiple sclerosis, and rheumatoid arthritis (Frieri, 2003). Cardiovascular disorders are linked to pro-inflammatory processes. For example IL-6 is highly relevant for cardiovascular disease processes (Ito & Ikeda, 2003). In a recent 7-year prospective large-scale study with well-functioning older adults, IL-6 was associated with significantly increased risk ratios for coronary heart disease, stroke, and congestive heart failure (Cesari et al., 2003).

CYTOKINE MEASUREMENT

Many methods exist for measuring cytokines and each has strengths and drawbacks (Banks, 2000; Bienvenu, Monneret, Gutowski, & Fabien, 1998).. Here we describe three of the approaches to cytokine measurement that are highly relevant and most commonly used by the behavioral medicine and stress researcher (specifically, ELISA, ELISPOT, and flow cytometry).

Types of Assays

When examining cytokines in biological fluids there are two broad categories for methods of measurement. *Immunoassays* measure the prevalence of cytokines or their soluble receptors by using either radioisotope tagged antibodies (i.e., radioimmunoassays or RIA), or enzyme-linked antibodies (i.e., enzyme-linked immunosorbant assays, or ELISAs) that are specific for specific peptides which are part of the cytokine structure. Strengths of immunoassays in general are their ease in use and relatively low cost, combined with relatively high specificity due to the use of monoclonal antibodies. However, these methods are not immune to methodological problems, as will be discussed below with respect to ELISAs. In addition, immunoassays do not provide information on functionality of the cytokine. *Bioassays* measure cytokine functionality as indexed by specific biological responses such as chemotaxis (movement through a chemical diffusion gradient), proliferation (increase in numbers of the particular cell line), cytotoxicity (ability of cells to kill pathogens), expression of cell surface molecules, or subsequent release of specific proteins. Bioassays thus give the researcher information not simply about soluble cytokine levels, but also about some aspect of their functionality. In addition, they are quite sensitive tests, with detection thresholds less than 1 picogram/milliliter (Bienvenu et al., 1998). However, they are generally less specific, less reliable (reported coefficients of variation are between 10-20%), and more time-consuming than immunoassays.

Other newer methods also exist for examining whole cell's capacities to produce and release cytokines. Two such notable methods are flow cytometry and ELISPOT, both of which measure the abilities of single cells to produce or release cytokines, respectively. These methods, in addition to ELISA, the extremely popular immunoassay technique, are described below.

ELISA

Perhaps the most well-known and used immunoassay is the enzyme-linked immunosorbant assay (ELISA). ELISAs have many variants, including indirect, sandwich, and competitive (Goldsby et al., 2003). An ELISA measures soluble protein in a solution, providing an assessment of cytokines in plasma, serum, or urine. The general procedure is as follows: Samples which presumably contain detectable amounts of soluble cytokine, are incubated in microtiter wells that have enzyme-linked antibodies for the cytokine of interest bound to them. When the solution is passed through the wells, the cytokine is then immobilized when it binds to its antibody. If the "sandwich" procedure is used, a second enzyme-linked antibody specific to a different epitope (arrangement of amino acids) on the cytokine is added and binds to the immobilized cytokine. After washing free these secondary antibodies from their enzymes, a chromogenic (color-inducing) substrate is added that binds to the enzyme and induces the enzyme to generate color that will differ in intensity based on the amount of enzyme, and thus cytokine. The optical density of this color is then read and compared to a standard curve for inferring concentration values. Thus, ELISA measures integrated amounts of soluble protein, not single-cell or frequency amounts.

Because ELISAs generally use monoclonal antibodies that bind very specifically to the epitope in question, and often use a sandwich procedure in which two different epitopes of the cytokine must be bound in order to be recognized, they are able to provide a more accurate measure of integrated protein levels as compared to other techniques (Pala et al., 2000). This specificity for peptides, combined with the fact that no radioactive substances are required, as well as the relatively low cost and ease of use, make the ELISA very popular for assessing soluble cytokine levels. ELISAs are also capable of measuring soluble receptors of cytokines. This can be considered both a strength and a weakness of the ELISA method, depending on the study methodology, as described below.

Because of the penchant of monoclonal-antibody based immunoassays to detect very small peptide fragments, ELISAs may detect fragments of cytokines as well as structurally whole cytokines. Thus, ELISAs hardly provide an error-free estimate of whole soluble cytokines or their receptors. In addition, because new isoforms of cytokines and some of their soluble receptors are continuously being discovered, it is not clear whether the integrative protein amounts detected in an ELISA truly reflect amounts of cytokine that may be biologically active and/or as relevant for the population of interest (Banks, 2000). Although this has been a common complaint with bioassays as well, it is important to note that ELISAs are also susceptible to this error in the following manner: If the cytokine that the ELISA has been specified to measure has a soluble receptor (for example, IL-6, TNF, or IFN-γ), it will be unclear how much of the integrated protein measured by the ELISA is actually reflecting cytokines that are already bound to what is in many cases an inhibitory soluble receptor. Because the soluble receptors of a cytokine often exist in concentrations 100-1000 fold higher than the cytokine itself, the effect of this interference could be sizable, especially for clinical populations in which soluble receptor amounts are different from those of a healthy population (Banks, 2000).

Relating ELISA-measured cytokine levels to biologically active levels thus may be questionable; however, certain methodological actions may render these issues less problematic. For example, there are ELISAs for some but not all soluble receptors. If possible, conducting assays of both the cytokine and its soluble receptors will give more information about potential circulating active levels of cytokine vs. soluble receptor bound, often-inhibited cytokine. In addition, attention paid to the cytokine isoforms that are most clinically relevant for the population of interest will guide the researcher in selecting the ELISA that utilizes monoclonal antibodies most suitable for the purpose of the research. It is also suggested that validation studies, including, for example, the assessment of spiked cytokine recovery be conducted to better estimate the amount of error induced while measuring cytokine levels in a particular population (Banks, 2000). Additionally, while ELISAs generally display good to adequate interassay variability (with coefficients of variation less than 10%), assays of cytokines with very low soluble levels will inflate variability or potentially render undetectable amounts of the cytokine. Thus, it is important to examine whether the soluble cytokine of interest is present in high enough amounts to be detected by an ELISA and whether the range of the amount is adequate to infer proper values by using standard curve estimates. If cytokines that have markedly low soluble levels have soluble receptors, measuring the soluble receptor levels via ELISA may yield more accurate results and give some indication of cytokine level, though admittedly not flawless interpretation.

ELISPOT

ELISPOT is essentially a modification of the ELISA procedure and as such is susceptible to similar methodological issues inherent in the ELISA. The ELISPOT was initially developed in order to obtain information about early activation of lymphocyte populations at the level of single cells (Meierhoff et al., 2002). ELISPOT can be thought of as a combination of a bioassay and an immunoassay in that cloned *in-vitro* cells or fresh *ex-vivo* cells are first stimulated with an antigen and then placed on plates coated with antibodies (termed *capture antibodies*) specific for the cytokine of interest. As the cells settle onto the surface of the plate during the incubation, they react with the capture antibodies on the plate, secreting the cytokine of interest and producing a spot or ring of peptide-antibody complexes that reflects both the kinetics and quality of cytokine production by individual cells during the test period. The cells are removed and an enzyme-linked antibody is added that binds to the cytokine. Chromogenic substrate is then added to identify the cytokine producing cells as colored points and reveal their position on the plate.

ELISPOTS are advantageous for situations in which it may be important to estimate the frequency of stimulated cytokine producing cells rather than resting levels of integrated amounts of secreted protein. Although in principle a similar methodology could be (and often is) employed with ELISA (i.e., first stimulating the cells and then conducting an ELISA with the resulting supernatant), one still faces the methodological issues inherent in ELISA mentioned above. Indeed, ELISPOTs are reported to be substantially more sensitive than ELISAs used for similar purposes (Meierhoff et al., 2002). ELISPOTs also provide the advantage of reflecting functionally active cytokine secretion from different cell subsets and in principle may even be used to measure cytokine co-expression in cells, though such detection is more difficult than using methods like flow cytometry (Pala et al., 2000). In addition, ELISPOT is substantially less expensive than flow cytometry that measures frequency of cytokine-producing cells. The ELISPOT method has been used successfully in a variety of clinical research paradigms, including those examining the immunomodulatory effects of agents such as dexamethasone and hydrocortisone on cytokine release, as well as helping monitor treatment effects and disease status for many different patient populations (Meierhoff et al., 2002).

Flow Cytometry

A widely used method for examining frequencies of cytokine producing cells is flow cytometry with intracellular staining for cytokines. In general, the technique of flow cytometry affords extremely specific information about cell subsets, including depiction of important cell markers, cellular adhesion molecules, and intracellular contents. In the general process of flow cytometry, cells that have been stained or tagged with particular fluorescent antibodies specific to the cell surface or intracellular marker of interest are passed one at a time through a laser which detects and identifies the cells based on the intensity of fluorescence. This technique requires that cells first be "fixed" or inactivated and made permeable. In the case of detecting intracellular cytokine content, the cells must first be activated either *in vivo* or *in vitro* before inactivation. Flow cytometry provides the advantage of detecting different cytokine-producing cell phenotypes; indeed, the technique of flow cytometry was essential in testing the T_H1/T_H2 cytokine subset theory (Prussin, 1997). This approach to detection and comparison of cytokine-producing cell subtypes has been used to examine changes in cell subsets that occur in specific patient populations.

Flow cytometry also allows one to detect cytokine co-expression in a single cell with relative ease as compared with the ELISPOT (Pala et al., 2000) and may be considerably less time-consuming than the ELISPOT (Prussin, 1997). However, there are certain drawbacks inherent in the use of flow cytometry, including the high price tag of a flow cytometer instrument. Second, while flow cytometry requires that cells be activated, the analysis itself is conducted with cells that have been killed or immobilized, thus providing only a snapshot of cytokine production at a given point in time. In addition, although in principle stimulated cells can be obtained *ex vivo*, only a relatively small percentage of such cells will accurately stain for intracellular cytokines, perhaps due to differences in kinetics of expression, and this may limit the investigative utility of the technique (Pala et al., 2000).

Assay Methods Summary

The techniques described above are perhaps the most common methods of assessing cytokine levels for the purposes of stress and behavioral medicine research. Each technique provides distinct advantages as well as potential drawbacks. Decisions on the specific cytokine assessment methodology used will likely be primarily informed by cost-effectiveness and practicality. As the assessment techniques discussed above provide different vantage-points and sensitivities for examining cytokine prevalence and function, a thorough review of the literature that is pertinent to the population of interest will help to inform the researcher of the best cytokine assessment methodology to utilize. Finally, as with other assessments of relevant behavioral medicine biological outcome markers, potential confounding factors should always be carefully considered and controlled for by study design and/or statistical analytic techniques, including, but not limited to, age, gender, ethnicity, diurnal variation characteristics such as menstrual cycle and circadian rhythm, health behaviors such as physical activity, medication use, smoking and alcohol consumption. Such considerations will ultimately strengthen potential findings and interpretations.

CYTOKINES AND THE CENTRAL NERVOUS SYSTEM (CNS)

As noted earlier, cytokines mediate more than local cellular immune responses. Cytokines and their receptors are present in many other types of cells besides peripheral immune cells. In the past decade, a growing body of research has demonstrated that cytokines play both direct and indirect active roles within the CNS. For example, it is now known that cytokines are secreted by certain classes of brain cells, including microglial cells and astrocytes (Kronfol & Remick, 2000). The endogenous expression of cytokines and their receptors have been found in the hypothalamus, basal ganglia, cerebellum, circumventricular sites, and brainstem nuclei (Anisman & Merali, 2002). Included in the considerably large list of brain-active cytokines are interferons alpha and gamma, tumor necrosis factors alpha and beta, and interleukins 1, 2, 3, 4, 5, 6, 8, 10, and 12 (Kronfol & Remick, 2000). Studies involving systematic administration of cytokines in some of the brain regions mentioned above indicate that cytokines promote the release of neurotransmitters, including norepinephrine, dopamine, and serotonin (Anisman & Merali, 2002). Thus, in addition to their immunoprotective effects within the brain, cytokines may promote neurochemical cascades that directly affect mood and behavior.

Cytokines also affect the CNS via peripheral mechanisms. Though cytokines are too large to effectively cross the blood-brain barrier, there are several posited indirect mechanisms of action. One hypothesis is that cytokines might enter the brain via passive transport in areas where the blood-brain barrier is not present (e.g., circumventricular sites). Another is that cytokines might bind to cerebral vascular endothelium, facilitating the release of active second messengers such as nitric oxide. Yet another hypothesis is that cytokines might be transported across the blood-brain-barrier via carrier-mediated transport. Finally, it has been posited that cytokines might affect the CNS indirectly via stimulation of peripheral afferent nerve terminals (Kronfol & Remick, 2000).

Though none of these hypotheses necessarily precludes the other, there may be certain explanations that are more plausible than others for how cytokines indirectly affect brain activity. Cytokines have relatively shorter half-lives than hormones, making it unlikely that peripheral cytokines transported via the blood to the brain are a primary force in affecting the CNS (Maier & Watkins, 1998). Thus, it has been posited that the main indirect effects of cytokines on the CNS may occur via stimulation of afferent nerve fibers. One such nerve fiber that has received considerable attention for this potential function is the vagus (Aronson, Mittleman, & Burger, 2001; Floto & Smith, 2003; Maier & Watkins, 1998). Among its many functions the vagus nerve promotes parasympathetic end-organ activity (such as slowing of the heart beat), primarily via acetylcholine release. Although the vagus has been long appreciated for its efferent nerve activity, it may be less well appreciated that the vagus nerve, in addition to innervating secondary and tertiary lymph organs such as the spleen, gut, thymus, and lymph nodes, receives afferent stimulation from these organs as well. The hypothesis that cytokines might affect brain function via peripheral end-organ stimulation of the vagus has been posited since at least the 1990s (Kapcala, He, Gao, Pieper, & DeTolla, 1996; Maier & Watkins, 1998; Watkins, Maier, & Goehler, 1995). The plausibility of such a hypothesis at the time was partially fueled by the discovery that receptors for IL-1 were found on paraganglia, which surround the terminals of the vagus (Goehler et al., 1997; X. Wang, Wang, Duan, Liu, & Ju, 2000). Subsequent studies indicated that direct stimulation of the vagus resulted in inhibition of release of pro-inflammatory cytokines TNF-α, IL-1β and IL-18 in response to endotoxin but that this vagal stimulation did not inhibit the release of the anti-inflammatory cytokine IL-10 (Borovikova et al., 2000). A recent study (Floto & Smith, 2003) demonstrated that blockade of nicotinic acetylcholine α-receptors on vagal terminals prevents this cytokine antagonism, suggesting that the cholinergic system is indeed an important constituent of this anti-inflammatory process.

These findings support the notion that the vagus is indeed intimately tied to the effects of cytokines on the CNS in the following manner: macrophages in lymphoid structures may release cytokines that bind to their respective receptors in paraganglia near the vagal terminals. Such stimulation may induce acetylcholine release from paraganglia neurons, activating afferent vagal fibers, which then send signals via neural impulses to the brain.

Further, vagal activity may play an important role in dampening pro-inflammatory cytokine release within the CNS. Studies with heart patients that have examined relations between heart period variability and pro-inflammatory cytokine activity have shown significant negative associations, though it is not completely clear that these associations are due to vagal contributions (Aronson et al., 2001; Malave, Taylor, Nattama, Deswal, & Mann, 2003).

CYTOKINE AND THE HYPOTHALAMIC-PITUITARY ADRENAL AXIS (HPA)

Considerable progress has been made in understanding the complex interactions between cytokines and the HPA. This has been the focus of several recent in-depth reviews (Haddad, Saade, & Safieh-Garabedian, 2002; John & Buckingham, 2003). Briefly, it is now well understood that complex and dynamic interactive communication exists between cytokines and the HPA and that the regulation of cytokine release, as well as HPA responses to immune insults, are governed in part by positive and negative feedback loops between the two systems. In particular, pro-inflammatory cytokines have been shown to stimulate HPA stress responses while T_H2 cytokines can inhibit this activation (Frieri, 2003). For example, pro-inflammatory cytokines appear to activate corticotropin releasing hormone (CRH) and arginine vasopressin neurons in the parvocellular paraventricular nucleus within the hypothalamus. This activation results in a downstream HPA cascade in which CRH is released from the hypothalamus, promoting release of corticotrophin (ACTH) from the anterior pituitary gland and resulting in release of the glucocorticoids corticosterone and cortisol from the adrenal cortex. There are several postulated mechanisms of action for how this cascade is initiated by pro-inflammatory cytokines, some of which involve mediating effects of cytokines on the HPA via afferent vagal fiber activity (Haddad et al., 2002; John & Buckingham, 2003).

In addition to effects on the anterior pituitary and adrenal cortex via CRH release from the hypothalamus, pro-inflammatory cytokines may also affect the anterior pituitary and adrenal cortex directly, resulting in similar end-organ effects (release of corticosterone from the adrenal cortex). For example, IL-6 is synthesized and released within the human adrenal gland itself, promoting glucocorticoid release (Path, Scherbaum, & Bornstein, 2000). The multitude of sites of action allows pro-inflammatory cytokines several pathways of promoting a similar end-organ response so that even if higher-level actions of cytokines on hypothalamic or anterior pituitary structures are inhibited (for example, via antagonism by a T_H2 cytokine such as IL-10), some level of glucocorticoid release into the circulation is preserved. In turn, glucocorticoid actions on cytokines help to maintain homeostasis via negative feedback loops. For example, cortisol inhibits cellular synthesis and release of pro-inflammatory cytokines, thus acting to preserve homeostasis in the system. However, the effects of glucocorticoids on maintaining this homeostasis are dampened in cases of chronic stress, possibly due to the ability of the pro-inflammatory cytokines to promote receptor desensitization, downregulation, or prevalence of negative isoforms of the glucocorticoid receptor, causing glucocorticoid resistance (Haddad et al., 2002; John & Buckingham, 2003). Thus, cytokines are intimately intertwined with HPA responses, providing a potent influence on stress responses and appearing to play a very active role in HPA modulations during chronic stress.

Cytokines, Stress, Depression, and Fatigue

While evidence from animal research has long generally supported that cytokines are altered during psychological experiences of stress, depression and fatigue, human studies focusing on cytokine regulation during these states have emerged mostly within the last decade. As is common in more developing research areas, findings have not always been consistent, due in part to a host of factors, including heterogeneity of subject populations and varying sophistication of cytokine assessment methodologies. We present a synopsis of human studies in these areas, as well as provide data from our laboratory that elaborate on cytokine connections with experiences of stress, depression, and fatigue. Finally, we highlight the potential relevance of these cytokine alterations to disease processes. Further reading on these topics can be found in the following reviews and books (Anisman & Merali, 2002; Kim & Maes, 2003; Plotinikoff, Faith, Murgo, & Good, 1999).

Cytokines and Acute Stress

Studies examining cytokine responses to acute stressors have been conducted with both laboratory and naturalistic stressors. Laboratory stressors include mental stress tasks such as the Stroop test and mirror star tracing, social-mental stress tasks such as public speeches, and physiological stress paradigms such as exercise and administration of pharmacological challenges. The majority of these studies have generally focused on examining potential changes in pro-inflammatory, not anti-inflammatory cytokines. Thus far, the literature indicates that acute stress may increase levels of certain pro-inflammatory cytokines while leaving others unchanged. There is some evidence to suggest that such increases in cytokine levels are correlated with sympathetic nervous system activity, and that the cytokine increases are modulated by the HPA axis response to stress.

Steptoe and colleagues (Steptoe, Willemsen, Owen, Flower, & Mohamed-Ali, 2001) reported increases in plasma IL-6 and IL-1 receptor antagonist (IL1Ra) but not TNF-α as compared to a control group after participation in Stroop tasks and mirror star tracing. A follow-up study using a similar protocol examining effects for plasma IL-6 and TNF-α and potential relations to cardiac measures reported replications of increased IL-6 at recovery with no significant differences from baseline in TNF-α (Owen & Steptoe, 2003). Further, the recovery levels of IL-6 correlated with heart rate measures taken at recovery. These latter findings suggest a link between sympathetic nervous system activity and the IL-6 response to mental stressors.

Importantly, Owen and Steptoe (2003) noted that not all individuals show increases in pro-inflammatory cytokines in response to these stressors. Indeed, in their study, only 54% of the subjects showed an increase in TNF-α and 61.2% showed an increase in IL-6. Such findings have been somewhat replicated in another recent study that offered a potential explanation for these individual differences. Using a similar protocol, (Kunz-Ebrecht,

Mohamed-Ali, Feldman, Kirschbaum, & Steptoe, 2003) examined cortisol responses to the mental stress tasks as well as plasma levels of IL-6 and IL-1Ra. Based on the cortisol responses to the stressor, they divided the participants into cortisol responders and non-responders (the two groups did not significantly differ on initial cortisol levels). Cortisol non-responders had significantly higher resting IL-6 levels and greater IL-1Ra increases during the stressor than cortisol responders, as well as significantly greater stress-induced inhibition of heart rate variability during the stressors. These findings are consistent with cortisol's known action of inhibiting effects on pro-inflammatory cytokines. In addition, the indication of decreased vagal activity for the cortisol non-responders may also provide an explanation for why pro-inflammatory cytokines are increased in this group, given that vagal activity is known to decrease pro-inflammatory cytokine activity (Borovikova et al., 2000; H. Wang et al., 2003). Perhaps most importantly, these recent studies indicate that inter-individual differences play an important role in determining cytokine responses to stressors.

Our and other laboratories have used speech and exercise challenges to examine the effects of stressors on circulating cytokine levels of IL-6, TNF-alpha and IFN-γ (Ackerman, Martino, Heyman, Moyna, & Rabin, 1998; Buske-Kirschbaum, Gierens, Hollig, & Hellhammer, 2002; Goebel, Mills, Irwin, & Ziegler, 2000; Larson, Ader, & Moynihan, 2001). We examined the effects of a speech stressor, an exercise challenge, and infusion of the beta-adrenergic agonist isoproterenol. We were interested in how these 3 different acute challenges to the sympathetic nervous system would affect circulating white blood cells and their stimulated cytokine levels. In addition to an expected leukocytosis, including increases in lymphocyte, monocyte and granulocyte populations, we found that the lipopolysaccharide (LPS)-induced IL-6 response was increased by both the speaking task and exercise whereas LPS-stimulated TNF-α production was elevated in response to exercise (Figure 2). The isoproterenol challenge led to a reduction in TNF-α levels. We concluded from this study that in response to the challenges, IL-6 and TNF-α production show different profiles. Purely β-agonist stimulation leads to a down-regulation of TNF-α production, giving evidence for the anti-inflammatory effect of in vivo β-receptor activation. The enhanced production of both cytokines upon exercise and for IL-6 following the speech task could be best explained by a simultaneous up-regulation of pro-inflammatory and inflammation-responding mediators.

Another approach to studying the more acute effects of stress on cytokines is the naturalistic stressor of academic examinations. Findings from these studies have been disappointing in their inconsistency. For example, while some studies have reported a decrease in IFN-γ immediately following examinations (Dobbin, Harth, McCain, Martin, & Cousin, 1991; Kang & Fox, 2001), at least one study has reported an increase (Maes et al., 1998). Similarly, while a few studies have reported increases in IL-1β following academic stress (Dobbin et al., 1991; Guidi et al., 1999; Paik, Toh, Lee, Kim, & Lee, 2000), another study has reported a decrease (Kiecolt-Glaser, Marucha, Atkinson, & Glaser, 2001). Other studies have more consistently reported increases in IL-6 (Kang & Fox, 2001; Maes et al., 1998; Paik et al., 2000) and decreases in IL-2 (Guidi et al., 1999; Kang & Fox, 2001; Uchakin, Tobin, Cubbage, Marshall, & Sams, 2001) following academic stress. Thus, results from the literature on the effects of academic stress on cytokines and subsequent T_H1/T_H2

balance are less clear perhaps due to assessment of cytokines at slightly different time points and with slightly different populations. It is an area that merits further careful research.

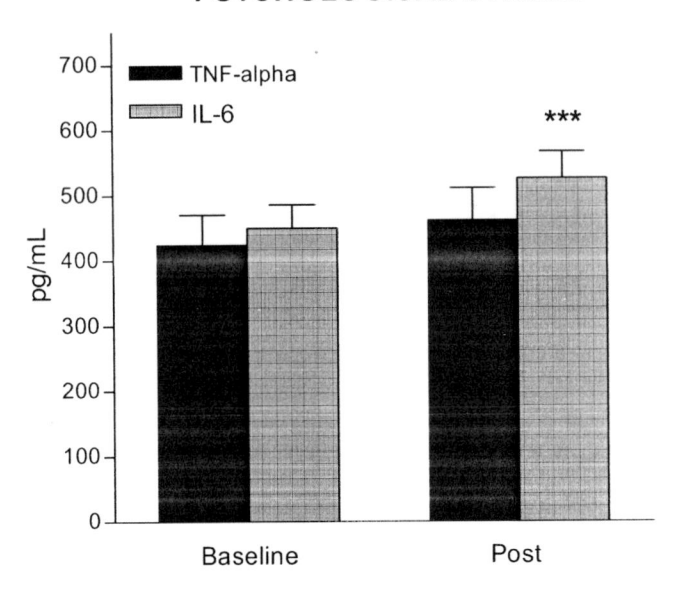

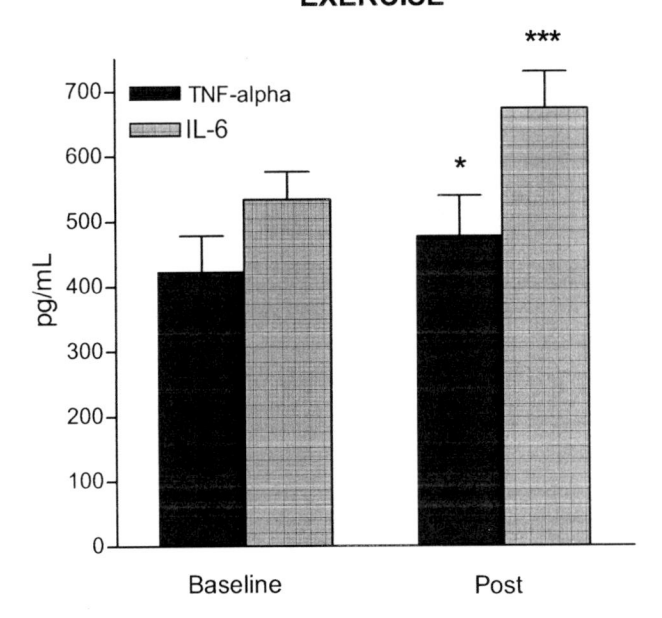

Figure 2: Levels of lipopolysaccharide-induced TNF-α and Il-6 production in response to a stressful public speaking task and a bicycle ergometer exercise. IL-6 increased significantly upon the speech and exercise task (p's< .001). TNF-α production did not change significantly upon the speech, but was moderately elevated following exercise (p< .05).

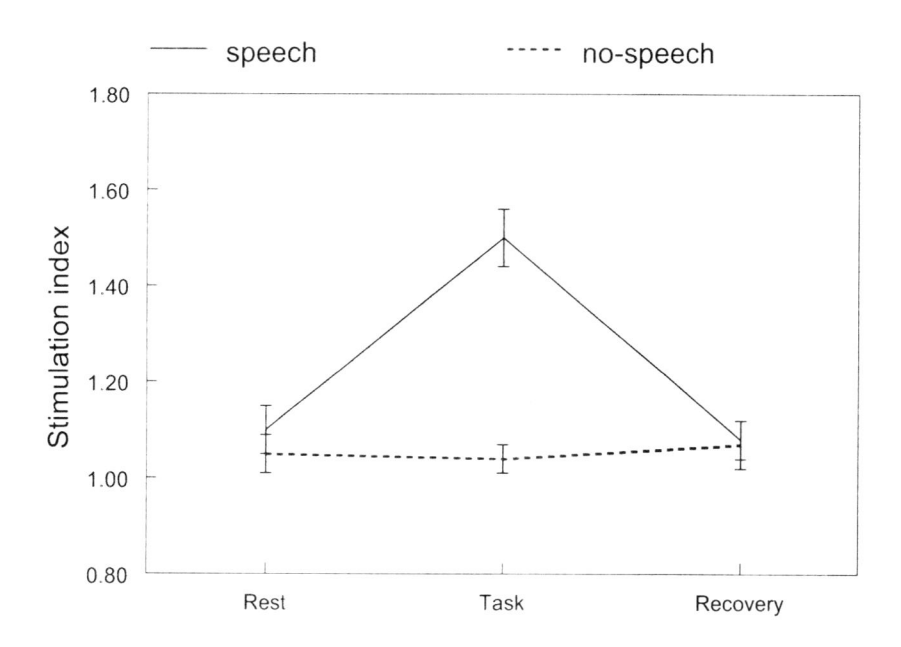

Figure 3: Chemotaxis of peripheral immune cells in subjects performing a stressful public speaking task (speech) or sitting quietly reading a magazine (no speech). Cells were sampled at rest, immediately following speech/ reading and 20 minutes later. Chemokine-mediated (FMLP) chemotaxis increased significantly in response to the speech (p<0.04).

In addition to cytokines themselves, two other related and meaningful approaches to exploring the effects of acute stressors on cytokine-related physiology is examining stressor effects on *in vivo* leukocyte trafficking and *in vitro* leukocyte adhesion and/or chemotaxis. Regarding the former, there is a large literature on the effects of acute stressors on immune cell redistribution (Mills et al., 1995). The relevance to cytokines is that stressors affect the expression of cellular adhesion molecules (including L-selectin, ICAM-1 and LFA-1) and chemokine receptors that are important to immune cell actions. Recall that chemokines are a family of structurally related cytokines that support chemotaxis and that chemotaxis is the process whereby leukocytes migrate to sites of inflammation. Work from our laboratory has shown that public speech stress leads to a significant decrease of L-selectin expression and increase of LFA-1 expression on circulating lymphocytes (Mills et al., 2003). Bosch and colleagues (Bosch, Berntson, Cacioppo, Dhabhar, & Marucha, 2003) showed that public speech stress leads to an increase in the number of circulating lymphocytes expressing the chemokine receptors CXCR2, CXCR3, and CCR5, the ligands of which are chemokines secreted by activated endothelial cells. These phenomena of stressors effects on adhesion molecules and chemokine receptors have a significant bearing on the actual trafficking and adhesion of immune cells, effects which are born out by *in vitro* studies. For example, we examined the effects of a public speech on chemokine-induced leukocyte chemotaxis (Redwine, Snow, Mills, & Irwin, 2003). Compared to a non-stress control condition, the speech led to a significant increase of leukocyte chemotaxis to two important chemotactic chemokines (FMLP and SDF-1) (Figure 3). We have also shown that exercise stress leads to an increase in immune cell adhesion to cytokine-activated endothelial cells, but only in patients with high blood pressure (Mills et al., 2000). Together, these related findings indicate that acute stressors can lead to a circulating environment where immune cells have characteristics that lead to increased responsiveness and adhesion to the endothelium (Figure 1). These phenomena provide insight into how stressors alter the cytokine-regulated migration and recruitment properties of immune cells that are important for responses to infection and inflammation, including the inflammatory process known to underlie the development of atherosclerotic plaque formation.

Cytokines and Chronic Stress

A few studies have examined effects of chronic stress on cytokines in humans, and appear equivocal in their findings that chronic stress is associated with a shift in T_H1/T_H2 responses towards T_H2 dominance. In an early study examining chronic stress and wound healing, Kielcolt-Glaser and colleagues (Kiecolt-Glaser, Marucha, Malarkey, Mercado, & Glaser, 1995) demonstrated that compared to matched controls, Alzheimer's caregivers showed a decrease in IL-1 mRNA secretion in response to LPS stimulation of peripheral blood leukocytes, which may have contributed to slower wound healing in this group. A further study by this group with the same population indicated lower IL-1β and IL-2 responses to virus-specific stimulation for Alzheimer's caregivers versus controls (Kiecolt-Glaser, Glaser, Gravenstein, Malarkey, & Sheridan, 1996). More recently, studies from this group report increased intracellular IL-10 (but no change in INF-γ or IL-2) levels in T-helper and T-cytotoxic cells for Alzheimer's caregivers versus controls, with the difference between these groups being significantly greater for younger subjects (Glaser et al., 2001). Finally, recently reported findings from a longitudinal study where IL-6 levels for Alzheimer's caregivers and controls were tracked over six years showed an almost fourfold rate of increase in Alzheimer's caregivers in IL-6 compared to matched controls. This result was consistent even for caregivers whose spouses had died during the six-year period (Kiecolt-Glaser et al., 2003). Another study examining IL-6 associations with aging and chronic stress in women indicated that Alzheimer's caregivers showed significantly higher levels of IL-6 compared to age-matched women who were experiencing moderate forms of stress (i.e., moving), as well as compared to older and younger control subjects (Lutgendorf et al., 1999).

Some of these findings suggest that chronic stress associated with Alzheimer's caregiving in the elderly promotes increases in T_H2 cytokines and inhibition of T_H1 cytokines. Findings from our laboratory looking at L-selectin expression (CD62L) support this contention (Mills, Yu, Ziegler, Patterson, & Grant, 1999). T_H1 and T_H2 cells can be differentiated according to CD62L expression, with the T_H1 subset being CD62L⁻ and the T_H2 subset being CD62L⁺. We examined CD62L expression in T lymphocytes in elderly stressed and non-stressed spousal caregivers and found that the more stressed vulnerable caregivers had 60% fewer L-selectin negative (CD62L⁻) T lymphocytes. We also found that plasma epinephrine levels were 44% higher in the vulnerable caregivers; this was likely a contributing mechanism to the loss of CD62L⁻ because epinephrine suppresses the T_H1 phenotype. In summary, a shift in T_H1/T_H2 cytokine balance may explain prior observations of immunologic decrements associated with chronic stress in caregivers. The findings also suggest pathways by which caregiving in the elderly leads to significantly increased risk for deleterious health outcomes even well after the death of the spouse being cared for.

Cytokines and Depression

Perhaps the psychological disorder most often discussed in terms of its links to cytokine imbalance is depression. Theories of cytokine underpinnings in depression include speculations that cytokines function as trait markers of depression (Anisman, Ravindran, Griffiths, & Merali, 1999b), that cytokines play an important mechanistic role in stress-induced depression (Connor & Leonard, 1998), and that cytokines are simply associated with certain aspects of depression due to a general medical condition (i.e., sickness behavior due to cytokine therapy) and not to "typical depression" (de Beaurepaire, 2002). The heterogeneity in theories linking cytokines and depression stems from the diverse sources of information about cytokines and depression, including animal studies, studies with exogenous administration of cytokines as treatment for patients, administration of cytokines in controlled studies, and cross-sectional studies examining cytokine levels in depressed patients (Anisman & Merali, 2002, 2003; Capuron & Dantzer, 2003; Dantzer, Wollmann, & Yirmiya, 1999; de Beaurepaire, 2002). A synopsis of conclusions from human studies as well as their potential relevance to disease processes and outcomes will be discussed here.

Perhaps the strongest evidence linking causal cytokine action with depressive states comes from studies where exogenous cytokines are administered for therapeutic purposes in humans. Many patients undergoing cytokine therapy (for example, IFN-α, IL-2, or IFN-γ therapy) for the treatment of cancer show a "sickness behavior" response. This "sickness syndrome" includes neurovegetative symptoms of depression such as fatigue, loss of appetite, and disturbed sleep, as well as depressed neurocognitive functioning and hallmark symptoms of depression such as anhedonia and feelings of sadness (Capuron et al., 2002; Capuron, Ravaud, & Dantzer, 2000). These symptoms seem directly linked to the presence of the exogenous cytokines, as symptoms remit after cessation of cytokine therapy (Anisman & Merali, 2002). Indeed, it has been reported that depression is prevalent in nearly 50% of cancer patients who receive chronic, high dose IFN-α therapy (Musselman et al., 2001). Interestingly, administration of paroxetine helps buffer against the depressive effects of cytokine therapy for cancer patients (Musselman et al., 2001). Antidepressant medication has been found in depressive patients to ameliorate depressive symptoms while having no significant effect on cytokine levels (Anisman, Ravindran, Griffiths, & Merali, 1999a; Kubera et al., 2000; Maes, 1999). This may be due to these antidepressants' ability to normalize serotonin levels that have been decreased due to increased activity of pro-inflammatory cytokines. For example, it is known that certain pro-inflammatory cytokines (such as IL-1β, TNF-α, and IFN-γ) decrease production of serotonin by stimulating activity of an enzyme (indoleamine 2, 3 dioxygenase or IDO) that degrades tryptophan, the precursor to serotonin. Thus, selective serotonin reuptake inhibitors may help to restore serotonin levels, while not directly affecting cytokines themselves.

Relatively few controlled studies exist that compare cytokine levels in depressed patients versus healthy, non-depressed controls. However, the majority of the studies reported so far indicate increases in several cytokines in depressed persons versus healthy controls, including IFN-γ and IL-1β as well as IL-1, and IL-2 and their respective soluble receptors (see Anisman & Merali, 2002 for review). However, not all studies have shown such a relationship. A recent study found no difference in stimulated IL-2 production between dysthymic patients and controls (Irwin, Clark, Kennedy, Christian Gillin, & Ziegler, 2003). Another study reported no statistically significant difference between depressed patients and controls in resting serum IL-6 and IL1Ra levels (Kubera et al., 2000). The heterogeneity in findings thus far may be due to examining different aspects of cytokine levels or production, as well as due to studying different depressive populations at different times. For example, one study reported differences in IL-6 between depressed patients and controls during acute illness, but not after remission (Frommberger et al., 1997). In addition, it appears that the strongest association between pro-inflammatory cytokines and depression are found for more severe, melancholic depression (Anisman & Merali, 2002; Maes, 1995).

Cytokines and Fatigue

Perhaps the most important area of research examining the relationship between cytokines and fatigue is within cancer. Fatigue is one of the most frequent complaints of cancer patients, with studies showing incidence rates of 40% to 75% of patients reporting feeling tired and weak and with rates up to 95% during chemotherapy and/or radiotherapy treatment (Smets, Garssen, Cull, & de Haes, 1996; Winningham et al., 1994). As with depression, there are many components of fatigue, including physiological (such as pain and anemia), psychological (including depression), social, and chronobiological (such as circadian rhythms disorders and sleep disruption). The growing literature demonstrating the role of cytokines in sleep maintenance and disruption (Mills & Dimsdale, 2004) points to a clear linkage between increased fatigue and sleep problems (Ancoli-Israel, Moore, & Jones, 2001). IL-6 and TNF-α, for example, are fatigue-inducing cytokines that are elevated during the day in disorders of excessive daytime sleepiness (Vgontzas et al., 2000; Vgontzas et al., 1997) and in healthy subjects following sleep deprivation (Irwin, 2002).

However, much of the fatigue that cancer patients experience is likely attributed to not simply sleep loss but also to cytokines that are elevated either by the cellular damage from the cancer itself or by its treatment (Kurzrock, 2001; Mills et al., 2004). High levels of endogenous cytokines are seen in many malignancies (Argiles, Busquets, & Lopez-Soriano, 2003). Significantly higher serum levels of IL-1 receptor antagonist (IL-1Ra) and soluble TNF-receptor II (sTNF-RII) are found among breast cancer survivors who report a high level of fatigue as compared to low-fatigued breast cancer patients (Bower, Ganz, Aziz, & Fahey, 2002).

We used the Multidimensional Fatigue Symptom Inventory-Short Form (MFSI-SF) (Stein, Jacobsen, Blanchard, & Thors, 2004) to determine total fatigue ratings in 21 women with breast cancer stages I-III and 18 healthy women of similar age without breast cancer.

Consistent with the literature, we found that ratings of total fatigue were significantly elevated in women with breast cancer (Figure 4). We also examined plasma IL-6 levels in these patients. We found that that IL-6 was significantly elevated in these breast cancer patients as compared to the healthy women without breast cancer (Figure 4). IL-6 levels correlated significantly with the MFSI-SF total fatigue scores (r=0.56). These data provide further support that pro-inflammatory cytokines, at least in breast cancer may be related to the degree of self-reported fatigue.

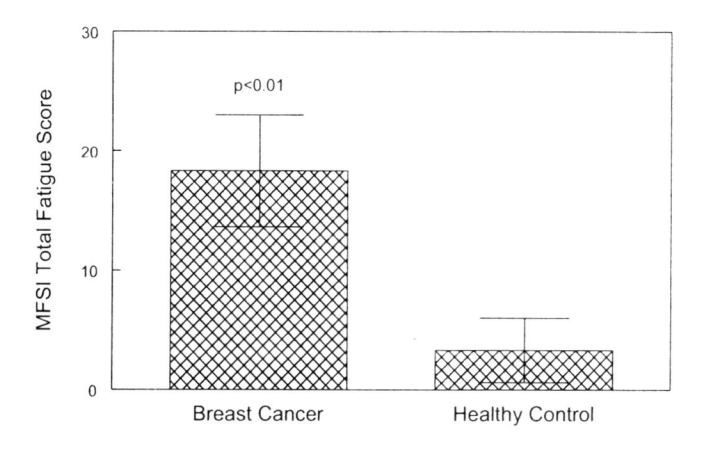

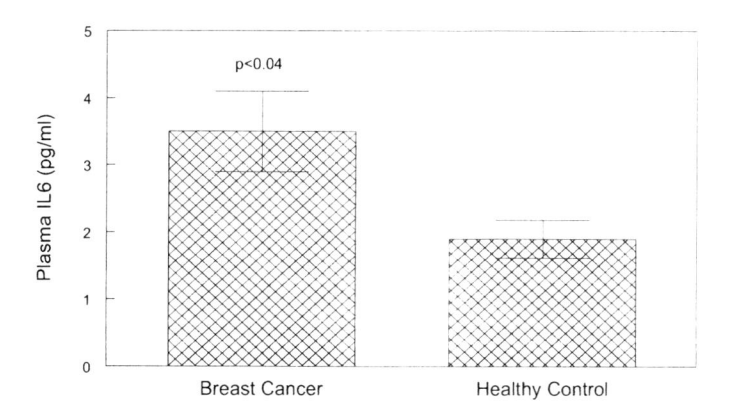

Figure 4: Total fatigue scores (using the Multidimensional Fatigue Symptom Inventory-Short Form (MFSI-SF) and plasma IL-6 levels in 21 women with breast cancer stages I-III and 18 healthy women of similar age without breast cancer. Ratings of total fatigue (p<0.01) and IL-6 levels (p<0.04) were elevated in women with breast cancer. IL-6 levels correlated with total fatigue scores (r=0.56, p=0.031).

Fatigue has also been linked to enhanced inflammatory responses in non-cancer patients. Vital exhaustion is a syndrome marked by persistent fatigue often stemming from an inability to cope with one or more chronic stressors and has been implicated as an independent risk factor for negative cardiovascular events. Vital exhaustion in women has been linked to elevated circulating TNF-alpha levels (Grossi, Perski, Evengard, Blomkvist, & Orth-Gomer, 2003). A recent study comparing vitally exhausted middle-aged males with controls indicated that vital exhaustion was associated with increased IL-6, IL-1ra, and IL-10 levels, as well as increased procoagulant activity (van der Ven et al., 2003). Similarly, a recent study examining vital vs. non-vital exhaustion in male industrial workers (Wirtz et al., 2003) showed decreased glucocorticoid sensitivity for highly exhausted men, both by dexamethasone inhibition of LPS-stimulated IL-6 release and by the IC_{50} (a measure of glucocorticoid sensitivity that is independent of absolute cytokine release). In addition, vitally exhausted workers showed significantly increased resting levels of C-reactive protein. Together, the findings suggest that excessive fatigue in otherwise healthy women and men may be associated with a shift towards a pro-inflammatory profile.

Stress, Depression, Fatigue and Cytokines: Relevance for Disease Outcomes

The potential increase in pro-inflammatory cytokines in depression, stress and possibly fatigue may have implications for certain disease processes. There is considerable evidence, for example, that depression and other negative affect states confer a sizable increased risk for negative cardiovascular incidents for patients already suffering from cardiovascular illnesses, as well as for otherwise healthy individuals (Carney & Freedland, 2003; Joynt, Whellan, & O'Connor, 2003; Musselman, Evans, & Nemeroff, 1998; Smith & Ruiz, 2002). However, the mechanisms by which depression exacerbates cardiovascular disease processes are still not completely clear. There are many potential physiological pathways by which depression may increase cardiovascular risk (Joynt et al., 2003), among them being increased pro-inflammatory cytokine levels. Increases in basal levels of pro-inflammatory cytokines IL-1, IL-6, and TNF-α found in stressed and depressed patients may exacerbate the inflammatory response to endothelial damage and speed along the process of atherosclerosis (Joynt et al., 2003). Pro-inflammatory cytokines such as IL-1 and TNF-α promote procoagulant activity in part by stimulating tissue factor expression on endothelial cells and monocytes (Grignani & Maiolo, 2000) and thus increases in these cytokines in depressed patients might further alter homeostasis in the direction promoting increased clot formation. In addition, as noted earlier, elevated IL-6 levels in depression and distress may exacerbate humoral inflammatory processes associated with its activity, including increased acute phase protein synthesis and release as well as increased HPA stimulation. Indeed, the elevated pro-inflammatory cytokines that are associated with stress and depression (i.e., TNF-α, IL-6, and IL-1Ra) have been associated with clinical instability and markedly poorer prognosis for patients with coronary artery disease (Cesari et al., 2003; Denollet et al., 2003; Patti et al., 2002).

There is a possibility that the chronic prevalence of fatigue in otherwise healthy individuals may also increase risk for cardiovascular disorders via a cytokine-mediated response. We already reviewed that vital exhaustion is characterized by a generalized increased inflammatory profile. Not surprisingly, individuals who experience vital exhaustion also report a general lack of energy and some symptoms of depression, such as hopelessness. A relatively recent large-scale study indicated that vital exhaustion was independently associated with a twofold risk of mortality from coronary heart disease in older men (Cole, Kawachi, Sesso, Paffenbarger, & Lee, 1999). In addition, a recent study reports that vital exhaustion is a significant independent risk indicator for first stroke in middle aged men and women (Schuitemaker, Dinant, Van Der Pol, Verhelst, & Appels, 2004), implying that this state of persistent and excessive fatigue (and its negative effects) is not necessarily a consequence of existing cardiovascular disorders. Longitudinal studies with younger, chronically stressed men and women will help to elucidate the potential effects of vital exhaustion on glucocorticoid resistance, cytokine balance and subsequent immune response over time.

Obviously, alterations in cytokines that are associated with stress, depression and fatigue affect more than cardiovascular disease progression. Increases in pro-inflammatory cytokines associated with acute stress and depression may directly affect disease progression for disorders such as rheumatoid arthritis, multiple sclerosis, and diabetes (Frieri, 2003). In addition, increases towards T_H2 activity and possible suppression of T_H1 activity in chronic stress might directly exacerbate immune processes already aberrant in cancer, asthma, and other allergic disorders.

The Potential for Behavioral Interventions

The importance for treating stress, fatigue and depression for patients of these various disorders becomes even more pressing given the considerable physiological as well as psychological risks at stake. We've already noted that patients who receive intensive exogenous pro-inflammatory cytokine therapy as part of their treatment protocol run a high risk for developing depressive symptoms (Raison & Miller, 2003). While antidepressant medication may help to alleviate certain aspects of the phenomenological states of depression, it does not appear to alleviate neurovegetative aspects of depression that are most closely associated with pro-inflammatory cytokine increases (Capuron et al., 2002). Thus, other forms of interventions, including those more preventative in nature, deserve attention.

Currently there are only a handful of studies examining the effects of mind-body interventions on cytokines, though some findings are promising. These studies vary in their methodological rigor and thus only a select number of studies are reviewed here. Several studies have examined the effects of acupuncture on cytokines for various patient groups. Of these, a recent study examined the effects of real acupuncture, sham acupuncture, or no treatment with chronic allergic rhinitis patients. This study also included a comparison group of healthy controls that received real acupuncture. The results indicated that one 20-min session of acupuncture resulted in decreased IL-10 but only for the rhinitis patients who received real acupuncture. Both groups (rhinitis and healthy controls) who received real acupuncture also showed decreases in IL-2. Interestingly, both the sham acupuncture and real acupuncture chronic rhinitis groups showed decreases in self-reported symptom severity following treatment (Petti, Liguori, & Ippoliti, 2002). Another study examined the effects of four weeks of real vs. sham acupuncture in bronchial allergic asthma patients. The authors reported significant pre-post decreases in IL-6 and IL-10, increases in IL-8, and increased self-report of general well-being for the real acupuncture group but not the sham acupuncture group. Another study reported that acupuncture resulted in decreased IL-2 for rheumatoid arthritis patients, but not healthy controls (Xinlian et al., 1993).

Two studies have examined the effects of hypnosis on cytokine levels, both with healthy hypnotizable subjects. One examined the effects of hypnosis versus no treatment on distress levels as well as IL-1β levels in hypnotically susceptible medical and dental students. Although there was no group by time interaction, significantly less students in the hypnosis group showed maintenance of initial IL-1β levels over time compared to those in the no-treatment group. However, no differences were found in self-reported distress (Kiecolt-Glaser et al., 2001). The other study reported decreased IFN-γ and IL-2 in a very small sample of highly hypnotizable subjects after two session of hypnosis; however, no control group or measure of distress or well-being was utilized in this study (Wood, Bughi, Morrison, Tanavoli, & Zadeh, 2003).

Other studies utilizing strategies for reducing distress and/or depression in patient groups have reported changes in cytokines as well. One study examined the effects of progressive muscle relaxation (PMR) versus no treatment in chronic tinnitus sufferers, with a comparison group of healthy subjects who also participated in the intervention. Results showed reductions in TNF-α for chronic tinnitus sufferers who participated in PMR as well as decreases in perceived stress, depression, and anger; changes were not found for the no-treatment or healthy comparison group (Weber, Arck, Mazurek, & Klapp, 2002). Another study indicated that individual cognitive-behavioral or group therapy was as efficacious as sertraline in reducing antigen-stimulated IFN-γ levels in patients with multiple sclerosis and comorbid depression (Mohr, Goodkin, Islar, Hauser, & Genain, 2001). Importantly, reductions in depression were associated with this decrease in IFN-γ. Finally, a recent study examining the effects of mindfulness-based stress reduction in breast and prostrate cancer patients (Carlson, Speca, Patel, & Goodey, 2003) reported increased T-cell production of IFN-γ and IL-4 and decreased NK cell production of IL-10, as well as decreased perceived stress, increased quality of life, and increased appetite. However, this study did not have a control group or comparison group.

Another promising behavioral intervention approach that would target cytokines and have significant potential for reducing associated symptoms of depression and fatigue, particularly in cancer, is exercise. Regular aerobic exercise intervention programs in cancer patients are shown to increase functional/physical capacity (MacVicar, Winningham, & Nickel, 1989) and decrease symptoms (Winningham & MacVicar, 1988). A six-week walking exercise program during radiation therapy was shown to lead to an enhanced exercise capability and reduced self-reported fatigue, depression, and anxiety in breast cancer patients (Mock et al., 1997). The fatigue-relieving effect of aerobic exercise has been shown in cancer patients both during (Sarna & Conde, 2001; Schwartz, Mori, Gao, Nail, & King, 2001) and after (Burnham & Wilcox, 2002; Carr, Goudas, & Lawrence, 2002) active cancer treatments. Given the known profound effects of exercise on the cytokine axis (Nemet et al., 2002; Shephard, 2002) examining cytokines as potential mediators of these positive outcomes remains a logical and we believe promising area of research.

CONCLUSIONS

Over the past 25 years, the field of behavioral medicine has made great strides, deepening our understanding of behavioral mediators of disease and wellness. Cytokines have emerged as not only important mediators of immune function but also as immunotransmitters that have widely varying and far-reaching effects on other physiological systems, including the central nervous system and hypothalamic-pituitary axis. Imbalances in cytokines and their effects on psychosocial and physiological functioning are reflected in numerous populations of relevance to stress, including but not limited to, cancer, asthma, cardiovascular disorders, allergic disorders, multiple sclerosis, and rheumatoid arthritis. In addition, because of their far-reaching effects, it is becoming clearer that cytokines play an important role in the psychophysiological states of stress, depression and fatigue. It is our hope that continued rigorous research in these areas will at once further elucidate the linkages between cytokines and these psychological states as well as identify effective interventions aimed at relieving the associated symptomatology.

REFERENCES

Ackerman, K. D., Martino, M., Heyman, R., Moyna, N. M., & Rabin, B. S. (1998). Stressor-induced alteration of cytokine production in multiple sclerosis patients and controls. *Psychosom Med, 60*(4), 484-491.

Ancoli-Israel, S., Moore, P., & Jones, V. (2001). The relationship between fatigue and sleep in cancer patients: A review. *European Journal of Cancer Care, 10*, 245-255.

Anisman, H., & Merali, Z. (2002). Cytokines, stress, and depressive illness. *Brain Behav Immun, 16*(5), 513-524.

Anisman, H., & Merali, Z. (2003). Cytokines, stress and depressive illness: brain-immune interactions. *Ann Med, 35*(1), 2-11.

Anisman, H., Ravindran, A. V., Griffiths, J., & Merali, Z. (1999a). Endocrine and cytokine correlates of major depression and dysthymia with typical or atypical features. *Molecular Psychiatry, 4*(2), 182-188.

Anisman, H., Ravindran, A. V., Griffiths, J., & Merali, Z. (1999b). Interleukin-1 beta production in dysthymia before and after pharmacotherapy. *Biol Psychiatry, 46*(12), 1649-1655.

Argiles, J. M., Busquets, S., & Lopez-Soriano, F. J. (2003). Cytokines in the pathogenesis of cancer cachexia. *Curr Opin Clin Nutr Metab Care, 6*(4), 401-406.

Aronson, D., Mittleman, M. A., & Burger, A. J. (2001). Interleukin-6 levels are inversely correlated with heart rate variability in patients with decompensated heart failure. *J Cardiovasc Electrophysiol, 12*(3), 294-300.

Banks, R. E. (2000). Measurement of cytokines in clinical samples using immunoassays: problems and pitfalls. *Crit Rev Clin Lab Sci, 37*(2), 131-182.

Bienvenu, J. A., Monneret, G., Gutowski, M. C., & Fabien, N. (1998). Cytokine assays in human sera and tissues. *Toxicology, 129*(1), 55-61.

Borovikova, L. V., Ivanova, S., Zhang, M., Yang, H., Botchkina, G. I., Watkins, L. R., et al. (2000). Vagus nerve stimulation attenuates the systemic inflammatory response to endotoxin. *Nature, 405*(6785), 458-462.

Bosch, J. A., Berntson, G. G., Cacioppo, J. T., Dhabhar, F. S., & Marucha, P. T. (2003). Acute stress evokes selective mobilization of T cells that differ in chemokine receptor expression: a potential pathway linking immunologic reactivity to cardiovascular disease. *Brain Behav Immun, 17*(4), 251-259.

Bower, J. E., Ganz, P. A., Aziz, N., & Fahey, J. L. (2002). Fatigue and proinflammatory cytokine activity in breast cancer survivors. *Psychosom Med, 64*(4), 604-611.

Burnham, T. R., & Wilcox, A. (2002). Effects of exercise on physiological and psychological variables in cancer survivors. *Med Sci Sports Exerc, 34*(12), 1863-1867.

Buske-Kirschbaum, A., Gierens, A., Hollig, H., & Hellhammer, D. H. (2002). Stress-induced immunomodulation is altered in patients with atopic dermatitis. *J Neuroimmunol, 129*(1-2), 161-167.

Capuron, L., & Dantzer, R. (2003). Cytokines and depression: The need for a new paradigm. *Brain, Behavior, and Immunity, 17*(1, Supplement 1), 119-124.

Capuron, L., Gumnick, J. F., Musselman, D. L., Lawson, D. H., Reemsnyder, A., Nemeroff, C. B., et al. (2002). Neurobehavioral Effects of Interferon-[alpha] in Cancer Patients*1: Phenomenology and Paroxetine Responsiveness of Symptom Dimensions. *Neuropsychopharmacology, 26*(5), 643-652.

Capuron, L., Ravaud, A., & Dantzer, R. (2000). Early depressive symptoms in cancer patients receiving interleukin 2 and/or interferon alfa-2b therapy. *Journal Of Clinical Oncology: Official Journal Of The American Society Of Clinical Oncology, 18*(10), 2143-2151.

Carlson, L. E., Speca, M., Patel, K. D., & Goodey, E. (2003). Mindfulness-based stress reduction in relation to quality of life, mood, symptoms of stress, and immune parameters in breast and prostate cancer outpatients. *Psychosom Med, 65*(4), 571-581.

Carney, R. M., & Freedland, K. E. (2003). Depression, mortality, and medical morbidity in patients with coronary heart disease. *Biol Psychiatry, 54*(3), 241-247.

Carr, D., Goudas, L., & Lawrence, D. (2002). *Management of cancer symptoms: pain, depression, and fatigue*. Rockville, MD: Agency for Healthcare Research and Quality.

Cesari, M., Penninx, B. W., Newman, A. B., Kritchevsky, S. B., Nicklas, B. J., Sutton-Tyrrell, K., et al. (2003). Inflammatory markers and onset of cardiovascular events: results from the Health ABC study. *Circulation, 108*(19), 2317-2322.

Cole, S. R., Kawachi, I., Sesso, H. D., Paffenbarger, R. S., & Lee, I. M. (1999). Sense of exhaustion and coronary heart disease among college alumni. *Am J Cardiol, 84*(12), 1401-1405.

Connor, T. J., & Leonard, B. E. (1998). Depression, stress and immunological activation: The role of cytokines in depressive disorders. *Life Sciences, 62*(7), 583-606.

Dantzer, R., Wollmann, E., & Yirmiya, R. (1999). *Cytokines, stress and depression*. New York: Kluwer Academic/Plenum Publishers.

de Beaurepaire, R. (2002). Questions raised by the cytokine hypothesis of depression. *Brain, Behavior, and Immunity, 16*(5), 610-617.

Denollet, J., Conraads, V. M., Brutsaert, D. L., De Clerck, L. S., Stevens, W. J., & Vrints, C. J. (2003). Cytokines and immune activation in systolic heart failure: the role of Type D personality. *Brain Behav Immun, 17*(4), 304-309.

Diehl, S., & Rincon, M. (2002). The two faces of IL-6 on Th1/Th2 differentiation. *Mol Immunol, 39*(9), 531-536.

Dobbin, J. P., Harth, M., McCain, G. A., Martin, R. A., & Cousin, K. (1991). Cytokine production and lymphocyte transformation during stress. *Brain Behav Immun, 5*(4), 339-348.

Feinberg, B., Kurzrock, R., Talpaz, M., Blick, M., Saks, S., & Gutterman, J. U. (1988). A phase I trial of intravenously-administered recombinant tumor necrosis factor-alpha in cancer patients. *J Clin Oncol, 6*(8), 1328-1334.

Floto, R. A., & Smith, K. G. (2003). The vagus nerve, macrophages, and nicotine. *Lancet, 361*(9363), 1069-1070.

Frieri, M. (2003). Neuroimmunology and inflammation: implications for therapy of allergic and autoimmune diseases. *Ann Allergy Asthma Immunol, 90*(6 Suppl 3), 34-40.

Frommberger, U. H., Bauer, J., Haselbauer, P., Fraulin, A., Riemann, D., & Berger, M. (1997). Interleukin-6-(IL-6) plasma levels in depression and schizophrenia: comparison between the acute state and after remission. *European Archives Of Psychiatry And Clinical Neuroscience, 247*(4), 228-233.

Glaser, R., MacCallum, R. C., Laskowski, B. F., Malarkey, W. B., Sheridan, J. F., & Kiecolt-Glaser, J. K. (2001). Evidence for a shift in the Th-1 to Th-2 cytokine response associated with chronic stress and aging. *J Gerontol A Biol Sci Med Sci, 56*(8), M477-482.

Goebel, M. U., Mills, P. J., Irwin, M. R., & Ziegler, M. G. (2000). Interleukin-6 and tumor necrosis factor-alpha production after acute psychological stress, exercise, and infused isoproterenol: differential effects and pathways. *Psychosom Med, 62*(4), 591-598.

Goebel M. U. and Mills P. J. (2000). Lymphocyte Trafficking, in *Encyclopedia of Stress* (Editor, G. Fink), Academic Press, San Diego, volume 2, 646-655.

Goehler, L. E., Relton, J. K., Dripps, D., Kiechle, R., Tartaglia, N., Maier, S. F., et al. (1997). Vagal paraganglia bind biotinylated interleukin-1 receptor antagonist: a possible mechanism for immune-to-brain communication. *Brain Res Bull, 43*(3), 357-364.

Goldsby, R. A., Kindt, T. J., Osborne, B. A., & Kuby, J. (2003). *Immunology* (5th ed.). New York: W.H. Freeman and Company.

Grignani, G., & Maiolo, A. (2000). Cytokines and hemostasis. *Haematologica, 85*(9), 967-972.

Grossi, G., Perski, A., Evengard, B., Blomkvist, V., & Orth-Gomer, K. (2003). Physiological correlates of burnout among women. *J Psychosom Res, 55*(4), 309-316.

Guidi, L., Tricerri, A., Vangeli, M., Frasca, D., Riccardo Errani, A., Di Giovanni, A., et al. (1999). Neuropeptide Y plasma levels and immunological changes during academic stress. *Neuropsychobiology, 40*(4), 188-195.

Haddad, J. J., Saade, N. E., & Safieh-Garabedian, B. (2002). Cytokines and neuro-immune-endocrine interactions: a role for the hypothalamic-pituitary-adrenal revolving axis. *J Neuroimmunol, 133*(1-2), 1-19.

Irwin, M. (2002). Effects of sleep and sleep loss on immunity and cytokines. *Brain Behav Immun, 16*(5), 503-512.

Irwin, M., Clark, C., Kennedy, B., Christian Gillin, J., & Ziegler, M. (2003). Nocturnal catecholamines and immune function in insomniacs, depressed patients, and control subjects. *Brain Behav Immun, 17*(5), 365-372.

Ito, T., & Ikeda, U. (2003). Inflammatory cytokines and cardiovascular disease. *Curr Drug Targets Inflamm Allergy, 2*(3), 257-265.

John, C. D., & Buckingham, J. C. (2003). Cytokines: regulation of the hypothalamo-pituitary-adrenocortical axis. *Curr Opin Pharmacol, 3*(1), 78-84.

Joynt, K. E., Whellan, D. J., & O'Connor, C. M. (2003). Depression and cardiovascular disease: mechanisms of interaction. *Biol Psychiatry, 54*(3), 248-261.

Kang, D. H., & Fox, C. (2001). Th1 and Th2 cytokine responses to academic stress. *Res Nurs Health, 24*(4), 245-257.

Kapcala, L. P., He, J. R., Gao, Y., Pieper, J. O., & DeTolla, L. J. (1996). Subdiaphragmatic vagotomy inhibits intra-abdominal interleukin-1 beta stimulation of adrenocorticotropin secretion. *Brain Res, 728*(2), 247-254.

Kiecolt-Glaser, J. K., Glaser, R., Gravenstein, S., Malarkey, W. B., & Sheridan, J. (1996). Chronic stress alters the immune response to influenza virus vaccine in older adults. *Proc Natl Acad Sci U S A, 93*(7), 3043-3047.

Kiecolt-Glaser, J. K., Marucha, P. T., Atkinson, C., & Glaser, R. (2001). Hypnosis as a modulator of cellular immune dysregulation during acute stress. *J Consult Clin Psychol, 69*(4), 674-682.

Kiecolt-Glaser, J. K., Marucha, P. T., Malarkey, W. B., Mercado, A. M., & Glaser, R. (1995). Slowing of wound healing by psychological stress. *Lancet, 346*(8984), 1194-1196.

Kiecolt-Glaser, J. K., McGuire, L., Robles, T. F., & Glaser, R. (2002). Emotions, morbidity, and mortality: new perspectives from psychoneuroimmunology. *Annu Rev Psychol, 53*, 83-107.

Kiecolt-Glaser, J. K., Preacher, K. J., MacCallum, R. C., Atkinson, C., Malarkey, W. B., & Glaser, R. (2003). Chronic stress and age-related increases in the proinflammatory cytokine IL-6. *Proc Natl Acad Sci U S A, 100*(15), 9090-9095.

Kim, Y.-K., & Maes, M. (2003). The role of the cytokine network in psychological stress. *Acta Neuropsychiatrica, 15*(3), 148-155.

Kronfol, Z., & Remick, D. G. (2000). Cytokines and the brain: implications for clinical psychiatry. *Am J Psychiatry, 157*(5), 683-694.

Kubera, M., Kenis, G., Bosmans, E., Zieba, A., Dudek, D., Nowak, G., et al. (2000). Plasma levels of interleukin-6, interleukin-10, and interleukin-1 receptor antagonist in depression: comparison between the acute state and after remission. *Pol J Pharmacol, 52*(3), 237-241.

Kunz-Ebrecht, S. R., Mohamed-Ali, V., Feldman, P. J., Kirschbaum, C., & Steptoe, A. (2003). Cortisol responses to mild psychological stress are inversely associated with proinflammatory cytokines. *Brain Behav Immun, 17*(5), 373-383.

Kurzrock, R. (2001). The role of cytokines in cancer-related fatigue. *Cancer, 92*(6 Suppl), 1684-1688.

Kurzrock, R., Quesada, J. R., Rosenblum, M. G., Sherwin, S. A., & Gutterman, J. U. (1986). Phase I study of i.v. administered recombinant gamma interferon in cancer patients. *Cancer Treat Rep, 70*(12), 1357-1364.

Larson, M. R., Ader, R., & Moynihan, J. A. (2001). Heart rate, neuroendocrine, and immunological reactivity in response to an acute laboratory stressor. *Psychosom Med, 63*(3), 493-501.

Lutgendorf, S. K., Garand, L., Buckwalter, K. C., Reimer, T. T., Hong, S. Y., & Lubaroff, D. M. (1999). Life stress, mood disturbance, and elevated interleukin-6 in healthy older women. *J Gerontol A Biol Sci Med Sci, 54*(9), M434-439.

MacVicar, M. G., Winningham, M. L., & Nickel, J. L. (1989). Effects of aerobic interval training on cancer patients' functional capacity. *Nurs Res, 38*(6), 348-351.

Maes, M. (1995). Evidence for an immune response in major depression: a review and hypothesis. *Prog Neuropsychopharmacol Biol Psychiatry, 19*(1), 11-38.

Maes, M. (1999). Major depression and activation of the inflammatory response system. *Adv Exp Med Biol, 461*, 25-46.

Maes, M., Song, C., Lin, A., De Jongh, R., Van Gastel, A., Kenis, G., et al. (1998). The effects of psychological stress on humans: increased production of pro-inflammatory cytokines and a Th1-like response in stress-induced anxiety. *Cytokine, 10*(4), 313-318.

Maier, S. F., & Watkins, L. R. (1998). Cytokines for Psychologists: Implications of bidirectional immune-to-brain communication for understanding behavior, mood, and cognition. *Psychological Review, 105*(1), 83-105.

Malave, H. A., Taylor, A. A., Nattama, J., Deswal, A., & Mann, D. L. (2003). Circulating levels of tumor necrosis factor correlate with indexes of depressed heart rate variability: a study in patients with mild-to-moderate heart failure. *Chest, 123*(3), 716-724.

Meierhoff, G., Ott, P. A., Lehmann, P. V., & Schloot, N. C. (2002). Cytokine detection by ELISPOT: relevance for immunological studies in type 1 diabetes. *Diabetes Metab Res Rev, 18*(5), 367-380.

Meltzer, E. O. (2003). The role of the immune system in the pathogenesis of asthma and an overview of the diagnosis, classification, and current approach to treating the disease. *J Manag Care Pharm, 9*(5 Suppl), 8-13.

Mills, P. J., Berry, C. C., Dimsdale, J. E., Ziegler, M. G., Nelesen, R. A., & Kennedy, B. P. (1995). Lymphocyte subset redistribution in response to acute experimental stress: effects of gender, ethnicity, hypertension, and the sympathetic nervous system. *Brain Behav Immun, 9*(1), 61-69.

Mills, P. J., & Dimsdale, J. E. (2004). Sleep Apnea: A model for studying cytokines, sleep and sleep disruption. *Brain Behav Immun,* 18(4):298-303.

Mills, P. J., Farag, N. H., Hong, S., Kennedy, B. P., Berry, C. C., & Ziegler, M. G. (2003). Immune cell CD62L and CD11a expression in response to a psychological stressor in human hypertension. *Brain Behav Immun, 17*(4), 260-267.

Mills, P. J., Maisel, A. S., Ziegler, M. G., Dimsdale, J. E., Carter, S., Kennedy, B., et al. (2000). Peripheral blood mononuclear cell-endothelial adhesion in human hypertension following exercise. *J Hypertens, 18*(12), 1801-1806.

Mills, P. J., Parker, B., Jones, V., Adler, K. A., Perez, C., Johnson, S., et al. (2004). The effects of standard anthracyline-based chemotherapy on soluble ICAM-1 and VEGF levels in breast cancer. *Clinical Cancer Research,* 10(15):4998-5003).

Mills, P. J., Yu, H., Ziegler, M. G., Patterson, T., & Grant, I. (1999). Vulnerable caregivers of patients with Alzheimer's disease have a deficit in circulating CD62L- T lymphocytes. *Psychosom Med, 61*(2), 168-174.

Mire-Sluis, A. R. (1999). The development of non-animal-based bioassays for cytokines and growth factors. *Dev Biol Stand, 101,* 169-175.

Mock, V., Dow, K. H., Meares, C. J., Grimm, P. M., Dienemann, J. A., Haisfield-Wolfe, M. E., et al. (1997). Effects of exercise on fatigue, physical functioning, and emotional distress during radiation therapy for breast cancer. *Oncol Nurs Forum, 24*(6), 991-1000.

Mohr, D. C., Goodkin, D. E., Islar, J., Hauser, S. L., & Genain, C. P. (2001). Treatment of depression is associated with suppression of nonspecific and antigen-specific T(H)1 responses in multiple sclerosis. *Arch Neurol, 58*(7), 1081-1086.

Musselman, D. L., Evans, D. L., & Nemeroff, C. B. (1998). The relationship of depression to cardiovascular disease: epidemiology, biology, and treatment. *Arch Gen Psychiatry, 55*(7), 580-592.

Musselman, D. L., Lawson, D. H., Gumnick, J. F., Manatunga, A. K., Penna, S., Goodkin, R. S., et al. (2001). Paroxetine for the prevention of depression induced by high-dose interferon alfa. *The New England Journal Of Medicine, 344*(13), 961-966.

Naka, T., Nishimoto, N., & Kishimoto, T. (2002). The paradigm of IL-6: from basic science to medicine. *Arthritis Res, 4 Suppl 3,* S233-242.

Nemet, D., Hong, S., Mills, P. J., Ziegler, M. G., Hill, M., & Cooper, D. M. (2002). Systemic vs. local cytokine and leukocyte responses to unilateral wrist flexion exercise. *J Appl Physiol, 93*(2), 546-554.

Owen, N., & Steptoe, A. (2003). Natural killer cell and proinflammatory cytokine responses to mental stress: associations with heart rate and heart rate variability. *Biol Psychol, 63*(2), 101-115.

Paik, I. H., Toh, K. Y., Lee, C., Kim, J. J., & Lee, S. J. (2000). Psychological stress may induce increased humoral and decreased cellular immunity. *Behav Med, 26*(3), 139-141.

Pala, P., Hussell, T., & Openshaw, P. J. (2000). Flow cytometric measurement of intracellular cytokines. *J Immunol Methods, 243*(1-2), 107-124.

Path, G., Scherbaum, W. A., & Bornstein, S. R. (2000). The role of interleukin-6 in the human adrenal gland. *Eur J Clin Invest, 30 Suppl 3,* 91-95.

Patti, G., D'Ambrosio, A., Dobrina, A., Dicuonzo, G., Giansante, C., Fiotti, N., et al. (2002). Interleukin-1 receptor antagonist: a sensitive marker of instability in patients with coronary artery disease. *J Thromb Thrombolysis, 14*(2), 139-143.

Petti, F. B., Liguori, A., & Ippoliti, F. (2002). Study on cytokines IL-2, IL-6, IL-10 in patients of chronic allergic rhinitis treated with acupuncture. *J Tradit Chin Med, 22*(2), 104-111.

Plotinikoff, N. P., Faith, R. E., Murgo, A. J., & Good, R. A. (1999). *Cytokines, Stress and Immunity.* Boca Raton: CRC Press.

Prussin, C. (1997). Cytokine flow cytometry: understanding cytokine biology at the single-cell level. *J Clin Immunol, 17*(3), 195-204.

Raison, C. L., & Miller, A. H. (2003). Depression in cancer: new developments regarding diagnosis and treatment. *Biol Psychiatry, 54*(3), 283-294.

Redwine, L., Snow, S., Mills, P., & Irwin, M. (2003). Acute psychological stress: effects on chemotaxis and cellular adhesion molecule expression. *Psychosom Med, 65*(4), 598-603.

Sakami, S., Ishikawa, T., Kawakami, N., Haratani, T., Fukui, A., Kobayashi, F., et al. (2002). Coemergence of insomnia and a shift in the Th1/Th2 balance toward Th2 dominance. *Neuroimmunomodulation, 10*(6), 337-343.

Sarna, L., & Conde, F. (2001). Physical activity and fatigue during radiation therapy: a pilot study using actigraph monitors. *Oncol Nurs Forum, 28*(6), 1043-1046.

Schuitemaker, G. E., Dinant, G. J., Van Der Pol, G. A., Verhelst, A. F., & Appels, A. (2004). Vital exhaustion as a risk indicator for first stroke. *Psychosomatics, 45*(2), 114-118.

Schwartz, A. L., Mori, M., Gao, R., Nail, L. M., & King, M. E. (2001). Exercise reduces daily fatigue in women with breast cancer receiving chemotherapy. *Med Sci Sports Exerc, 33*(5), 718-723.

Shah, S. H., & Newby, L. K. (2003). C-reactive protein: a novel marker of cardiovascular risk. *Cardiol Rev, 11*(4), 169-179.

Shephard, R. J. (2002). Cytokine responses to physical activity, with particular reference to IL-6: sources, actions, and clinical implications. *Crit Rev Immunol, 22*(3), 165-182.

Skinnider, B. F., & Mak, T. W. (2002). The role of cytokines in classical Hodgkin lymphoma. *Blood, 99*(12), 4283-4297.

Smets, E. M., Garssen, B., Cull, A., & de Haes, J. C. (1996). Application of the multidimensional fatigue inventory (MFI-20) in cancer patients receiving radiotherapy. *Br J Cancer, 73*(2), 241-245.

Smith, T. W., & Ruiz, J. M. (2002). Psychosocial influences on the development and course of coronary heart disease: current status and implications for research and practice. *J Consult Clin Psychol, 70*(3), 548-568.

Spath-Schwalbe, E., Hansen, K., Schmidt, F., Schrezenmeier, H., Marshall, L., Burger, K., et al. (1998). Acute effects of recombinant human interleukin-6 on endocrine and central nervous sleep functions in healthy men. *J Clin Endocrinol Metab, 83*(5), 1573-1579.

Stein, K. D., Jacobsen, P. B., Blanchard, C. M., & Thors, C. T. (2004). Further validation of the Multidimensional Fatigue Symptom Inventory-Short Form (MFSI-SF). *Journal of Pain Symptom Management, 27*(1):14-23.

Steptoe, A., Willemsen, G., Owen, N., Flower, L., & Mohamed-Ali, V. (2001). Acute mental stress elicits delayed increases in circulating inflammatory cytokine levels. *Clinical Science (London, England: 1979), 101*(2), 185-192.

Uchakin, P. N., Tobin, B., Cubbage, M., Marshall, G., Jr., & Sams, C. (2001). Immune responsiveness following academic stress in first-year medical students. *J Interferon Cytokine Res, 21*(9), 687-694.

van der Ven, A., van Diest, R., Hamulyak, K., Maes, M., Bruggeman, C., & Appels, A. (2003). Herpes viruses, cytokines, and altered hemostasis in vital exhaustion. *Psychosom Med, 65*(2), 194-200.

Vgontzas, A. N., Papanicolaou, D. A., Bixler, E. O., Hopper, K., Lotsikas, A., Lin, H. M., et al. (2000). Sleep apnea and daytime sleepiness and fatigue: relation to visceral obesity, insulin resistance, and hypercytokinemia. *J Clin Endocrinol Metab, 85*(3), 1151-1158.

Vgontzas, A. N., Papanicolaou, D. A., Bixler, E. O., Kales, A., Tyson, K., & Chrousos, G. P. (1997). Elevation of plasma cytokines in disorders of excessive daytime sleepiness: role of sleep disturbance and obesity. *J Clin Endocrinol Metab, 82*(5), 1313-1316.

Wang, H., Yu, M., Ochani, M., Amella, C. A., Tanovic, M., Susarla, S., et al. (2003). Nicotinic acetylcholine receptor alpha7 subunit is an essential regulator of inflammation. *Nature, 421*(6921), 384-388.

Wang, X., Wang, B., Duan, X., Liu, H., & Ju, G. (2000). The expression of IL-1 receptor type I in nodose ganglion and vagal paraganglion in the rat. *Chin J Neurosci, 16*, 90-93.

Watkins, L. R., Maier, S. F., & Goehler, L. E. (1995). Cytokine-to-brain communication: a review & analysis of alternative mechanisms. *Life Sci, 57*(11), 1011-1026.

Weber, C., Arck, P., Mazurek, B., & Klapp, B. F. (2002). Impact of a relaxation training on psychometric and immunologic parameters in tinnitus sufferers. *J Psychosom Res, 52*(1), 29-33.

Winningham, M. L., & MacVicar, M. G. (1988). The effect of aerobic exercise on patient reports of nausea. *Oncol Nurs Forum, 15*(4), 447-450.

Winningham, M. L., Nail, L. M., Burke, M. B., Brophy, L., Cimprich, B., Jones, L. S., et al. (1994). Fatigue and the cancer experience: the state of the knowledge. *Oncol Nurs Forum, 21*(1), 23-36.

Wirtz, P. H., von Kanel, R., Schnorpfeil, P., Ehlert, U., Frey, K., & Fischer, J. E. (2003). Reduced glucocorticoid sensitivity of monocyte interleukin-6 production in male industrial employees who are vitally exhausted. *Psychosom Med, 65*(4), 672-678.

Wood, G. J., Bughi, S., Morrison, J., Tanavoli, S., & Zadeh, H. H. (2003). Hypnosis, differential expression of cytokines by T-cell subsets, and the hypothalamo-pituitary-adrenal axis. *Am J Clin Hypn, 45*(3), 179-196.

Xinlian, L., Liquin, S., Jun, X., Shuying, Y., Chenggui, L., Qiushi, L., et al. (1993). Effect of acupuncture and point-injection treatment on immunologic function in rheumatoid arthritis. *Journal of Traditional Chinese Medicine, 13*(3), 174-178

In: Stress and Health: New Research
Editor: Kimberly V. Oxington, pp. 173-185

ISBN 1-59454-244-9
©2005 Nova Science Publishers, Inc.

Chapter VIII

EFFECT OF STRESS ON MALE AND FEMALE FERTILITY: LITERATURE REVIEW

Naomi Schneid-Kofman and Eyal Sheiner[*]

Department of Obstetrics and Gynecology, Faculty of Health Sciences, Soroka University Medical Center, Ben-Gurion University of the Negev, Beer-Sheva, Israel.

ABSTRACT

Many cultures consider reproduction to be of great importance, an obligatory achievement expected of any established couple. Infertility therefore may result in stress to a couple trying to conceive. This couple will undoubtedly experience feelings of frustration and disappointment if a pregnancy is not easily achieved. Labeled as having a fertility problem may result in a severe insult to self-esteem, body image, and self assessed masculinity or femininity. Despite the fact that various studies have demonstrated the importance of the mind-body connection and fertility, the psychosocial aspects of infertility have not been adequately addressed. The present review was aimed to determine the connection between psychological stress and both male and female infertility. Several studies addressing the psychological aspects of infertility will be discussed in this chapter, as well as evidence of infertility related to stress. More has been written regarding female stress and infertility and less was published about this evident body-mind connection regarding males. Psychological factors are risk factors of subsequent infertility among women. Moreover, the experience of the diagnosis and treatment of infertility causes subsequent psychological distress. A clear connection between stress and female infertility emerges from reading the presented research done in this field. It yet remains unclear as to what extent this connection is a predictor of failure or success, is it different among male and female individuals and what are the best intervention methods to improve fertility and psychological outcome. The knowledge existing today regarding the influence of emotional factors on male fertility is limited.

---

[*] Eyal Sheiner M.D.[1], Department of Obstetrics and Gynecology, Soroka Medical Center Ben Gurion University P.O. Box 151 Beer Sheva 84101, Israel. Phone: (972) 8 640-3524 Mob-Phone: (972) 54-874884 E-mail: sheiner@bgumail.bgu.ac.il

Psychological stress, in addition to being a result of infertility problems, may also be a cause for decreased fertility.

Further studies including intervention programs should be conducted in order to evaluate the true impact of stress upon male fertility. Meanwhile, stress parameters should be an important part of history taking and an integral parameter in regular follow up of patients diagnosed or treated for infertility.

INTRODUCTION

Many cultures consider reproduction to be of great importance, an obligatory achievement expected of any established couple. Infertility therefor may result in stress to a couple trying to conceive. This couple will undoubtedly experience feelings of frustration and disappointment if a pregnancy is not easily achieved. Labeled as having a fertility problem, the couple might experience a severe insult to self-esteem, body image, and self assessed masculinity or femininity [1,2].

Fertility treatments impose both a physical and an emotional burden on women and their partner [3]. Psychological factors such as depression, state anxiety, and stress induced changes of heart rate and blood cortisone level are predictive of a decreased probability of achieving a viable pregnancy. Hence, stress and infertility are closely related in different pathways: stress as a result of failure to reproduce, stress reducing the probability of achieving the goal of reproduction [4]. Psychological stress is connected with the measured levels of the following hormones: cortisone, prolactin, progesterone and testosterone [5].

Several studies addressing the psychological aspects of infertility will be discussed in this chapter. More has been written regarding female stress and infertility and less was published about this evident body-mind connection regarding males. Moreover, the vast majority of trials in this field regarded female subjects. Several studies have postulated a gender difference in the effect of stress upon fertility [6-8]. In some studies men were found to be less motivated than their female partners towards fertility treatments [8,9]. In one trial, fertility evaluation and treatment was regarded by female patients as the most stressful life event they have experienced more often than by male patients [10].

Further in this chapter the possible impact of job stress, as a usual cause of psychological stress, upon fertility, and the differences between male and female patients regarding the psychological effect of job parameters will be presented.

In developed nations, it is estimated that between 10-15% of couples suffer from infertility. The majority of studies have rejected the hypothesis of stress as a lone factor in the etiology of infertility. However, there is growing evidence supporting the assumption that stress stands as an additional, independent risk factor causing infertility [11]. A number of psychological factors were shown to differentiate between couples who conceive within a year and those who do not [12].

MALE STRESS AND INFERTILITY

Several studies have indicated that stress has a negative impact on sperm parameters [5,13-18]. In a study of 500 men, it was found that sperm quality was lower during their partners In Vitro Fertilization (IVF) treatment cycles than at other time [15]. Though the study did not examine stress directly, the author suggested the possibility that during psychological pressuring situations (in this case, the stress related to IVF treatments) sperm quality might be adversely affected. The first semen sample was collected in the couple's infertility work -up, and the second sample was given following ovum aspiration, in order to inseminate the eggs in vitro. Comparisons of samples revealed that sperm density, total sperm count, and both quantitative and qualitative sperm motility were found to be significantly lower in the second sample presented for IVF. For 91% of cases, there was no change across samples in assigned fertility index categories. However, 14 cases revealed quality deterioration, falling from normal to pathologic, and in 21 cases a vital change in semen characteristics from normal in IVF work -up to severely pathologic in IVF treatment, was found. For these cases, the incidence of total fertilization failure of the procedure also dramatically increased. The investigators suggested the possibility that during pressuring psychological situations, sperm quality may be adversely affected [14]. An additional study demonstrated a decline in sperm quality in 40 men, during IVF treatments, during the stage of treatment in which the embryo was transferred to their partner's uterus [15]. An apparent association between emotional stress and quality of sperm was demonstrated in 28 men followed every 2 weeks for one half of a year measuring stress parameters and sperm analysis [16]. Concurrent self-reports were obtained on abstinence, frequency of ejaculation, health behavior and status, experienced stress, social support, and life events. A single assessment of characteristic adaptability (ego resiliency) also was obtained. Significant between-subject positive correlation was reported among selected semen measures, abstinence, and ego-resiliency. Increased stress was found in an inverse relation with sperm volume and percent of normal morphological shape [16].

Occupational stress, studied in the past regarding the aspects of occupational exposure to substances or sources of energy and the impact of short and long term exposure upon fertility, has received some attention lately in the literature. The findings regarding male patients will be mentioned briefly at this stage, while other aspects will be later discussed in this chapter.

Approached in the latest researches, occupational stress is an important factor in most of our daily stress, measured by burnout and cognitive weariness was found to be associated with male infertility. Comparing men with diagnosed infertility problems with men attending an infertility clinic for their spouse's infertility problem it appears to be associated with infertility. Burnout was defined as a combination of emotional exhaustion, physical fatigue and cognitive weariness. The patients were asked to fill-out a questionnaire, after having received an explanation about the purpose of the study. The attending physician filled-out another questionnaire including detailed medical history and laboratory test results. The study population consisted of 202 consecutive male patients attending a fertility clinic. Of those 106 patients had attended the clinic due to a male infertility problem (case group), 66 patients had attended the clinic due to a female infertility problem (control group). High reliability was found, as demonstrated by Cronbac's alpha of 0.85-0.91 for the four-burnout parameters.

Male infertility was statistically related to higher marks in all measures of burnout, using the Mann-Whitney test. The largest difference was obtained in the measure of cognitive weariness (mean: 2.9 among the male infertility group vs. 2.1 in the control group, p<0.05). In a multiple logistic regression analysis, cognitive weariness (OR=1.8, 95% CI 1.03-4.6) was found to be an independent risk factor in male infertility problems [18].

A male partner's decreased mood and low self-esteem was found to influence pregnancy outcome in a prospective study [13].

In a recent study the results challenge some of the data presented. Investigating 430 Danish couples who were trying to conceive for the first time, no correlation was found between stress (assessed by a questionnaire) and semen quality, and no correlation between stress and levels of luteinizing hormone (LH), follicle-stimulating hormone (FSH), Inhibin, Testosterone or estradiol was found. In this study, a pregnancy rate of 14% was found within the group of couples with the highest stress scores, and a pregnancy rate of 18% in the group with the lowest stress scores. Odds of pregnancy decreased moderately with increasing score. The effect was confined to 77 men with a sperm density below 20 million/ml (adjusted odds ratio = 0.06; 95% confidence interval = 1.01-0.58 for highest distressed quartile vs. lowest distressed quartile in this low sperm density group). High absolute stress scores were associated with a lower frequency of sexual intercourse [19]. According to within-subject analyses, cycle-specific changes in male stress did not alter the odds of pregnancy. The authors concluded that the effect of a man's daily life psychological stress on his semen quality is small.

In another recent study published, among 399 Danish couples who were trying to become pregnant for the first time, odds for pregnancy were not associated with job strain. These patients were observed for up to 6 menstrual periods. Job demand and job control were measured by a self-administered questionnaire at entry, and in each cycle the participants recorded changes in job control or job demand during the preceding 30 days. In this study a probable effect of stress upon fecundity was suggested in the sub-group of couples with sperm analysis with a low sperm concentration [20].

In summary, the knowledge existing today regarding the influence of emotional factors on male fertility is limited. Psychological stress, in addition to being a result of infertility problems, can also be a cause for decreased fertility, perhaps by altering sperm quality. Further studies including intervention programs should be conducted in order to evaluate the true impact of stress upon male fertility.

FEMALE STRESS AND INFERTILITY

From investigating the relationship between stress and infertility, emerge various possible forms of association between these topics. Indeed, different explanations as to the nature of the connection between psychological factors and infertility were published [21]. These include on one hand, a hypothesis that psychological factors are risk factors of subsequent infertility, and on the other hand, the contrasting hypothesis that the experience of the diagnosis and treatment of infertility causes psychological distress [1,22].

Psychological Factors are Risk Factors of Subsequent Infertility

Supporting data of the first hypothesis that psychological factors are predictors of infertility emerges from the studies that demonstrate the correlation between childhood sexual abuse, adult sexual abuse, domestic violence and a higher prevalence of gynecological problems and chronic pelvic pain in women [23-26].

Women who have suffered of depression in the past were more likely to report infertility than women with no such history [27] were. Furthermore, among couples seeking treatment for infertility, those with higher positive expectations related to motherhood, and men whose wishes for a child was integrated with their sexual relations were significantly more fertile than couples with no such beliefs [11].

In a prospective study that examined healthy women who became pregnant for the first time, without a history of infertility, the following psychosocial and behavioral factors predicted greater than average fertility rates. Low scores of psychosomatic symptoms, few negative life events, low consumption of coffee (less than 5 cups a day), having phobic traits, no fluctuations in body weight prior to pregnancy, and having regular religious practice. One more predictor was looking younger than one's actual age (evaluated in 7% of women by a psychiatrist) which probably reflected a combination of biological vitality and transmission of youthful positive affect [28].

In a methodologically unique study, 13 healthy women from the community were asked to keep diaries concerning mood during months in which they were trying to conceive. During months in which women did conceive, they reported more favorable mood states and being less "hassled" than during months of efforts that did not result in conception. Interestingly, frequency of coital activity did not increase during months of conception when mood was better suggesting that the elevated mood itself may have exerted its influence on fertility via other psycho-physiological pathways. In contrast to these findings, by using standard self-report measures, no relation was found between conception and various urinary measures including adrenaline, nor-adrenaline and cortisone [29] which are hormones of a known relation to psychological states. A possible restriction to the value of this conclusion is that these biological measures were only taken twice during a monthly cycle, and thus may have missed cyclical fluctuations of stress hormones that may predict conception.

An additional study found that high levels of distress were significant predictors of lower odds of conception per cycle, especially among women with long (> 35 days) menstrual cycles [30].

One other study deserves mention because it ties physiological stress indicators to fertility outcomes. Facchinetti and colleagues found that high stress responses detected in an experimental trial to a strop-task (a cognitive stress test of the ability to disregard irrelevant stimuli) using blood pressure and heart rate responses predicted outcomes from IVF treatments [31]. Women with lower systolic blood pressures and heart rate responses were more likely to become pregnant from the IVF treatment, indicating a cardiovascular stress response that interacts with fertility.

The existing literature includes studies of variable methodological strengths, and based on the prospective studies, there is some evidence to suggest that certain psychological variables predict fertility or infertility.

The Experience of the Diagnosis and Treatment of Infertility Causes Psychological Distress

Some studies support the second hypothesis mentioned above, of psychological effects as a consequence of infertility problems.

Many couples feel that fertility treatment is a serious psychological strain and that the health care systems do little to ease this psychological burden [32]. One study found that approximately half of the women undergoing fertility treatment rate the problem of infertility as the most stressful experience of their life. This severe rating was not as striking in the male partners, and consisted of 15% of men undergoing the same treatment [9].

A comparative international survey conducted among women awaiting IVF treatment demonstrated that these women had four times the level of depressive symptoms than a control group of women without fertility problems. Furthermore, their scores on self-assessed attractiveness, anxiety, memory or concentration were also less favorable than those of the control group [33]. Another study reported that infertile women had depression levels twice as high when compared with a group of control women. Furthermore, women with a 2 to 3 year history of infertility had the highest levels of depression compared to those experiencing problems either less than one year or more than six years [34]. This U-shape pattern implies that initially, women's hope for positive results may protect them from depressive symptoms, and that prolonged experience with infertility and fertility-treatments may then increase depressive symptoms among women who experience treatment failure. Although, six years of such experience derives an acceptance of the situation, which seems to have a protective affect against depressive symptoms.

One methodologically unique study examined the psychological sequel of infertility and treatment failure among Chinese women in Hong Kong. The prevalence of distress (assessed by the General Health Questionnaire) increased from 33% to 43% after treatment failure while prevalence of depression remained constant (8%). Finally, the severity of depression following treatment failure was predicted by duration of infertility [35]. This dose-response relation between duration of infertility and depression is in contrast to the U-shape relation presented previously [34]. The different results may result from use of different instruments to assess depression or perhaps from cultural difference.

The levels of anxiety and depression observed among infertile women are comparable to women with cancer, or with Congestive heart disease, but are lower than the levels of anxiety and depression among women with chronic pain syndromes or Human immunodeficiency virus (HIV) [36]. In one study, self-blame and an avoidance coping were the best predictors of psychological distress in infertile men and women. Furthermore, in men, older age and conceiving for the first time were also predictors of distress [37].

Last, studies supporting the reciprocal relations between psychological distress and infertility.

A MUTUAL ASSOCIATION BETWEEN STRESS AND INFERTILITY

Most often it is not clear what comes first- the infertility or the stress, as the chicken or the egg dilemma. In order to examine a reciprocal relation between psychological factors and the consequences of fertility treatments, more studies investigating this issue included patients who proceeded to IVF. A significant difference between the level of depressive symptoms observed among women entering IVF for the first treatment and women who have already treated by repeated cycles was reported [38]. Clinically elevated depression scores were highest among repeaters (25%), high among first time patients (15%) and both groups were higher than the rate of depression in the community (12%) [39]. Furthermore, among the first cycle women, those with symptoms of depression were less likely to achieve a pregnancy than non-depressed women were. This study clearly demonstrates the reciprocal relation between depression and IVF outcome and its subsequent psychological effects.

Following failure of an IVF treatment, a substantial increase was found in the prevalence of mild to moderate levels of depression reported in women [22]. Predisposition toward anxiety, pre-IVF levels of depression and the attempt to conceive for the first time, predicted adverse psychological reactions to IVF-failure.

JOB PARAMETERS, PSYCHOLOGICAL STRESS AND RESULTING INFERTILITY

The possible relationship between job induced psychological stress and infertility was lately discussed in the literature, one drawback in such research is the difficulty to differentiate between sources of emotional stress at work and outside work [21]. This approach to stress through occupation psychological stress was associated with a poor outcome of IVF and an embryo transfer fertility treatment [18].

In a prospective cohort study, including 75 couples admitted for a female infertility problem, a correlation was found between infertile women conceiving after treatment and job characteristics of a less mentally stressful job, and less simultaneous obligatory tasks at work. Women who conceived held less mentally stressful jobs (stress scores ± S.D. 1.00±0.70 (n=33) vs. 1.40±0170 (n=41), respectively; p<0.025). In this sub-group of working women, delivery rates were higher (1.00±0.75 (n=20) vs. 1.40±0.70 (n=52); p<0.042). A non-significant statistical tendency towards a higher pregnancy rate in women who had more freedom to determine their personal schedule during working hours was noted (Odds ratio = 2.4, 95% confidence interval 0.7-8.3, p=0.110). In this study no significant association was found between job strain and job satisfaction and women's fertility outcomes [40]. The authors concluded that during an 18- month follow up, an inverse ratio between a more demanding and mentally stressful job and the success of fertility treatments exists.

Interestingly, another study has not found a relation between job-strain (many work demands and little job control) and pregnancy in a prospective study of 6 cycles among Danish women. However, when restricting the sample to those with idiopathic infertility, job-strain did emerge as a predictor of unsuccessful pregnancy [38].

In another study comparing 64 working women with infertility problems with 106 working women whose husbands were infertile, the level of occupational stress was assessed by measurements of job strain, job satisfaction and burnout. (8 parameters investigating physical fatigue and emotional exhaustion). The infertile women were older, worked more hours per week and participated in more sports activities and reported lower levels of burnout on one sub-scale (listlessness) than women with an infertile husband [21]. It is interesting to note that infertility due to a male problem was related to higher burnout scores as compared to patients admitted due to their partner's reproductive impairment.

The opposite was found in another study [21], as was demonstrated by the trend of female patients towards lower burnout scores. A possible explanation might be that under nearly any condition it is considered to be sterility of the couple, and the burden of being sterile mainly lays upon the female, regardless of the reason of sterility [18]. One study postulated that in men occupational stress was an etiological factor whereas in female patients it might be a consequence of the fertility status [7].

It is yet unclear whether there is an impact of sport activity and prolonged working hours upon female infertility and if it is the cause or the result [41]. It is to say that women who feel "guilty" in the infertility status may tend to search for some type of personal compensation such as over-involvement in physical and working activities. It may be suggested that the social responsibility for the conception and care rests much more upon the shoulders of women than men, and hence it is possible that as a defense mechanism they tend to participate in more job events and sport activities.

On the other hand, it is possible that the career choice of these women is conducive to an intense working schedule, which brought them to try to conceive at a more advanced age and thus to the acknowledgment of their infertility later in life [41-44]. Within the past few decades a new and far reaching phenomenon has been observed in which an increasing number of women begin a realization of the family - unit relatively late in their reproductive lives. Today this delay in childbearing is socially accepted and relates primarily to increased opportunities for education, career choices and effective birth control means [9,41-43]. Importantly, advanced age is a well-known risk factor for infertility [43-44]. Moreover, the success rates of elderly women in programs of assisted reproductive techniques are relatively lower in comparison to younger women [44].

INTERVENTION STUDIES

Several studies have examined the effects of psychological interventions on a number of outcome measures in infertile women and couples. While they demonstrate positive potential in relation to psychological outcomes, many of these studies do not report findings in relation to achievement of pregnancy [45-46].

A group who compared personality factors among couples who have conceived after IVF treatment and the couples who have conceived naturally, have found different emotional responses and further suggested that IVF couples might need emotional support in early pregnancy [47]. Likewise another author recommended that psychological services should be available for patients whose infertility causes them much strain [48].

Concluding from the data presented above, it seems requisitioned that psychological intervention be a part of fertility treatment. Investigating the benefits of such intervention, Domar and her colleagues have worked with groups of infertile women and found that a cognitive behavioral treatment mode reduced psychological distress and resulted in greater numbers of viable pregnancies than usual care [49]. Statistical significance of the pregnancy rate was problematic owing to the much higher number of dropouts in the control group [50]. However, Domar's work excluded women with clinical levels of depression and there were high rates of demoralized dropouts in the control condition. It seems important to include depressed women in intervention studies given the high prevalence of depression among infertile women. It was concluded that it is important to offer psychological interventions at an earlier point of fertility treatment in conjunction with initiation of medical treatment [51].

In a preliminary randomized-controlled study, Sarrel et al. [52] provided 10 infertile couples with a psychotherapeutic interview and additional 10 women were provided with usual care. They found a 60% pregnancy rate in the interviewed group compared to a 10% rate in the controls. A 24 week program on coping with infertility and developing healthy eating patterns designed for obese, infertile women (mean initial weight 98 kilograms) was successful in helping them both to lose weight, improve self esteem and reduce anxiety and depression [53]. Over 80% of group participants became pregnant.

In another study, 17 infertile couples underwent cognitive-behavioral therapy (CBT) which included reducing helpless thoughts, increasing marital communication and expressing fears concerning with performance and outcome. Compared to pregnancy rates found in other studies with various forms of idiopathic infertility (7.2-14.3%), one third of the CBT group became pregnant [54]. However, neither a control group, nor randomization was included in this study, making it difficult to interpret its findings. Nevertheless, significant reductions in helplessness, ruminative thoughts about infertility and marital distress were reported.

Kupka et al [55] have evaluated characteristics of couples with spontaneous conceptions following non-successful treatment with assisted reproductive technologies. Data from 254 couples who underwent 1127 therapy cycles between were analyzed. Spontaneous pregnancies occurred in 14% of all treated couples. Psychological counseling was performed in only 21%, but was observed more frequently among patients without later spontaneous conception. The authors concluded that the positive input of psychological counseling for stress relief during infertility treatments should be noted, although a statistical significant impact could not be demonstrated in their study [55].

Finally, a recent randomized-controlled trial among infertile women demonstrated that five weekly 90-minute sessions of CBT (relaxation, guided imagery and stress management) resulted in a significant reduction in emotional distress and natural-killer cell activity (47.7% to 34.1%). Further, increased pregnancy rates (37.8% versus 13.5%) were noted in the CBT group compared to the control group [56].

In summary, a clear relationship between stress and female-infertility emerges from reading the presented research done in this field. It yet remains unclear as to what extent this connection is a predictor of failure or success, is it different among male and female individuals and what are the best intervention methods to improve fertility and psychological outcome.

REFERENCES

[1] Cwikel, J; Gidron, Y; Sheiner, E. Psychological interactions with infertility among women: a review. *Europ J Obstet Gynecol Reprod Biol* 2004, (in press).

[2] Sheiner, EK; Sheiner, E; Hammel, RD; Potashnik, G; Carel, R. Effect of occupational exposures on male fertility: literature review. *Ind Health*, 2003. 41, 55-62

[3] Greil, AL. Infertility and psychological distress: a critical review of the literature. *Soc Sci Med.* 1977. 45, 1679-704

[4] Csemiczky, G; Landgerm, BM; Collins, A. The influence of stress and state anxiety on the outcome of IVF treatment, psychological and endocrinological assessment of Swedish women entering IVF treatment. *Acta Obstet Gynecol Scand.* 2000. 79, 113-118

[5] Bonde, JP. Semen quality and sex hormones among mild steel and stainless steel welders: a cross sectional study. *Br J Ind Med.* 1990. 47, 508-14.

[6] Wright, J; Duchesne, C; Sabourin, S; Bissonnette, F; Benoit, J; Girard, Y. Psychosocial distress and infertility, men and women respond differently. *Fertil Steril,* 1991. 55,100-8.

[7] Stoleru, S; Teglas, JP; Spira, A; Magnin, F; Fermanian, J. Psychological characteristics of infertile patients, discriminating etiological factors from reactive changes. *J Psychosom Obstet Gynaecol*, 1996. 17,103-18.

[8] Jordan, C; Revenson, TA. Gender differences in coping with infertility, a meta-analysis. *J Behav Med.* 1999. 22, 341-358.

[9] Fonteyn, VJ; Isada, NB. Nongenetic implications of childbearing after age thirty-five. *Obstet Gynecol Survey.* 1988. 43, 709-20.

[10] Freeman, EW; Boxer, AS; Rickels, K; Tureck, R; Mastoinni, L. Psychological evaluation and support in a program of in vitro fertilization and embryo transfer. *Fertil Steril.* 1985. 43, 48-53.

[11] Stoleru, S; Teglas, JP; Fermanian, J; Spira, A. Psychological factors in the aetiology of infertility: a prospective cohort study. *Hum Reprod.* 1993. 8, 1039-46.

[12] Viau, V. Functional cross-talk between the hypothalamic-pituitary-gonadal and -adrenal axes. *J Neuroendocrinol.* 2002. 14, 506-13.

[13] Slade, P; Raval, H; Buck, P; Lieberman, BE. A 3-year follow-up of emotional, marital and sexual functioning in couples who were infertile. *J Reprod Inf Psychol.* 1992. 10, 233-43.

[14] Harrison, KL; Callan, VJ; Hennessey, JF. Stress and semen quality in an in-virto fertilization program. *Fertil Steril.* 1987. 48, 633-6.

[15] Clarke, RN; Klock, SC; Geoghegan, A; Travassos, DE. Relationship between psychological stress and semen quality among in-vitro fertilization patients. *Hum Reprop.* 1999. 14, 753-8.

[16] Gilbin, PT; Poland, ML; Moghissi, KS; Ager, JW; Olson, JM. Effects of stress and characteristic adaptability on semen quality in healthy men. *Fertil Steril.* 1988. 49, 127-32.

[17] Clarke, RN; Klock, SC; Geoghegan, A; Travassos, DE. Relationship between psychological stress and semen quality among in- vitro fertilization patients. *Hum Reprod.* 1999. 14, 733-8.

[18] Sheiner, EK; Sheiner, E; Carel, R; Potashnik, G; Shoham-Vardi, I. The potential association between male infertility and occupational psychological stress. *J Occup Envir Med.* 2002. 44, 1093-9.

[19] Hjollund, NH; Bonde, JP; Henriksen, TB; Giwercman, A; Olsen J. The Danish first pregnancy planner study team. Reproductive effects of male psychological stress. *Epidemiology.* 2004. 15(1), 21-7.

[20] Hjollund, NH; Bonde, JP; Henriksen, TB; Giwercman, A; Olsen J. The Danish first pregnancy planner study team. Job strain and male infertility. *Epidemiology.* 2004. 15(1), 114-7

[21] Sheiner, E; Sheiner, EK; Potashnik, G; Carel, R; Shoham- Vardi, I. The relationship between occupational psychological stress and female infertility. *Occup Med* (Lond). 2003. 53, 265-269.

[22] Newton, CR; Sherrard, W; Glavac, I. The Fertility Problem Inventory, measuring perceived infertility-related stress. *Fert Steril.* 1999, 72:54-62.

[23] Wright, J; Allard, M; Lecours, A; Sabourin, S. Psychosocial distress and infertility, a review of controlled research. *Int J Fertil.* 1989. 34, 126-142.

[24] Plichta, SB. Violence and abuse, implications for women's health. In *Women's Health, The Commonwealth Fund Survey*, ed. M.M. Falik & K.S. Collins, Baltimore, MD, Johns Hopkins Univ. Press. 1996. p. 237-270.

[25] Harrop-Griffiths, J; Katon, W; Walker, E; Holm, L; Russo, J; Hickok, L. The association between chronic pelvic pain, psychiatric diagnoses, and childhood sexual abuse. *Obstet Gynecol.* 1988. 71, 589-594.

[26] Walker, EA; Katon, WJ; Hansom, J; Harrop-Griffiths, J; Holm, L; Jones, ML; Hickok, LR; Russo J. Psychiatric diagnoses and sexual victimization in women with chronic pelvic pain. *Psychosomatics.* 1995. 36, 531-540.

[27] Lapane, LK; Zierler, S; Lasatar, TM; Stein, M; Barbout, MM; Hume, AL. Is a history of depressive symptoms associated with an increased risk of infertility in women? *Psychosom Med.* 1995. 57, 509-513.

[28] Vartiainen, H; Saarikoski, S; Halonen, P; Rimon, R. Psychosocial factors, female fertility and pregnancy, a prospective study – Part I, Fertility. *J Psychosom Obstet Gynaecol.* 1994. 15, 67-75.

[29] Sanders, KA;. Bruce, NW. Psychosocial stress and treatment outcome following assisted reproductive technology. *Hum Reprod.* 1999. 14, 1656-1662.

[30] Hjollund, NH; Jensen, TK; Bonde, JP; Henriksen, TB; Andersson, AM; Kolstad, HA; Ernst, E; Giwercman, A; Skakkebaek, NE; Olsen, J. Distress and reduced fertility, A follow-up of first pregnancy planners. *Fertil Steril.* 1999. 72, 47-53.

[31] Facchinetti, F; Matteo, ML; Artini, GP; Volpe, A; Genazzani, AR. An increased vulnerability to stress is associated with a poor outcome of in vitro fertilization-embryo transfer treatment. *Fertil Steril.* 1997. 67, 309-14.

[32] Schmidt, Lp. Infertile couples' assessment of infertility treatments. *Acta Obstet Gynecol Scand.* 1998. 77, 649-653.

[33] Oddens, BJ; den Tonkelaar, I; Nieuwenhuyse, H. Psychosocial experience in women facing fertility problems – a comparative survey. *Hum Reprod.* 1999. 14, 255-261.

[34] Domar, AD; Broome, A; Zuttenmeister, PC; Seibel, M; Friedman, R. The prevalence and predictability of depression in infertile women. *Fertil Steril.* 1992. 58, 1158-1163.

[35] Lok, IH; Lee, DT; Cheung, WS; Lo, WK; Haines, CJ. Psychiatric morbidity amongst infertile Chinese women undergoing treatment with assisted reproductive technology and the impact of treatment failure. *Gynecol Obstet Invest.* 2002. 53, 195-9.

[36] Domar, AD; Zuttermeister, PC; Friedman, R. The psychological impact of infertility, a comparison with patients with other medical conditions. *J Psychosom Obstet Gynaecol.* 1993.14 (suppl), 45-52.

[37] Morrow, KA; Thoreson, RW; Penney, LL. Predictors of psychological distress among infertility clinic patients. *J Consult Clin Psychol.* 1995. 63, 163-167.

[38] Hjollund, NH; Kold-Jensen, T; Bonde, JP; Henriksen, TB; Kolstad, HA; Andersson, AM; Ernst, E; Giwercman, A; Skakkebaek, NE; Olsen, J. Job strain and time to pregnancy. *Scand J Work Environ Health.* 1998. 24, 344-50.

[39] Thiering, P; Beaurepaire, J; Jones, M; Saunders, D; Tennant, C. Mood state as a predictor of treatment outcome after in vitro fertilization/embryo transfer technology (IVF/ET). *J Psychosom Res.* 1993 . 37, 481-491.

[40] Barzilay-Pesach, V; Sheiner, EK; Sheiner, E; Potashnil, G; Shoham-Vardi, I. Women's occupational psychological stress affects the outcome of fertility treatments. Presented at the *Second Congress of Women's Mental Health*, Beer-Sheva, Israel, October, 2003.

[41] Stein, ZA. A woman's age: childbearing and child rearing. *Am J Epidemiol.* 1985. 121, 327-42.

[42] Sheiner, E; Shoham-Vardi, I; Hershkovitz, R; Katz, M; Mazor, M. Infertility treatment is an independent risk factor for cesarean section among nulliparous women aged 40 and above. *Am J Obstet Gynecol.* 2001. 185, 888-92.

[43] Speroff, L; Glass, RH; Kase, NG. *Clinical gynecologic endocrinology and infertility.* Sixth ed. Lippincott Williams and Wilkins. 1999. 1013-42.

[44] Meldrum, DR. Female reproductive aging-ovarian and uterine factors. *Fertil Steril.* 1993. 59,1-5.

[45] Stewart, DE; Boydell, KM; McCarthy, K; Swedlyk S; Redmond, C; Cohrs, W. A prospective study of brief professionally led support groups for infertility patients. *Int J Psychiatry Med.* 1992. 22, 173-182.

[46] McNaughton-Cassill, ME; Bostwick, JM; Vanscoy, SE; Arthur, NJ; Hickman, TN; Robinson, RD; Neal, GS; Bostwick, M. Development of brief stress management support groups for couples undergoing in vitro fertilization treatment. *Fertil Steril.* 2000. 74, 87-93.

[47] Hjelmstedt, A; Widstrom, AM; Wramsby, H; Matthiesen, AS; Collins, A. Personality factors and emotional responses to pregnancy among IVF couples in early pregnancy: a comparative study. *Acta Obstet Gynecol Scand.* 2003. 82, 152-61.

[48] Schmidt, L; Holstein, BE; Boivin, J; Sangren, H; Tjornhoj-Thomsen, T; Blaabjerg J; Hald F; Andersen AN; Rasmussen, PE. Patients' attitudes to medical and psychosocial aspects of care in fertility clinics: findings from the Copenhagen Multi-center Psychosocial Infertility (COMPI) Research Program. *Hum Reprod.* 2003. 18, 628-37.

[49] Domar, AD; Seibel, MM; Benson, H. The mind/body program for infertility, A new behavioral treatment approach for women with infertility. *Fertil Steril.* 1990. 53, 246-249.

[50] Domar, AD; Clapp, D; Slawsby, EA; Kessel, B; Orav, J; Freizinger, M. The impact of group psychological interventions on distress in infertile women. *Health Psychol.* 2000. 19, 568-575.

[51] Domar, AD; Clapp, D; Slawsby, EA; Dusek, J; Kessel, B; Freizinger, M. Impact of group psychological interventions on pregnancy rates in infertile women. *Fertil Steril.* 2000. 73, 805-811.

[52] Sarell, PM; DeCherney, AH. Psychotherapeutic intervention for treatment of couples with secondary infertility. *Fertil Steril.* 1985. 43, 897-900.

[53] Galletly, C; Clark, A; Tomlinson, L; Blaney, F. Improved pregnancy rates for obese, infertile women following a group treatment program. An open pilot study. *Gen Hosp Psychiatry.* 1996. 18, 192-195.

[54] Tuschen- Caffier, B; Florin, I; Krause, W; Pook, M. Cognitive-behavioral therapy for idiopathic infertile couples. *Psychother Psychosom.* 1999. 68, 15-21.

[55] Kupka, MS; Dorn, C; Richter, O; Schmutzler, A; Van der ven, H; Kuczycki, A. Stress relief after infertility treatment – spontaneous conception, adoption and psychological counseling. *Eur J Obstet Gynecol Reprod Biol.* 2003. 110, 190-5.

[56] Hosaka, T; Matsubayashi, H; Sugiyama, Y; Izumi, S; Makito, T. Effect of psychiatric group intervention on natural- killer cell activity and pregnancy rate. *Gen Hosp Psychiatry.* 2002. 24, 353-6.

In: Stress and Health: New Research
Editor: Kimberly V. Oxington, pp. 187-201
ISBN 1-59454-244-9
©2005 Nova Science Publishers, Inc.

Chapter IX

BRIEF COGNITIVE-BEHAVIORAL COUPLES SUPPORT GROUPS DEVELOPED TO MANAGE THE STRESS OF IVF TREATMENT

Mary Ellen McNaughton-Cassill[*]

University of Texas at San Antonio Division of Behavioral and Cultural Sciences 6900 N. Loop 1604 West San Antonio, Texas, 78249

John Michael Bostwick

Mayo Clinic 200 First Street Southwest Rochester, Minnesota 55905

Nancy J. Arthur and Randal D. Robinson

Wilford Hall Medical Center 59th Medical Wing Department of OB/GYN (MMNO) 2200 Berquist Drive, Suite 1 San Antonio, Texas 78236-5300

Gregory S. Neal

Fertility Center of San Antonio 4499 Medical Drive, Suite 200 San Antonio, TX 78229

ABSTRACT

Couples who have difficulty conceiving a child frequently seek extensive, costly medical solutions to their infertility. Such treatments often involve the use of medication, surgery, and other high technology interventions and can involve the sharing of intimate personal details of one's sexual activities with medical personnel. Psychologically, infertility can be associated with the experience of stress, anxiety, and depression, and may result in relationship difficulties, and even divorce. This article describes the development and evaluation of a brief, Cognitive-behavioral group therapy approach offered to both members of a couple while they were undergoing in vitro fertilization. Couples were recruited from an infertility center at a military hospital and either volunteered to participate in the groups and complete two sets of surveys, or to serve as controls by

---

[*] Mary Ellen McNaughton-Cassill 210-458-4353 phone 210-458-4347 fax mmcnaughton-cassill@utsa.edu

completing the two surveys but not attending the group sessions. Group facilitators used Cognitive-behavioral techniques to help participants process their feelings and cognitions about their infertility. Emotional and cognitive factors were assessed both before and after group attendance. Women who attended the groups were significantly less depressed and anxious after the IVF treatment than they were before the cycle. Men who attended the group were more optimistic than non-group males or the females at the completion of the IVF cycle, but endorsed greater numbers of irrational beliefs. These results suggest couples can benefit psychologically from participating in an IVF specific couples therapy group.

EPIDEMIOLOGY, ETIOLOGY OF INFERTILITY

Infertility is typically defined as the inability to conceive a child after actively trying to do so for at least one year. It has been estimated that infertility affects 10-15% of couples of childbearing age in the United States (Speroff, Glass, & Kase, 1999; McQuillan, Greil, White, & Jacob, 2003). This complex disorder can be attributed to a number of causes including delayed marriage and childbearing, the increasing incidence of sexually transmitted diseases, and possibly smoking and alcohol use (Rosenthal & Goldfarb, 1997). Among women, disorders involving the fallopian tubes, disruptions in ovulation, damage to the ovaries, poor cervical mucous production and endometriosis have also been implicated as causes of infertility. Disorders of the hypothalamus and the pituitary may also disrupt fertility (Reed, 2001). Male factor infertility accounts for 40-50% of infertility and may be due to impotence, ejaculatory failure, the disruption of pituitary hormone production, or testicular dysfunction (Sultan, Grifo, & Rosenwaks, 1995).

MEDICAL APPROACHES TO INFERTILITY

Although advances in medical treatment for infertility have greatly increased the number of options available to infertile couples, the process of seeking, receiving and financing medical treatment is still quite stressful (McNaughton-Cassill, Bostwick, Arthur, Robinson, & Neal, 2002). The diagnosis and initial treatment of infertility may include planning intercourse according to basal body temperature, undergoing postcoital examinations of cervical mucus, and collecting semen specimens by masturbation. Couples often report both anxiety and embarrassment when undergoing such procedures Treatments may also require the ingestion or injections of medications, which can have significant side effects (Reed, 2001). One or both members of the couple may also require surgical procedures, which although generally safe, can lead to health complications as well as stress, and depression (Gerrity, 2001; Lalos, Lalos, Jacobsson, & vonShoultz, 1985). In addition, pursuing medical approaches to infertility often requires travel, time off from work, and can generate extensive financial debt as treatments are not always covered by insurance.

When initial treatments for infertility are unsuccessful couples may elect to try advanced reproductive technologies such as in vitro fertilization (IVF). IVF is a complex and invasive process which involves hormonal manipulation consisting of the use of injectable fertility drugs to stimulate the development of multiple oocytes, oocyte retrieval, fertilization of gametes, and embryo transfer (Reed, 2001). Such procedures are costly (Collins, Bustillo, Visscher, & Lawrence, 1995), may only be partially covered by insurance, and have success rates ranging from 20-40% (Reed, 2001). Consequently, couples may be forced to seek treatment over extended periods of time, potentially experiencing repeated cycles of hope and failure (Daniluk, 2001). The use of high technology treatments can also engender practical and ethical concerns including: the dispensation of eggs or embryos not used in procedures, the use of donor sperm and/or eggs, debate about whether to use donor sperm, donor eggs or the use of a surrogate, and questions about the impact of the use of these procedures on families (Greenfield, 1997). Arthur Greil (1991) suggests that the medicalization of infertility treatment can result in couples engaging in successively painful and costly infertility treatments, often with little understanding or formal consideration of the medical and psychological impacts of such approaches.

PSYCHOLOGICAL APPROACHES TO INFERTILITY

In addition to generating numerous medical concerns, infertility has also been strongly related to psychological distress (Downey 1993; McQuillan, Greil, White, & Jacob, 2003). Infertility is often considered a life crisis (Berk & Shapiro, 1984), and has been shown to be a cross cultural crisis (Burns, 1993). Members of infertile couples often experience depression, anxiety, isolation, anger, guilt, and shame (Golombok, 1992; Domar, Broome, Zuttermeister, Seibel, & Friedman, 1992). Such stress may persist for years, and be exacerbated each time a treatment or procedure is unsuccessful (Domar et al. 1992). Marital distress is also a common sequelae of infertility, and can even result in divorce (Raval, Slade, Buck, & Lieberman, 1987; Hirsch & Hirsch, 1995). Causes of marital dissatisfaction can include the impact of infertility concerns and treatment on sexual functioning (Black & Greenfield, 1993). Differences in emotional distress and coping styles may also contribute to communication problems within the couple (Burns & Covington, 1999; Meyers, Weinshel, Scharf, Kezur, Diamond, & Rait,1995; Hsu & Kuo, 2002). For men acceptance of a childless lifestyle results in increased marital adjustment, but for women the stress of infertility influences their perception of the marriage, and may diminish marital adjustment as the course of treatment for infertility lengthens (Ulbrich, Coyle, & Llabre, 1990). When the members of a couple perceive equal levels of infertility related stress they may exhibit better marital adjustment than couples who differ in their perception of the stress caused by their infertility (Peterson, Newton, & Rosen, 2003).

Given the rising number of couples dealing with infertility, and the increasing complexity of available medical treatments, some investigators have begun to suggest that infertility treatment programs should include a psychological treatment component (Connolly et al. 1993). Such treatment may take the form of individual therapy addressing the relationship between infertility and grief work (Daniels, 1993), long-term adjustment to infertility, and acute reactions to failed treatment procedures (Connolly, Edelman, Cooke, & Robson, 1992). Couples approaches may address communications issues, marital adjustment, and sexual satisfaction. Domar and colleagues (Domar et al., 2000) used a relatively long-term (6-12 month) group format and reported psychological benefits to female participants.

Stewart et al., (1992) also offered 8 week support groups for individual patients entering an infertility program. Few studies however, have emphasized the provision of group therapy for both members of the couple while they are actually undergoing infertility procedures (Connolly et al. 1993; Daniels, 1993).

The lack of research on the utility of group formats in working with couples undergoing infertility treatment is surprising given the mounting evidence that acute psychological treatment benefits people undergoing other complex medical treatments (Redd et al. 1991). For example, group therapy for women undergoing somatic treatments for breast cancer has been shown to enhance survival rates, presumably by helping patients cope with the stress of their illness (Spiegel et al. 1989). Although infertility is not typically life threatening, it is clearly stressful, has a negative impact on the psychological well-being of the individuals involved, and may undermine the strength of their relationship (Pengelly, Inglis, & Cudmore, 1995). This suggests that the psychological benefit of helping patients to understand and cope with their medical procedures, and to manage cognitive and emotional responses to their difficulties conceiving a child, should be considered in any approach to the treatment of infertility (Greenfeld, 1997). Consequently, we decided to develop a couples support group specifically for people undergoing IVF treatment, and to formally evaluate the efficacy of the groups (McNaughton-Cassill, Bostwick, Arthur, Robinson, & Neal, 2002).

DEVELOPMENT OF A BRIEF COUPLES SUPPORT GROUP

Wilford Hall Medical Center (WHMC) in San Antonio, Texas is a United States Air Force Medical Center. The infertility treatment program at WHMC provides services to members of all five military branches throughout the United States. In order to participate in the program patients must be 40 years old or younger, be married, and have undergone fewer than 4 lifetime IVF cycles. Couples accepted into the program are typically on a waiting list for about a year, which can be a source of stress since people who are stationed or transferred overseas are specifically excluded from IVF treatment in the program. This program is partially covered as a military benefit, therefore a typical treatment cycle costs approximately one-third as much as comparable services in the civilian sector. As a result, the treatment population is probably more diverse than that of typical IVF clinics where self-selection occurs based on socioeconomic status.

The program requires women to spend 2-3 weeks in the San Antonio area for the stimulation phase of the IVF cycle as well as the oocyte retrieval and embryo transfer procedures. In some cases, both the husband and wife are present for the entire cycle, while in other cases the woman arrives first, and her husband joins her later. Still others choose to commute various distances, some up to 6 hours, to keep appointments while continuing to reside at home.

IVF procedures at WHMC are only offered to 100 couples a year, in four one-month long cycles. This structure makes it possible to avoid some of the logistic difficulties often experienced when forming couples groups because we were able to recruit enough couples per cycle to form viable groups. This scheduling format allowed us to develop a brief couples support group model that coincided with treatment, while generating a large enough sample size per cycle to form viable groups. The sessions were offered twice a week, in the morning, in order to insure all patients had the opportunity of attending the groups throughout their treatment period. However, because women were required to remain in or near San Antonio for the cycle and men were not, more women actually participated in the groups.

Participants

Couples were recruited by the nurse coordinating their IVF treatment. The test group consisting of at least one member of 26 couples (26 females and 17 males) undergoing treatment participated in the group version and completed two surveys during the study period. The control group consisted of at least one member of 19 other couples (19 females and 18 males) undergoing IVF treatment who did not participate in group sessions, but did complete two surveys. While both of the groups received routine support from their physicians and nurses, no other specific psychological support was provided to either group.

The average age of women in the program was 34 years old, with a range of 25-40 years. The average age of men was 35.78 with a range of 27 to 42 years old. None of the subjects exhibited significant clinical levels of depression or anxiety upon entry to the study, and therefore we did not choose to exclude any willing participants. However, there was no penalty for subjects who chose not to participate.

Although this pool of 45 couples is comparable in number to those reported in the literature, it does represent only about a third of the patients undergoing IVF treatment during the study period. Several logistic factors affected group attendance. Individuals who were commuting to their appointments were less likely to attend group sessions than those who were visiting from out of state and staying on or near the military base. In addition, many potential subjects reported to the nursing staff that they felt too stressed or too busy to devote time to anything other than required procedures.

Procedure

Institutional Review Board approval was obtained for this project from both the University of Texas at San Antonio and WHMC. Groups met twice a week for 1.5 hours and were facilitated by either a Psychiatrist, a Clinical Psychologist or both. The group size in this study ranged from 4 to 7 couples. Females who participated in the group attended an average of 3.23 times (range 1-6) and males 3.35 times (range 1-7). During each group session, there was a constant flow of patients in and out of the group based on the timing of their menstrual cycles and treatment schedule. This meant group membership overlapped but was not constant across the cycle. On two occasions, couples who were attending group sessions were dropped from the IVF cycle because of a failure to respond to medications. They were offered the chance of returning for a later cycle, but did not continue in the current group (McNaughton-Cassill, et al., 2000).

GROUPS

The groups used a Cognitive-behavioral format (Beck, 1976). Within this framework, cognitions, or thought patterns, are believed to play a major role in one's evaluation of stressful events and perceived coping resources (Ellis, 1977). Learning to recognize and alter such cognitions has been shown to be an effective means of ameliorating emotional stress in a variety of context (Beck, 1976). Consequently, the facilitators encouraged members to identify their own cognitions regarding their infertility, and to explore the links between their irrational beliefs and expectations and emotional distress in this context. They also introduced techniques for reframing attributions and generating constructive thoughts and solutions for common problems. Alternative solutions to childlessness were also discussed.

Rational and Measures Used to Assess Group Efficacy

Couples completed the questionnaires described below at the beginning of their treatment cycle, and upon the completion of their IVF treatment. A variety of measures were used to assess the efficacy (or effectiveness) of this group. Socioeconomic and infertility background information was collected from all participants completing the survey.

Depression is known to be a key response to stressful life events (Lomranz, Hobfoll, Johnson, Eyal, & Zemach, 1994), and has been associated with infertility in numerous studies (Reed, 2001; Burns, 1993). In this study depression was assessed using the Beck Depression Inventory (BDI), a 21-item test which evaluates depression by asking participants to respond to questions regarding the cognitive, emotional, and physiological aspects of depression. The BDI has been shown to be a reliable measure of depression using a 4-point scale (Beck & Beamsdorfer, 1974).

Another common response to infertility is anxiety (Burns, 1993). Anxiety can be conceptualized both as a stable individual tendency towards anxiety, called trait anxiety, and as an immediate response to a particular situation or time, called state anxiety (Speilberger, 1983). Anxiety was measured using the Beck Anxiety Inventory, a 21-item measure used to assess current symptoms of anxiety (Beck, Epstein, Brown, & Steer, 1988). This measure has been shown to be reliable, and to correlate well with other measures of anxiety and is structured much like the Beck Depression Inventory.

Cognitions of a rigid, inflexible nature, sometimes called irrational beliefs, have been related to the negative appraisal of a number of stressful situations (Alloy & Abramson, 1979; Olinger, Kuiper & Shaw, 1987) and to depression and anxiety (Malouff, Schutte, & McClelland, 1992; Hayslip, Galt, Lopez, & Nation, 1994; McNaughton, Patterson, Smith, & Grant, 1995). Indeed, research suggests the endorsement of irrational beliefs is associated with both state and trait measures of anxiety (Malouff, Schutte, & McClelland, 1992). Irrational beliefs' data were studied using an 11-item scale developed by Alden and Safran (1978). Each item is based on one of the irrational beliefs identified by Ellis (1977). Subjects are asked to indicate how much they agree or disagree with each statement using a 9-point scale that ranges from strong disagreement to strong agreement. This measure has been shown to assess 3 separate factors: dependence on others, over-reactivity to undesirable events and the inability to accept current circumstances (Dubvosky & Smith, 1983).

Optimism is typically defined as the tendency to view the world in a positive light, and to anticipate good outcomes from situations, and is seen as a relatively stable attributional style (Seligman, 1991). Conversely, pessimism, or the opposite attributional style, is defined as the tendency to believe that bad events will last for a long time, have far reaching effects and are one's own fault (Seligman, 1991). The lack of optimism has been shown to contribute to the prediction of depression and diminished life satisfaction (Plomin et al., 1992), and to result in distress in response to physical symptoms (Scheier & Carver, 1987). It has also been shown to predict diminished rates of postpartum depression, to be a risk factor for illness (Peterson, 1988; Cutrona, 1982), and to be related to the use of an active coping style (Scheier & Carver, 1985). Optimism/Pessimism was measured using the Life Orientation Test (LOT) which has been shown to have adequate internal consistency and test-retest reliability (Scheir & Carver, 1985).

Social Support was evaluated using the Social Provisions Scale (SPS) developed by Cutrona & Russell (1987). This self-report scale evaluates six components of social support which include guidance, reliable alliance, reassurance of worth, social integration, attachment, and the opportunity to provide nurturance, and generates a total support score. It has been shown to be a reliable measure which correlates strongly with other measures of social support (Cutrona & Russell, 1987; 1990).

Group Themes

During the course of the group sessions, couples shared their infertility histories and emotional responses to their situation. Such conversations seemed to have a normalizing function, which enabled couples to talk about their problems in an accepting environment. All of the groups were characterized by animated conversations about medical procedures, and ways of managing the logistical challenges of attempting IVF. The bonds formed among the groups were strong, and members often exchanged email and telephone information, and in some cases, reported staying in touch well after the groups ended.

The couples also discussed the stress infertility placed on their marriages, and differences in how men and women experienced this stress. Frequently men stated they did not wish to talk about their feelings as much as their wives did, and some said they felt they had to remain calm and rational to balance their wives stress levels. Wives frequently reported feeling guilty about not being able to conceive or carry a child to term, and expressed the feeling they were letting their spouse down. In some cases they even reported offering the spouse the option of divorce, since they could not "give him a child." Men often reported they coped by focusing on the specifics of the treatment, learning to give their wives shots, and other practical aspects of the process which gave them a sense of control.

Group members also reported feeling jealous and/or inadequate when watching other people with children, attending baby showers or holiday gatherings, or seeing babies or pregnant women in shopping malls or in the media. Several participants even commented on how often babies and children are featured in print and television advertisements. Another topic of interest was the fact friends, family, and co-workers frequently failed to recognize their stress, misunderstood the medical procedures they were undergoing, or expressed disapproval of infertility treatment decisions they had made. Comments from people with children implying having children was stressful, or indicating the childless couple somehow deserved their fate were especially upsetting. Family holiday celebrations were cited as being particularly stressful, since the decision not to go to avoid exposure to children, or unwanted input, often resulted in family discord, and/or feelings of sadness about being left out.

Ethical, religious, and moral issues also entered the conversations as couples discussed their options for achieving parenthood, and the many decisions they had to make. Some reported they received support from their religious beliefs, but others felt conflicted or angry over their inability to conceive a child, and felt this interfered with the strength of their religious convictions. Concern about what to tell family and friends about the use of technology, and how to respond to negative reactions from others also arose. Some members indicated that attendance at support groups such as RESOLVE, or using web-based chat groups helped since it did give them the opportunity to converse with people going through similar process and stressors. Couples also reported distress about what to tell future children about how they were conceived, and worry about how they would handle the prospect of a multiple pregnancy (McNaughton- Cassill et al. 2002).

EFFICACY OF THE GROUPS

Comparisons of those individuals who participated in the groups to those who did not indicated no significant differences in age, income, education level, or the number of previous IVF attempts made. In addition, group members did not differ from non-group members (compared by gender) in any significant ways on measures of irrational beliefs, social support, depression, or anxiety before the groups started, although males who did not attend the group reported less optimism than males who did participate. Pregnancy rates did not differ significantly between the group participants and non-participants.

However, comparisons of males and females own measures before and after IVF treatment told a different story. Those women who had participated in the group sessions were significantly less anxious and depressed than they were initially, but there were no other significant differences in measures of optimism, irrational beliefs, or social support for women. Men who attended the group were actually more optimistic, but also reported more irrational beliefs upon completion of the group.

The relationship between gender and group participation was also evaluated. The results suggested males who attended the group were more optimistic afterwards than either males who did not attend the group, or females in either category. In addition both males and females valued the social support provided by the group, reported that the groups were helpful in dealing with the stress of the IVF procedure, and indicated they thought the group would be useful to others undergoing IVF treatment. Taken together, this data suggests attending the groups did have a positive affect on participants.

DISCUSSION

After attending the group sessions women reported significantly less anxiety and depression, and men who attended the groups were more optimistic. Although the participants in this study were not clinically depressed or anxious, it is clear that participating in the group helped them to manage their emotions while participating in a complicated, anxiety provoking medical procedure spread over a period of three weeks. While it has long been known that infertility can cause anxiety and depression (Domar et al., 1992; Hirsch & Mosher, 1987), most group treatment approaches have involved long-term groups, which include individuals in all stages of treatment, rather than an acute stress management model. The focus of this project was on the acute psychological needs of both men and women undergoing IVF treatment, which differs a great deal from the more traditional long-term, ongoing psychological approaches to chronic mental health problems. In fact, the timing of these groups actually seemed to give couples a chance to seek specific support during a particularly stressful point in their infertility experience, much the way Lamaze groups often function during pregnancy.

We did not find a significant difference in perceived social support between either women or men at the outset of the study, or as a function of group participation, despite the fact members reported the group was useful, and they would recommend it to others. It is not clear whether this is due to the short-term nature of this intervention, or to the fact the measure, which assessed global social support, was not sensitive enough to detect differences resulting from this design. Previous research does suggest that in general women see infertility as a stigma which they feel reluctant to talk about to others, and men frequently report that they do not talk to anyone other than their partners about their infertility (Pengelly, Inglis, & Cudmore, 1995). Future longitudinal studies might do well to assess the degree of social support group members derive from each other, whether they stay in touch following the termination of the group, and whether they do report greater satisfaction with support specific to infertility issues.

The fact that male participants reported slightly more irrationality after group participation is puzzling. Perhaps men attending the group sessions were exposed to aspects of infertility they had not previously considered, thus altering their outlook. It is also possible the instrument used failed to capture the benefits of this specific, structured group intervention. Men who attended the group sessions became more optimistic than either males who did not attend the group, or any of the females. Since optimism is known to be strongly correlated with positive mental and physical health (Seligman, 2000), this finding should be explored further. Perhaps optimism in the face of infertility requires the suspension of realistic or pessimistic assessments of the situation, and so contributes to the small, observed increase in irrationality observed in males.

Fewer males than females were able to participate in the groups, but it is not clear whether this is actually a gender-based difference, or the result of the fact the study was conducted among a military population, many of whom had to travel out of state to participate in the program. Evaluating participation rates in a similar program among a civilian population in a stable geographic area would be of use to clarify this issue. Nevertheless, the fact that the group targeted both females and males is a departure from many other IVF interventions, and the data do indicate that men can derive psychological benefit from such an approach.

The number of group sessions individuals attended did vary, as did the combinations of the three participating therapists. However, the measures of change reported reflect aggregated group measures, and so should actually reveal less change if someone attended fewer sessions, and/or there was variability in how sessions were conducted. Conversely, if group membership indeed had a negative effect on outcome then those members who attended the group the most should have actually contributed to change scores in a negative direction.

It should be noted that group membership in this study did not result in differential pregnancy rates between those who attended the group and those who did not. Although numerous attempts have been made to determine whether stress or psychological factors affect pregnancy rates, the results have been equivocal (Strauss, Hepp, Staeding, & Mettler, 1998;

Csemiczky, G., Landgren, B.M., & Collins, 2000). The fact this intervention did not affect pregnancy rates should not be surprising given this intervention coincided with actual IVF treatment and may well have been too brief to impact the neuroendocrinological effects presumed to mediate a possible stress/pregnancy relationship. Facchinetti, Tarabusi, &Volpe (2002) do suggest that Cognitive-behavioral treatment decreased the cardiovascular and neuroendocrine reactions of women exposed to a stressful task while waiting for assisted reproduction. Domar et al. (2000) and (Tuschen-Cafier, Florin, Drause, & Pook (1999) also suggest the use of Cognitive-behavioral treatment techniques may impact conception rates in infertile women. Consequently, the Cognitive-behavioral techniques employed to assist couples undergoing IVF treatments in this study suggests the use of this practical, time limited approach should be explored further.

This study did not specifically explore couple's responses to failed IVF attempts. Research does suggest that both members of infertile couples, but particularly women, are likely to experience either mild or moderate depression after a failed cycle, and those women without any children are most likely to become depressed (Newton, Hearn, & Yuzpe, 1990). Infertile women have also been shown to have lower self-confidence than fertile women in general, and to show decreased self-esteem after a failed treatment cycle (Hynes, Callan, Terry, & Gallois, 1992). Tracking such trends, and the impact of group participation in this process would be of interest in future studies, particularly in regard to how people who participate in the group handle unsuccessful cycles relative to those who failed to conceive, but were not part of a group.

Participants who attended the group may have derived extra benefit from discussions of alternative ways to resolve infertility issues including the use of a surrogate option, adoption, and the conscious decision to remain childless. Such a result would be consistent with the work of Edelmann, Connolly, and Bartlett, (1994) who demonstrated that some acceptance of infertility was a positive coping strategy, for both men and women. This possibility suggests it might be useful to contact study participants at a much later date, for example 2 years following treatment, to assess how those couples who failed to get pregnant during this IVF cycle were resolving or had resolved their desire to have a child.

Working with couples seeking IVF treatment does result in a number of practical and logistical difficulties in recruiting group participants. Infertility is a complex life stress, superimposed on people's other financial and time constraints. The complexity of the treatments can be prohibitive, and many couples were unable or unwilling to add a therapy group to their stressful schedules. In other cases, one or both members of a couple missed several group sessions. While such differences may be inherent in working with this population, it may also mean the couples in our sample were in fact less stressed than some of the subjects who opted not to participate in the study, and yet still derived benefit from the experience. We plan to evaluate some creative approaches to addressing these issues. Possibilities include developing an on-line chat room or a journaling paradigm in order to determine whether patients with time and geographical restraints could still benefit from specific focused psychological support while undergoing IVF. Certainly Pennebaker's (1991) work on journaling and improved health outcome suggests this might be a fruitful line of inquiry (Stewart et al., 1992).

Although this study was based on a relatively small number of participants, these findings suggest that a brief, cognitively based couples group, offered in conjunction with IVF treatment can be psychologically beneficial to both members of couples experiencing infertility. Both women and men experienced positive emotional changes, and reported the group experience was valuable to them as a means of coping with their infertility. Clearly, further research should be devoted to the study of the most effective and efficient ways to deliver such therapeutic support to the ever-increasing number of couples attempting to use a new, high technology treatment to deal with an age-old problem.

AUTHORS' NOTES

This project was not funded by any external or internal sources.

The opinions and assertions contained herein are the private views of the authors and not to be construed as official or as reflecting the views of the Department of the Army, Department of the Air Force or the Department of Defense.

REFERENCES

Alden, L., & Safran, J. (1978). Irrational beliefs and nonassertive behavior. *Cognitive Therapy and Research 2* (4), 357-364.

Alloy, L.B.,, & Abramson, L.Y. (1979). Judgement of contingency in depressed and nondepressed college students: Sadder but wiser? *Journal of Experimental Psychology: General, 108,* 441-485.

Beck, A.T., & Beamsdorfer, A. (1974). Assessment of depression: the depression inventory. *Pharmacopsychiatry, 7,* 151-69.

Beck, A.T. (1976). *Cognitive Therapy and the Emotional Disorders* New York: International Universities Press.

Berk, A., & Shapiro, J.L. (1984). Some implications of infertility on marital therapy. *Family Therapy, 11,* 37-47.

Beck, A.T., Epstein, N., Brown, G., & Steer, R. (1988). An inventory for measuring clinical anxiety: Psychometric properties. *Journal of Consulting and Clinical Psychology, 56,*(6) 893-897.

Black, R.B., & Greenfield, D.A., (1993). Pregnancy and pregnancy loss after infertility. *Psychological Issues in Infertility,* 4(3), 569-579.

Burns, L.H. (1993). An overview of the Psychology of infertility. *Psychological Issues in Infertility 4*, 433-453.

Burns, L.H., & Covington, S.N. (1999). *Infertility counseling: A comprehensive handbook for clinicians*. New York: Parthenon.

Collins, J.A., Bustillo, M., Visscher, R.D., & Lawrence, L.D. (1995). An estimate of the cost of in vitro fertilization services in the United States in 1995. *Fertility and Sterility, 64*, 538-554.

Connolly, K. J., Edelmann, R.J., Cooke, I.D., & Robson, J. (1992). The impact of infertility on psychological functioning. *Journal of Psychosomatic Research, 36*, 459-468.

Connolly, K.J., Edelmann, R.J., Bartlett, H., Cooke, I.D., Lenton. E., & Pike, S. (1993). An evaluation of counseling for couples undergoing treatment for in-vitro fertilization. *Human Reproduction, 8*, 1132-38.

Csemiczky, G., Landgren, B.M., & Collins, A. (2000). The influence of stress and state anxiety on the outcome of IVF-treatment: psychological and endocrinological assessment of Swedish women entering treatment. *Acta Obstetrics and Gynecology Scandanavia* 79(2), 113-18.

Cutrona, C.E. (1982). Nonpsychotic postpartum depression: a review of recent research. *Clinical Psychology Review, 2*, 487-503.

Cutrona, C.E., & Russell, D. (1987). The provisions of social relationships and adaptation to stress. In W.H. Jones & D. Perlman, (Eds). *Advances in personal relationships (Vol. 1*, pp.37-67). Greenwich, CT:JAI.

Cutrona, C., & Russell, D. (1990). Type of social support and specific stress: Toward a theory of optimal matching In: Sarason B.R., Sarason, I.G., et al. Eds. *Social support: An interactional view. New York NY: John Wiley & Sons,* 319-366.

Daniels, K.R. (1993). Infertility counseling: the need for a psychosocial perspective. *British Journal of Social Work*, 23, 501-515.

Daniluk, J.C. (2001). "If we had it to do over again..." Couple's reflections on their experiences of infertility treatments. *Family Journal,* 9 (2), 122-133.

Domar, A.D., Broome, A., Zuttermeister, P.C., Seibel, M., & Friedman, R. (1992). The prevalence and predictability of depression in infertile women. *Fertility and Sterility. 58* (6), 1158-63.

Domar, A.D., Clapp, D., Slawsby, E., Kesselm, B., Orav, J., & Freizinger, M. (2000). The impact of group psychological interventions on distress in infertile women. *Health Psychology, 9 (6), 568-75.*

Downey, J. (1993). Infertility and the new reproductive technologies. In: Stewart, D.E., & Scotland, N.L. (Eds), et al. *Psychological Aspects of Women's Health Care: The Interface Between Psychiatry and Obstetrics and Gynecology.* Washington, DC, USA: American Psychiatric Press, Inc., 193-206.

Dubvosky, A., & Smith, T.L. (1993). The impact of divorce, perceived parental hostility and family warmth on children's long-term adjustment. *Rocky Mountain Psychological Association.*

Edelmann, R.J., Connolly, K.J., & Bartlett, H. (1994). Coping strategies and psychological adjustment of couples presenting for IVF. *Journal of Psychosomatic Research,* 38 (4), 355-34.

Ellis, A,., & Grieger, R. (1977). *Handbook of Rational-Emotive Therapy.* Englewood Cliffs, N.J.: Prentice Hall.

Facchinetti, F., Tarabusi, M., & Volpe, A. (2004). Cognitive-behavioral treatment decreases cardiovascular and neuroendocrine reaction to stress in women waiting for assisted reproduction. *Psychoneuroendocrinology,* 29 (2), 162-173.

Gerrity, D.A. (2001). A biopsychosocial theory of infertility. *Family Journal, Alexandria,* 9, (2), 151-158.

Golombok, S. (1992). Psychological functioning in infertility patients. *Human Reproduction* 7, 208-212.

Greenfeld, D.A. (1997). Does psychological support and counseling reduce the stress experienced by couples involved in assisted reproductive technology. *Journal of Assisted Reproductive Genetics*, 14,4, 186-188.

Greil, A.L. (1991). *Infertile couples in contemporary America.* New Brunswick, New Jersey: Rutgers University Press.

Hayslip, B.l., Galt. C., Lopez, F., & Nation, P. (1994). Irrational beliefs and depression symptoms among younger and older adults: A cross-sectional comparison. *International Journal of Human Development, 88(* 4). 307- 326.

Hirsch, A.M., & Hirsch, S.M. (1995). The long-term psychosocial effects of infertility. *JOGNN Clinical Studies,* July/August, 517-522.

Hirsch, M.B., & Mosher, W.D. (1987). Characteristics of infertile women in the United States and their use of infertility services. *Fertility & Sterility* , *47*, 618-25.

Hsu, Y., & Kuo, B. (2002). *Journal of Nursing Research, 10* (4), 291-302.

Hynes, G.L. Callan, V.J., Terry, D.J., & Gallois, C. (1992). *British Journal of Medical Psychology 65,* 269-278.

Lalos, A., Lalos, O., Jacobsson, L., & vonSchoultz, B. (1985). Psychological reactions to the medicl investigation and surgical treatment of infertility. *Gynecologic and Obstetric Investigation, 20,* 209-217.

Lomranz, J., Hobfoll, S.E., Johnson, R., Eyal, N., & Zemach, M. (1994). A nation's response to attack: Israelis' depressive reactions to the Gulf War. *Journal of Traumatic Stress, 7* (1), 59-73.

Malouff, J., Schutte N., & McClelland, T. (1992). Examination of the relationship between irrational beliefs and state anxiety. *Personality and Individual Differences 9 (4),* 451-456.

McQuillan, J., Greil, A.L., White, L., & Jacob, M.C. (2003). Frustrated fertility: Infertility and psychological distress among women, *Journal of Marriage and Family* 65, 1007-1018.

McNaughton, M.E., Patterson, T.L., Smith, T.S., & Grant, I. (1995). The relationship among stress, locus of control irrational beliefs, social support, and health in Alzheimer's Disease Caregivers. *The Journal of Nervous and* Mental Disease, 183 (2), 78-85.

McNaughton-Cassill, M.E., Bostwick, J.M., Vanscoy, S.E., Arthur, N.J., Hickman T.N., Robinson, R.D., & Neal, G.S. (2000). Development of brief stress management support groups for couples undergoing in vitro fertilization treatment. *Fertility and Sterility 74 (1),* 87-93.

McNaughton-Cassill, M.E., Bostwick, J.M., Arthur, N.J., Robinson, R.D., &Neal, G.S. (2002). Efficacy of Brief Couples Support Groups Developed to Manage the Stress of In Vitro Fertilization Treatment. *Mayo Clinic Proceedings, 77,* 1060-1066.

Meyers, M., Weinshel, M., Scharf, C., Kezur, D., Diamond, R., & Rait, D.S. (1995). An infertility primer for family therapists: ii. Working with couples who struggle with infertility. *Family Process, 34,* 231-240.

Newton, C.R., Hearn, M.T., & Yuzpe, A.A. (1990). Psychological assessment and follow-up after in vitro fertilization: assessing the impact of failure. *Fertility and Sterility 54 (5),* 879-886.

Olinger, L.J., Kuiper, N.A., & Shaw, B.F. (1987). Dysfunctional attitudes and stressful life events: An interactive model of depression. *Cognitive Therapy and Research, 11* (1), 25-40.

Pengelly, P., Inglis, M., & Cudmore, L. (1995). Infertility Couple's experiences and the use of counseling in treatment centres. *Psychodynamic Counselling1*.4, 507-524.

Pennebaker, J.W. (1991). The effects of traumatic disclosure on physical and mental health: the values of writing and talking about upsetting events. *International Journal of Emergency Mental Health 1,* 9-20.

Peterson, C., Seligman, M.E.P., & Vallient, G. (1988). Pessimistic explanatory style as a risk factor for physical illness: A 35-year longitudinal study. *Journal of Personality and Social Psychology* 55, 23-27.

Peterson, B.D., Newton, C.R. & Rosen, K.H. (2003). Examining congruence between partners' perceived infertility-related stress and its relationship to marital adjustment and depression in infertile couples. *Family Process, 42* (1), 59-71.

Plomin, R., Scheier, M.F., Bergeman, C.S., Pedersen, N.L. Nesselroade, J.R., & McClearn, G.E., (1992). Optimism, pessimism and mental health: a twin/adoption analysis. *Personality and. Individual Differences, 15,* 921-929.

Raval, H., Slade, P., Buck, P., & Lieberman, B.E. (1987). The impact of infertility on emotions and the marital and sexual relationship. *Journal of Reproductive and Infertility Psychology, 5,* 221-34.

Reed, S.A. (2001). Medical and psychological aspects of infertility and assisted reproductive technology or the primary care provider. *Military Medicine,* 166 (11), 1018-1022.

Redd, W.H., Silberfarb, P.M., Andersen, B.L., Andrykowski, M.A., Bovbjerg, D.H., ,Burish, T.G., Carpenter, P.J., Cleeland, C., Dolgin, M., Levy, S.M. et al. (1991). Physiologic and psychobehavioral research in oncology. *Cancer,* 67, (3) 813-22.

Rosenthal, M.B., & Goldfarb J. (1997). Infertility and assisted reproductive technology: an update for mental health professionals. *Harvard Review of Psychiatry, 5,* 169-172.

Scheier, M. F., & Carver, C.S. (1985). Optimism, coping, and health: assessment and implications of generalized outcome expectancies. *Health Psychology, 4 (3),* 219-247.

Scheier, M.F., & Carver, C.S. (1987). Dispositional optimism and physical well-being: The influence of generalized outcome expectancies on health. *Journal of Personality, 55,* 169-210.

Seligman, M.E.P. (1991). *Learned Optimism.* New York: Alfred A. Knopf.

Seligman, M.E.P. (2002) *Authentic happiness*: Using the new positive psychology to realize your potential for lasting fulfillment. New York, NY, US: Free Press.

Speilberger C. (1983). *Manual to the State-Trait Anxiety Inventory*. Consulting Psychologists Press: Palo Alto, CA,

Speroff, L, Glass, R.H,, & Kase, N.G. (1999). *Clinical Gynecological Endocrinology Infertility*. Baltimore, MD Williams & Wilkins.

Spiegel, D., Draemer, H.C., Bloom, J.R., & Gottheil, E. (1989). Effect of psychosocial treatment on survival of patients with metastatic breast cancer. *Lancet ii* 888-891.

Stewart, D.E., Boydell, K., McCarthy, K,. Swerdlyk, S, , ,Redmond, C. & ,Cohrs, W.. (1992). A prospective study of the effectiveness of brief professionally-led support groups for infertility patients. *International Journal of Psychological Medicine* 22(1), 173-82.

Strauss, B., Hepp, U., Staeding, G., & Mettler, L. (1988). Psychological characteristics of infertile couples: can they predict pregnancy and treatment persistence. *Journal of Community Applications and Social Psychology 8,* 289-301.

Sultan, K.M.,Grifo,, J.A., & Rosenwaks, Z. (1995). The infertile couple. *Ambulatory Gynecology,* Nichols, D.H., & Sweeney, B. (eds). Philadelphia, PA:.Lippincott Company.

Tuschen-Caffier, B., Florin, I., Krause, W., & Pook, M. (1999). Cognitive–behavioral therapy for idiopathic infertile couples. *Psychotherapy and Psychosomatics 68,* 15-21.

Ulbric, P.M., Coyle, A.T., & Llabre, M.M. (1990). Involuntary childlessness and marital adjustment: His and hers. *Journal of Sex & Marital Therapy* 16(3), 147.

PSYCHOLOGICAL ADJUSTMENT OF SHORT INTERVAL FOLLOW-UP MAMMOGRAPHY- A FRENCH STUDY ABOUT 129 PATIENTS

B. Barreau[1], S. Tastet[2], A. Hubert[3]

[1] Department of Radiology, Institut Bergonié, Regional Cancer Center, 229 cours de l'Argonne, 33076 Bordeaux Cedex, France Email: beatrice.barreau@wanadoo.fr

[2] Laboratoire de Psychologie EA 526, Université Victor Segalen Bordeaux 2, 3 ter place de la Victoire, 33076 Bordeaux Cedex, France

[3] Centre National de la Recherche Scientifique (UMR 6578), Adaptabilité biologique et culturelle, Université de la Méditerranée, 27 boulevard Jean Moulin, 13385 Marseille Cedex, France

ABSTRACT

The objective is to investigate perceptions and perceived stress experience by women undergoing mammographic follow-up for probably benign lesions (registered category 3 according to Breast Imaging-Reporting And Data System of the American College of Radiology).

A near prospective study is carried out on women with diagnosed "probably benign" breast abnormalities. It is a multicentric study realised from March 1st to December 2002. The survey is performed at the first follow-up mammography and included questions about perceptions and perceived stress related to the follow-up experience. The response is analysed with chi-square test. One hundred twenty nine women (33-80 years) answered the questionnaire. All women are satisfied with reception. The mammographies are painful (56 cases). The time seemed too long during the follow up (24 cases), they are anxious (49 cases). Quality of life is affected (52 cases). Professional and social perturbations are not frequent (10 cases). Speaking about it with relatives is frequent (100 cases), but patients are not satisfied about it (33 cases). Medical information is appreciated (113 cases) but not satisfactory (38 cases). The median of the stress scale is 5. There are two peaks, one at 2 (19 cases), the second at 5 (28 cases). "Low-stressed" women could have a coping avoidance strategy. "High-stressed" women would use a helplessness-hopelessness strategy.

Women report a good informative medical support and a right comprehension of the short follow-up mammography. They are reassured by the medical care, but the evaluation of the stress level is high, probably due to the uncertainty of the diagnosis.

INTRODUCTION

The way "probably benign" mammograms and their follow-up are experienced by the patients has rarely been the subject of psychological investigations. It appears important however, to consider this theme empirically so as to evaluate quantitatively and qualitatively the way this type of clinical surveillance if felt by the women, so as to evaluate the stress level experienced at first examination. This would enable us to give better and more specific medical information, better adapted and more efficient, as specified in our French law on patient information of March 4th, 2002 [1].

POPULATION AND METHODS

This explorative and near prospective study was carried out from March to December 2002. The multicentered study involved two Cancer Prevention Centres, 3 specialised radiology centres and 2 neighbourhood radiology establishments. The questionnaire and accompanying letter were given at the end of the consultation to women having had a follow-up mammogram after the discovery of a probably benign anomaly (registered category 3 according to Breast Imaging Reporting and Data System) for which a close follow-up was advised [2-6]. The study started after the first follow-up consultation, i.e. the second mammogram. The women were invited to fill out the questionnaire right after consultation or could fill it out later and mail it (stamped envelope provided). The clinicians had to fill a medical form giving sociobiographic data such as age, profession, hormonal status (menopause, Hormonal Replacement Therapy) family or personal antecedents (previous microbiopsies, breast biopsies or breast cancer). The questionnaire was strictly anonymous.

The patient's questionnaires included 40 items with Likert type questions (4 possible answers positive, rather positive, rather negative, negative) as well as open questions. These cover the experience and feeling of stress as perceived by the patients and induced by the follow-up procedure. An analogical scale of perceived stress ranging from 0 (weak) to 10 (strong) completed the protocol. The answers were analysed through usual statistical methods of Chi 2 or Fisher test, according to the sample size.

RESULTS

The total number of women included was 129, with no refusals. The population came from various centres:

- two Cancer Prevention Centres (Centre Régional de Lutte Contre le Cancer): Bordeaux (30 women) and Nancy (2 women);
- three specialised radiology centres: Biarritz (61 women), La Rochelle (14 women) and Lyon (11 women);
- two neighbourhood radiology establishments: Cognac (6 women) and La Rochefoucauld (6 women).

Their age vary between 33 and 80, the average being 54 ($\sigma = 9.9$). Sixty-three were employed professionals (qualified as "active"), 36 were unemployed, 31 retired and 5 were seeking employment (qualified as "inactive") but 30 did not answer this question (NA).

Sixty-three were menopaused, 31 had HRT (NA = 35). In their medical past, 17 had undergone a breast biopsy, the results were malign for 7, benign for 10 and 4 of them qualified as atypical epithelial hyperplasia or lobular carcinoma in situ.

Thirty had family antecedents: 1 or 2 relatives of first or second degree with breast cancer.

QUESTIONNAIRE RESULTS

Qualitative Description of Each Item for the Whole Population

Mammogram Experience

Item 1: Were you happy with the welcome?
Positive = 122, rather positive = 7 (n = 129; 100%).

Item 2: Were you awed by the examination room?
Positive = 4, rather positive = 4 (n = 8; 6.2%) / Rather negative = 23, negative = 96 (n = 119; 93.8%); NA = 2.

Item 3: Was the breast compression painful?
Positive = 17, rather positive = 39 (n = 56; 43.8%) / Rather negative = 25, negative = 47 (n = 72; 56.2%); NA = 1.

Item 4: Did the examination seem long?
Positive = 4, rather positive = 10 (n=14; 10.9%) / Rather negative = 26, negative = 88 (n = 114; 89.1%); NA = 5.

Item 5: Did you appreciate the technician's explanations during the exam?
Positive = 97, rather positive = 21 (n = 118; 96.7%) / Rather negative = 2, negative = 2 (n = 4; 3.3%); NA = 7.

Item 6: What further explanations would you have wished for?
Open item: 15 patients answered (Bordeaux 6, Biarritz 2, Lyon 3, La Rochefoucauld 4). These answers will be analysed in the discussion.

Time Interval Between the Two Follow-Up Mammograms
Item7: Did the time interval between the two mammograms seem long?
Positive = 13, rather positive = 11 (n = 24; 19%) / Rather negative = 25, negative = 77 (n = 102; 81%); NA = 3.

The Waiting Experience Between the 2 Mammograms
Item 8: Did this wait worry you?
Positive = 17, rather positive = 31 (n = 49; 38.4%) / Rather negative = 28, negative = 49 (n = 77; 61.6%); NA = 3.

Item 9: Have you had trouble eating?
Positive = 4, rather positive = 2 (n = 6; 4.7%) / Rather negative = 13, negative = 109 (n = 122; 95.3%); NA = 1.

Item 10: Have you had trouble sleeping?
Positive = 17, rather positive = 16 (n = 33; 26.2%) / Rather negative = 12, negative = 81 (n = 93; 73.8%); NA = 3.

Item 11: Did you loose weight?
Positive = 4, rather positive = 5 (n = 9; 5.5%) / Rather negative = 9, negative = 110 (n = 119; 94.5%); NA = 1.

Item 12: Did your breasts hurt more than they usually do?
Positive = 10, rather positive = 14 (n = 24; 19.2%) / Rather negative = 15, negative = 86 (n = 101; 80.8%); NA = 4.

Did having had a control mammogram

Item 13: affect your professional life?
Positive = 3, rather positive = 2 (n = 5; 4.1%) / Rather negative = 8, negative = 103 (n = 111; 95.9%); NA = 13.

Item 14: affect your social life ?
Positive = 0, rather positive = 5 (n = 5; 3.9%) / Rather negative = 15, negative = 106 (n = 121; 96.1%); NA = 3.

Item 15: did you talk about it with people close to you
Positive = 92, rather positive = 8 (n = 100; 80.7%) / Rather negative = 6, negative = 18 (n = 24; 19.3%); NA = 5.

Item 16; to whom ?
Parents: husband = 41, sister = 16, daughter = 10, children = 16, mother = 9, sister in law = 2, brother (brother medical doctor) = 1.
Other: friends = 30, colleagues = 9.

Did having talked about it

Item 17: reassure you? Positive = 53 / negative = 20.

Item 18: worry you? Positive = 5 / negative = 43.

Item 19: satisfy you? Positive = 25 / negative = 33.

Item 20: did not matter? Positive = 38 / negative = 35.

Information on Follow-Up

Item 21: who informed you?
The radiologist = 74, gynaecologist = 13, doctor = 15, surgeon = 2; NA = 25.

Item 22: was this information satisfactory?
Positive = 98, rather positive = 15 (n = 113; 96.6%) / Rather negative = 3, negative = 1 (n = 4; 3.4%); NA = 12.

Did the given information

Item 23: reassure you? Positive = 82 / Negative = 15.

Item 24: worry you? Positive = 11 / Negative = 45.

Item 25: satisfy you? Positive = 30 / Negative = 38.

Item 26: did not matter? Positive = 4 / Negative = 49.

Item 27: What other information would you have wished for?
5 answers which will be treated in the discussion.
Your doctor has just told you that there is no change on your mammogram.

Are you

Item 28: reassure you? Positive = 94 / Negative = 8.

Item 29: worry you? Positive = 4 / Negative = 46.

Item 30: satisfy you? Positive = 29 / Negative = 34.

Item 31: did not matter? Positive = 2 / Negative = 48.
Your doctor has just told you that the following-up continues.
Are you

Item 32: reassure you? Positive = 61 / Negative = 18.

Item 33: worry you? Positive = 17 / Negative = 43.

Item 34: satisfy you? Positive = 29 / Negative = 36.

Item 35: did not matter? Positive = 1 / Negative = 49.

What has worried you most

Item 36: the mammogram = 4.

Item 37: the result = 89.

Item 38: both = 11.

Item 39: other = 5.

Perceived Stress Scale

Item 40: If you had to evaluate the intensity of your stress over this follow–up, giving a number between 0 (weak) and 10 (high), which number would you choose? (Table 1).

Table 1: Perceived stress

Stress level	Number of patients
0	5
1	4
2	19
3	16
4	5
5	28
6	9
7	12
8	9
8.5	3
10	8

NA: 11

The median is at 5 ($\sigma = 2.6$). Considering the whole population 59 women evaluate perceived stress at 5 or over.

Regrouping the stress level scale from:

- 0 to 2, the percentage of women with no or very little stress is of 23.8% (28 cases),

- 3 to 5, the percentage of women with medium stress is of 41.5% (49 cases),
- 6 to 7, the percentage of women with heavy stress is of 17.7% (21 cases).

Above or equal to 8, the percentage of women totally stressed is of 17% (20 cases).

The level of perceived stress according to the different centers where the follow-up took place:

	CPC	SRC	NRE
0 – 2	5	21	2
3 – 5	12	32	5
6 – 7	7	13	1
8 – 10	5	12	3

Cancer Prevention Centres (CPC), specialised radiology centres (SRC) and neighbourhood radiology establishments (NRE).

The perceived stress level is not significantly different in women consulting in cancer centres or clinics (p = 0.46).

The number of women having had the mammogram performed in neighbourhood specialised centres is too small to be statistically analysed (n = 11).

The perceived stress level is not significantly different between menopaused (M) and non-menopaused women (NM) (p = 0.022).

	M	NM
0 – 2	12	15
3 – 5	19	28
6 – 7	7	14
8 – 10	13	6

The perceived stress level is not significantly different between active (A) and non-active women (NA) (p = 0.03).

	A	NA
0 – 2	16	7
3 – 5	20	19
6 – 7	10	8
8 – 10	17	2

The perceived stress level is not significantly different between women having had previous biopsies (B) and those without antecedents of biopsies (NB) (p = 0.62).

	B	**NB**
0 – 2	7	20
3 – 5	7	39
6 – 7	1	17
8 – 10	2	17

The perceived stress level of women with breast cancer antecedents (C) and without previous breast cancer (NC) will not be analysed since the sample is too small.

	C	NC
0 – 2	1	27
3 – 5	2	46
6 – 7	3	18
8 – 10	0	19

We notice that the women with previous breast cancer do not have a very high level on the scale of perceived stress. They are normally statistically distributed on the perceived stress scores.

The perceived stress level is not significantly different between women with previous family breast cancer (F) and women without family antecedents of breast cancer (WF) ($p = 0.28$, regrouping the scores ≤ 5).

	F	WF
0 – 2	8	20
3 – 5	14	35
6 – 7	4	17
8 – 10	4	16

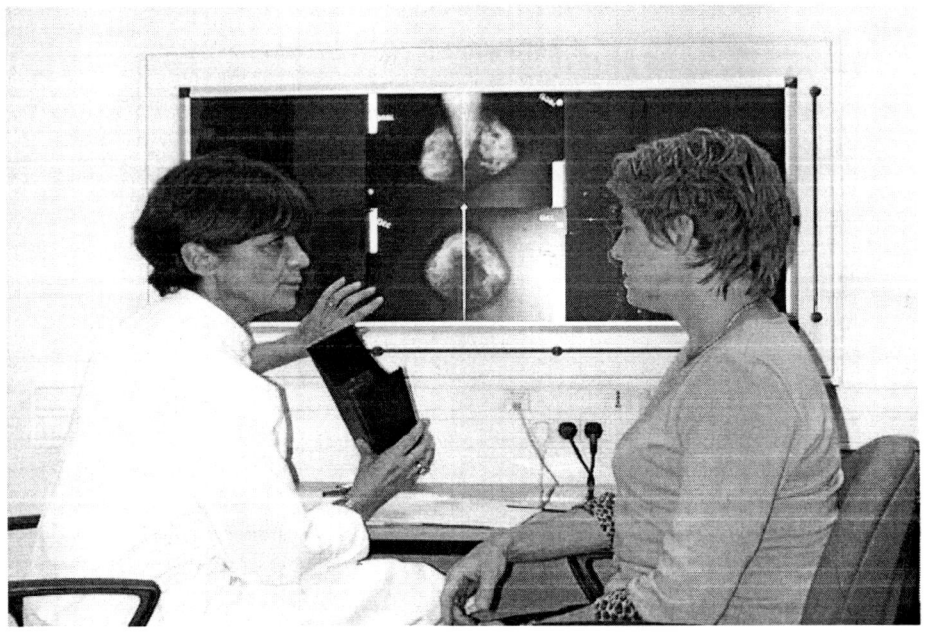

Photo : I. Brault

Fig. 1: Doctor–patient communication

DISCUSSION THE MAMMOGRAM EXPERIENCE

Admission into the radiology centre by a secretary is always satisfying (item 1: 100% positive or rather positive). This first contact with the centre's personnel is decisive, as it will condition the feasibility and quality of the mammography investigation. The patient must be relaxed while the examination is being carried out. Admission concerns entering the building, meeting with the personnel and entering the area where the mammogram will be taken. This is illustrated by a patient's comment: *"I think that the quality of admission, at least for the first exam, is essential, so that the anxiety, while waiting for the verdict, should not be amplified by an unpleasant admission. It was not the case, it was perfect"*.

This study confirms results from our first serie (50 cases) [7].

The women are but rarely awed by the examination area (item 2: 6.2% positive or rather positive). They have had this experience already when they had their first mammogram showing the anomaly. We could consider this as an "apprenticeship" facilitating the patient's adaptation. One woman gave the following comment: *"the room is too small, for me it increases the impressions, before and after"* (perceived stress 5).

In our previous study on the psychological experience of percutaneous macrobiopsy, the women were more awed, probably because the machines were more voluminous, although the space and material were common to both examinations [8]. We did show that it depended on the type of procedure. Only the women having had this type of procedure had a pre-positioning in this examination room. It could be explained as a phenomenon of habituation, erasing the "fear of the unknown".

The second factor explaining the acceptability is the care the radiologist takes to make this examination area agreeable and friendly. Particularly in private structures, the walls are decorated with poster of medical information or paintings and posters of "calming" landscapes of mountain, forests or sea.

The information given by the various media (women's magazines, television and radio) plays a central part in the vulgarisation of the act. Thanks to this intensive and progressive in-culturation, the individual experience and the perceptions of what these women experience are modified.

Mammal compression (item 3) is painful for 56 women (yes = 43.8%). During a preceding retrospective study on the psychological experience of percutaneaous mammal biopsy carried out on 99 cases, 38.8% of the women considered the compression painful. This compression for this type of biopsy lasts around 45 minutes (for a mammogram the compression lasts less than one minute). If we take the most recent published data, the pain felt during a mammography is studied essentially on series of organised detection. Keemers-Gels showed on a retrospective series of 945 women, that 689 (72.5%) describe mammography as painful [9]. The statistically significant factors influencing pain are breast sensitivity, antecedents of breast cancer in the family, education level, previous mammogram experience, anxiety, breast tenderness during the days preceding the exam, the "gentleness" of technicians. Hafsfund shows that pain during the mammography (170 women aged 40-69) is correlated to the anxiety level of the woman [10].

An American study on organised detection mentions a discomfort described by 933 of the women out of 1 800 (52%) [11]. It points to the part played by the technician in pain perceived during the mammography.

This act, generally well accepted can become disagreeable [12]. In a satisfaction study on care quality, Loken shows that it is mammography and double contrast examinations which provoke the most pain [13]. But, further than a plate, the mammogram is a particular experience. The woman is undressed, places her breast on a Plexiglas's tablet. The breast is pulled by the technician and compressed by an automatic compressor [14]. The absence of communication between the technician and the woman can induce pain felt as intolerable [15]. Thus, a study shows that an emotional and informative approach (psychological help) can lower the pain level felt by the patient [16]. This importance of informative help can be illustrated by the words of this woman, noted during an anthropological study on organised cancer detection [17]. *"The first time, it hurt very much, he was a brute, did not say anything, took my breast, pulled it, but pulled it, and I found myself stuck under this machine. It worse than the dentist...and this man... a bloc of ice, there is no other word, a bloc of ice...The next time, I went somewhere else, the people were very nice, the technician very gentle, she explained very well, and I felt no pain at all, she did not compress so quickly, which is why it didn't hurt".*

The exam seems long (item 4) to 14 women (positive 4, rather positive 10; 10.9%). The examination time varies between 2 and 20 minutes. It depends on the technique being used [numerical mammograms (Biarritz), analogical (other centres)]. There is no significative difference between the two techniques. This type of image can require complementary plates (magnifications for microcalcifications), and in certain cases an echogram of the breast.

The information given by the technician (item 5) during the examination is appreciated by 118 of the women (positive 97; rather positive 21; 96.7%); this exchange allows at the same time to communicate the necessary enquiries on the technique, acquire the good positioning and decreases anxiety by changing the woman's point of attention. It is always well appreciated, in a preceding study on percutaneous biopsies the woman had answered positively/rather positive [8]. This interactive communication allows them to "manage the fear". Loken shows that lack of information and the patient's distrust during the exam are factors of dissatisfaction [18].

Item 6 is an open question containing additional information desired during the taking of the mammogram. It illustrates several situations.

By their answers, 7 women corroborate the fact that the information is sufficient: *"Not"* *"It's OK"*; *"None"*. *"It was complete"*. *"All has been well explained"*. *"None, everything was perfectly well explained"*. *"Everything was perfect"*. *"The explanations were sufficient"*.

Eight women said they did not have the necessary information (or no information): *"I find that the breast examination by repeated mammograms during the same exam (several plates) is sometimes disagreeable and would benefit from previous information. Breast surveillance is very positive and encouraging"*. *"The technician did not explain anything. It is probably due to his youth. He will gain assurance. The first time it was an older man, very nice, who talked and explained what was to be done"*. This woman's mammogram was done by a trainee in a Cancer Centre. The centres taking in trainee technicians should follow them more closely. However, the women do accept the necessity to train health staff.

In their behaviour, the women are always interdependent and altruistic: *"I was not explained anything, only the positions to take. For me personally, none since I had had several mammograms taken and I know the principle, but perhaps some other women would wish to have technical explanations?"*.

When women have mammograms taken regularly, the technical aspect, by its frequent repetition can become a ritual. A different sequence in the exam can lead to questioning and fear. *"When there are plates taken over again on a breast, it would be nice to tell the patient the reasons why these plates are being taken once more, because this causes deep worry"*.

Some women would like to know the result from the very beginning of the exam: *"The technician at first did not give any explanation on what was going on. But the doctor, for the echogram, said there was an anomaly but he wasn't sufficiently reassuring"*.

Giving additional information is a real problem, because it involves an individual level. Some patients do not which for too much information. If the physician or the technician gives them more than they wish, it can increase their anxiety. Conversely, certain patients will wish as much information as possible, and the fact of not informing enough makes them anxious [19, 20]. It appears then that it is the clinician, thanks to his experience and the training he has, who has to measure the degree of information he gives (always respecting the law concerning patient information) and what the woman wishes, and this wish is rarely spoken.

TIME INTERVAL BETWEEN TWO FOLLOW-UP MAMMOGRAMS

The delay between mammograms seems long (item 7) to 24% of the women. This percentage remains low. Some ask for closer controls so as to decrease their anxiety: *"The control mammogram was done after 6 months. Couldn't she have done it before ? Six months is a long time!..."*. This wish of reducing the time interval is mostly motivated by a state of anxiety and anguish lasting all through the interval. A clear and precise information explaining the reason for the delay should be given so as to show the women that 6 months are necessary, medically speaking, but also that one understands and knows that waiting this long is difficult experience.

LIVING THROUGH THE INTERVAL

This waiting (item 8) worries 38.4% of the women. The amplitude of the worry varies in time and individually, it is therefore difficult to measure. It appears however, to evolve by cycles. It is greater during the days preceding the control. The expression of this comment is significative: *"The fortnight before the exam, sleep problems and worry by "flashes" during the day. Stress, and particularly the day of the exam, the waiting, the result"*.

Eating problems (item 9) are rare: 4.7%.

Sleeping problems (item 10) are more frequent: 26.2%.

Weight loss (item 11) is rare: 7%. Incurrent pathologies should be considered (flu, dental work).

Breast pain (item 12) is more frequent for 19.2% of the cases.

Consequences on professional activity and social activity is weak 4.1% (item 13) and 3.9% (item 14).

The social support is very present in this population since 80.7% of the women talked about it to close friends or family (item 15).

Family (item 16) is the first group of communication since 75 women shared this situation with their family. These exchanges are generally between female relatives since the words "father", "son", "brother in law" were never pronounced. One woman answered that she had talked about it with her brother but specified that he was a doctor (she was talking to the professional, not the brother). These verbal exchanges are thus limited to the women, excepting the husband who is informed (41 women). Friends and colleagues are part of the social web, 30 talked about it to friends, and 9 to their colleagues.

The fact of talking about it reassured (item 17) 53 of them, worried (item 18) 5, satisfied (item 19) 25, and had no importance (item 20) for 38.

This shows that in quantitative terms, social support is important, but qualitatively the women are not satisfied by this support (33 unsatisfied); these results allow us to say that the women have persons to whom they can talk about their situation (in quantitative terms: on how many persons can I count?) they are therefore satisfied by their social surroundings. However, in qualitative terms (that is "the psychological resource defining an individual's perception as to the quality of his social relations), they do not appear to be satisfied by the social support of their families, friends or colleagues [21].

INFORMATION ON CONTROL

The information on control (item 21) is given by the radiologist at the end of the examination. They then consult their doctor (gynaecologist, generalist); 74 women remembered that the information was given to them by the radiologist; The others remembered the information given by their generalist (15 cases) or gynaecologist (13 cases) and by the surgeon when surgical advice was asked for by their doctor (2 cases). Lindfors shows that the fact of talking about it with a doctor of different specialisations does not influence perceived stress [22]. The women however are very attentive to the clinician's opinion. *"The radiologist's attitude determines the way in which the patient will live the time interval until the next control. The two most important people involved in the patient's wait are the gynaecologist and radiologist. Family and friends are there to give support but the most important part remains that of the professionals who determine the information".*

The information is considered satisfactory by 96.6% of the women. We illustrate this by the comments of Mrs. R...: *"The answers to my questions satisfied us and reassured us. I leave feeling confident. Thank you".*

Eighty-two women are reassured (item 23), 11 are worried (item 24) 30 are satisfied (item 25), 4 women don't care (item 26). The informative medical support is felt as "good" in quantitative terms, but insufficient in proof of diagnosis (38 unsatisfied). These mammographical anomalies are said "probably benign" (Predictive Positive Value: $\leq 2\%$) [2, 4]. The results are given in terms of probability. The women have difficulties to understand this type of language where each human is defined as a mathematical equation; there is an inadequacy between the human person and the statistical subject-unit.

No complement of information (item 27) is asked for: *"I had all the explanations I wanted". "None". "Nothing to say"*. A time for listening is asked of the gynaecologist: *"He made it very ordinary and laughed at my worry. It was perhaps ordinary for him, but not for me. I would have wished him to give me an appointment, and a serious explanation as soon as I wished it"*. One woman has difficulties speaking French (the questionnaire is read and filled by an assistant) she tells of *"problems of relation with the radiologist"*

But does not explicit what it was about.

One woman did not comment this question, but at the end of the questionnaire writes: *"I prefer having an MRI taken than 2 mammograms, it's more precise"*. She did not ask the radiologist for information on controls, which could show an insufficient communication. The irradiation inherent to the mammography raises questions for the women. *"Before having had an explanations given by the doctor, my fear was that the frequency of mammograms would produce a high irradiation of the breasts, which could induce a cancer, going to a specialised center is reassuring"*.

The women use this space for free comments to mention their gratitude and their confidence towards the health professionals: *"It is good to have mammograms regularly taken, in a good context, with competent and serious people, it secures and reassures the patient". "I was not stressed because the staff is very nice and gives you confidence; After the exam; I leave reassured"*.

After this first control, the radiologist informs the patient on the absence of change in the mammograms. 94 women are reassured (item 28), 29 are satisfied (item 30) and 2 don't care (item 31). The number of unsatisfied is 34, which is high. It could be explained by the uncertainty of the diagnosis (the radiologist continues the controls) or to a difficulty to face the situation.

The controls are carried on. The doctor informs the patient. She is reassured (item 32) in 61 cases, worried (item 33) in 17 cases, satisfied (item 34) in 29 cases and always implicated (item 35). The high rate of dissatisfaction is probably due to the problem of uncertainty.

The ones satisfied and/or reassured express it by comments: *"I am satisfied with the prevention and control follow-ups". "I am reassured to be followed-up". "I am not worried, I find the control normal". "I was very satisfied with the doctor's explanations, he took time to explain and to reassure me". "The follow-up seems to me normal, as far as the preventive mammogram shows something. Completely reassured by the exam and particularly by full confidence in the radiologist"*.

They are rarely worried by the mammogram (item 36): 4 cases, often by the result of that exam (item 37): 89 cases, or by both (item 38): 11 cases. Other possibilities arise (item 39) but they are not explicit. Mrs C. expresses it in the free comments: *"The result is primordial for me"*. Comments express the women's worries about breast cancer. The word is not written, but suggested: "serious or not". One uses the word "illness" to talk about her mammogram presenting an anomaly "probably benign". *"At the beginning of the "illness" yes. Now I trust you"*.

Lindfors in a study of controls of mammal anomalies, shows that the anxiety level in not affected by the perception of the possibility of detecting a malign anomaly [22]. Contrary to this study, the women of our series show anxiety over the results. The concept of "pernicious disease" is not expressed, but implied [17]. *"When all goes well, all is too good". "Cancer does not hurt, if taken in time we can be cured, however".* Cancer remains a dreadful curse in our sample of women's popular beliefs.

STRESS SCALE OF PERCEIVED STRESS

Perceived stress level (item 40) goes from 0 (weak) to 10 (high). The histogram presents two peak levels. The first at 2: women qualified as "very little stress" (n = 19) and the second at 5: women "with average stress" (n = 28). The median 5 shows a stress going from average to high. In the results the regrouping of the scale level confirms this. These results could be influenced by the patient's various adjustment strategies. Lazarus and Folkman define adjustment or coping strategies as "cognitive and behavioural efforts, constantly changing, aimed at managing external and/or internal specific requirements perceived as menacing or overflowing a person's resources" [23].

Thus, on the one hand, the patients saying that they are "very" or "totally" stressed could easily preferentially use a strategy centered on emotion, called powerlessness–despair strategy [24]. Overwhelmed with despair and with little hope, they think they cannot do anything and therefore have a high level of perceived stress.

On the other hand, patients mentioning "low stress" could face controls and follow-up with a strategy called "avoidance strategy", with the aim of regulating emotions by distracting the subject from the source of stress. They avoid thinking about anything concerning control and follow-up and do all they can not to think about it. Thus their perceived stress score is low. All the patients with a low stress score do not have avoidance strategies. As one patient says: *"Honestly, I am not very worried with the follow-up, even if it was cancer; one has to face and trust the doctors, thus the capacity of managing and control the worry about surgery".*

Some trust themselves as well as the medical team. These patients are not overwhelmed by anxiety and distress: they establish a problem centred strategy with the aim at managing the impact of the situation by acting directly on it, through search for information, planning or direct action [23]. This type of strategy, aiming at solving the problem and affording the subject the impression of controlling the situation would reduce her emotional distress and her perceived stress level.

We note that the perceived stress level is not significantly different between the different types of care offered (cancer centres or clinics). The very low number of women followed-up by neighbourhood centres does not allow statistical comparison.

Perceived stress level is studied in function of hormonal status, since menopause is a particular phase of life and implies modification of identity. These transformations are at the same time biological, psychological and sociocultural [25]. Kaufert established cultural stereotypes to classify perceptions and representations [26]. In France, these representations are negative, neutral or both, and positive [27]. It would be interesting to find if this change of status will induce a different level of perceived stress. Regrouping the levels of perceived stress, only 13 are "completely" stressed in the group of menopaused women. However, there is no significative difference between the two populations "menopaused and not menopaused".

We also wondered if the level of perceived stress could be different according to different professional status (active versus non-active). Professional status as a variable does not allow to discriminate between the two. There is no significative difference between the "active" and the "non-active". Work does not influence the level of perceived stress and does not allow the patient to "think about something else" during her activity.

The level of perceived stress has also been examined in function of antecedents of breast biopsy. The fact of having undergone one could provoke a lowering of "self esteem" and a modification of the body pattern, which could influence stress level. In our society, based on "appearance", aesthetic norms are defined and powerful.

Having had a surgery experience could perhaps lower perceived stress by an habituation phenomenon. The stress level is not significantly different between women having had a benign biopsy and women without biopsy antecedents.

Stress level has also been considered in function of antecedents of breast cancer. Breast cancer is always considered as a mortal process, it remains an area of suffering in its material and immaterial dimensions. Surgery, radiotherapy and particularly chemotherapy are considered as therapeutic violence [28, 29]. This type of experience could induce a higher stress level. The scope of this population with breast cancer is low (since Agence Nationale d'Accréditation et d'Évaluation de la Santé recommendations [3] suggest an histological control of the anomalies. The women controlled had refused this proposition). This sample of 7 patients does not allow statistical evaluation. Their perceived stress shows a statistically normal distribution. This could be explained by the medicalisation of these patients or by a process of psychological adjustment about which we should remain prudent considering the small number in the sample.

Stress perceived has been also considered in function of family antecedents (non-genetic) of breast cancer. By the frequency of this illness, the women know or have shared the experience of a parent with cancer [30]. This can be illustrated by the comments of Mrs. C. (stress level 2): *"I think I managed this ordeal well, my daughter having died of breast cancer. I was with her throughout her illness which lasted seven years"*.

This experience builds sense and could modify the score of perceived stress. In our study the scores are not significantly different in both populations. It appears that the same women who have already experienced this situation with a parent, react like the other patients facing the illness or suspicion of illness for the first time. We can therefore assume that there is no "apprenticeship" of the illness and that each woman, even if they are familiar with the procedures by having accompanied a patient, does not manage any better than the others. It is therefore important to single out these women and to consider them completely as patients and not as patients having already had this experience.

CONCLUSION

This quantitative and qualitative study allowed us to examine in detail the experience of perceived stress by the women advised to submit to a close mammographical follow-up. The medical information support appears sufficient both qualitatively and quantitatively. The women are reassured buy this ritualised medical take over. The "human and technical" capabilities through interactive communication of health professionals warrant the acceptability of this surveillance. If common comprehension of the procedure is satisfactory, the lack of proof in the "probably benign" diagnosis induces a high stress level. In our western culture, biological life is at the heart of all health projects, the normative shift towards a "perfect" health, a "total" security presents a prescriptive character which induces inadequacy by the incertitude of the diagnosis.

AKNOWLEDGMENTS

I would like to thank Veronique Picot of the Statistics Department of the Institut Bergonié, and all the clinicians who have helped me to recruit patients for the study: Isabelle Brault in Lyon, José-Marie Gillet and Mourad Fawzi in Biarritz, Isabelle Audigey in Cognac, Thierry Pousse in La Rochefoucauld, Dominique Imbert in la Rochelle and Joseph Stinès in Nancy.

REFERENCES

[1] Loi n° 2002-2003 du 4 mars 2002 relative aux droits des malades et à la qualité du système de santé. *Journal Officiel*, 5 mars 2002.

[2] American College of Radiology. *Breast Imaging Reporting and Data System* (BI-RADS). Reston, VA: American College of Radiology, 1993-2003.

[3] ANAES (Agence Nationale d'Accréditation et d'Évaluation de la Santé). *Conduite à tenir diagnostique devant une image mammographique infraclinique anormale.* Paris, 1998.

[4] Varas X, Leborgne JH, Leborgne F, Mezzera J, Jaumandreu S, Leborgne F. Revisiting the mammographic follow-up of BI-RADS category 3 lesions. *Am J Roentgenol* 2002;691-5.

[5] Sickles EA. Probably benign breast lesions: when should follow-up be recommended and what is the optimal follow-up protocol? *Radiology* 1999;213:11-4.

[6] Barreau B, Stinès J. Conduite à tenir dans les lésions mammaires de catégorie BI-RADS 3 de la classification ACR. *J Le Sein* 2002;12:102-11.

[7] Barreau B, Tastet S, Stinès J, et al. Une étude exploratoire sur le vécu psychologique des femmes lors de la surveillance des anomalies mammographiques probablement bénignes. A propos de 50 cas. *Gynécol Obstét Fertil* 2003;31:629-38.

[8] Barreau B, Tastet S, Dilhuydy JM, Picot V, Henriquès C, Gilles R, et al. Le vécu psychologique des prélèvements percutanés mammaires: à propos de 99 cas. *J Le Sein* 2002;12:157-67.

[9] Keemers-Gels ME, Groenendijk RP, van den Heuvel JH, Boetes C, Peer PG, Wobbes TH. Pain experienced by women attending breast cancer screening. *Breast Cancer Res Treat* 2000;60:235-40.

[10] Hafslund B. Mammography and the experience of pain and anxiety. *Radiography* 2000;6: 269–72.

[11] Dullum JR, Lewis EC, Mayer JA. Rates and correlates of discomfort associated with mammography. *Radiology* 2000;214:547–52.

[12] Poulos A, Rickard M. Compression in mammography and the perception of discomfort. *Australas Radiol* 1997;41:247–52.

[13] Loken K, Steine S, Laerum E. Patient satisfaction and quality of care at four diagnostic imaging procedures: mammography, double–contrast barium enema, abdominal ultrasonography and vaginal ultrasonography. *Eur Radiol* 1999;9:1459–63.

[14] Netter E, Marelle P, Quinquis J, Séradour B, Stinès J. L'incidence oblique externe: nouvelle technique. *J Le Sein* 2000;10:165–70.

[15] Barreau B. La communication vers les femmes et leur information. In: Séradour B, ed. *Le dépistage des cancers du sein. Un enjeu de santé publique.* Paris: Springer, 2003: 139–151.

[16] Caruso A, Efficace F, Parrila A, Angelone L, Ferranti F, Grandinetti ML. Pain and anxiety related to mammography in breast cancer patients. Psychological evaluation in an experimental study. *Radiol Med* (Torino) 2001;102:335–9.

[17] Barreau B, Hubert A, Dilhuydy MH, Séradour B, Hoarau H, Dilhuydy JM. L'anthropologie comme interface entre la santé publique et les femmes invitées au dépistage de masse organisé des cancers du sein: étude qualitative des facteurs déclenchants, des contraintes et des variations bio–culturelles de la participation (les Bouches–du–Rhône et la Charente). In: *Société Française de Psycho–Oncologie (Association Psychologie et Cancers), Laboratoire Aventis,* éds. La Psycho–Oncologie pour le malade, son entourage, son équipe soignante. Les acteurs de la Psycho–Oncologie (travaux du XVIème Congrès de la SFPO). Paris: Éditions Dyk; 2001: p. 114–20.

[18] Loken K, Steine S, Laerum E. Mammography: influence of departmental practice and women's characteristics on patient satisfaction: comparison of six departments in Norway. *Qual Health Care* 1998;7:136–141.

[19] Sarason IG, Sarason BR, Shearin EN. Social support as an individual difference variable: its stability, origins and relational aspects. *J Pers Soc Psychol* 1986;50:845–855.

[20] Sarason BR, Sarason IG, Pierce GR. *Social support: an interactional view.* Wiley: New–York; 1990.

[21] Gentry WD, Kobasa SC. Social and Psychological ressources mediating stress–illness relationships in humans. In: Gentry WD, ed. *Handbook of behavioral medicine.* New–York: Guilford; 1984: p. 87–113.

[22] Lindfors KK, O'Connor J, Acredolo CR, Liston SE. Short interval follow–up mammography versus immediate core biopsy of benign breast lesions: assessment of patient stress. *AJR Am J Roentgenol* 1998;17:55–8.

[23] Lazarus RS, Folkman S. *Stress, coping and adaptation.* New York: Springer, 1984.

[24] Watson M, Law M, Santos M, Greer S, Baruchn J, Bliss J. The Mini–Mac: further development of the Mental Adjustment to Cancer Scale. *J Psychosoc Oncol* 1994;12:33–46.

[25] Barreau B, Fontanges M, Dilhuydy MH, Séradour B, Hoarau H, Hubert A. Approche anthropologique des représentations de la ménopause dans une population de femmes invitées au dépistage de masse organisé des cancers du sein (Bouches du Rhône et Charente). *Contracept Fertil Sex* 2000;28:309–16.

[26] Kaufert P. Anthropology and the menopause: the development of a theorical framework. *Maturitas* 1982;4:181–93.

[27] Delanoë D. Les représentations de la ménopause. Un enjeu des rapports sociaux d'âge et de sexe. *Contracept Fertil Sex* 1997;25:853–60.

[28] Lebeer G. La violence thérapeutique. *Sciences Sociales et Santé* 1997;15:69–95.

[29] Tastet S. *Approche biopsychosociale des cancers du sein: stratégies d'ajustement et immunocompétence. Une étude semi–prospective d'une cohorte de 85 patientes traitement [thèse]*. Université Victor Segalen Bordeaux 2, 2001: p. 1–388.

[30] Barreau B, Séradour B, Dilhuydy MH, Hubert A. L'anthropologie comme approche des faits bioculturels dans le dépistage de masse organisé des cancers du sein: une étude de terrain dans les Bouches–du–Rhône. *La Lettre du Sénologue* 2000; n° 7:27–30.

INDEX

A

Achenbach Child Behavior Checklist, 3, 18
acute stress, 43, 46, 58, 79, 120, 122, 127, 154, 157, 163, 168, 195
anxiety, vii, ix, 1, 2, 3, 4, 5, 6, 9, 10, 40, 43, 44, 47, 48, 56, 102, 104, 107, 109, 110, 114, 115, 116, 117, 118, 120, 121, 123, 164, 169, 174, 178, 179, 181, 182, 187, 188, 189, 191, 192, 194, 197, 198, 199, 211, 212, 213, 215, 216, 219
attentional problems, 126
attrition, 20, 98, 108, 119

B

bacterial invasions, 75
behavior problems, 2, 3, 4, 6, 8, 9, 10, 11, 12, 13, 14, 15, 16, 17, 22, 23, 25, 26, 28, 29, 30, 31, 33, 34, 35, 36, 37, 39, 41
birth defect, vii, 1, 2, 41
blood biochemistry, 63
blood pressure, 43, 44, 45, 46, 47, 48, 49, 50, 51, 52, 53, 54, 55, 56, 57, 58, 59, 64, 65, 83, 97, 100, 158, 177
blood viscosity, 44
body image, viii, 173, 174
breast abnormalities, 203

C

cardiac disorder, vii, 1, 2, 36
cardiac severity, 5, 6
child adjustment, vii, 1, 2, 6, 11, 15, 18, 26, 28, 33
child intelligence, vii, 1, 2, 16, 29
child language development, vii, 1

cognitive-behavioral techniques, 188, 196
coronary artery atherosclerosis, 43
coronary artery disease, 43, 44, 45, 46, 53, 54, 55, 162, 170
cortisol levels, viii, 118, 122, 125, 126, 127, 134, 135, 136, 137, 155
cortisol response, viii, 125, 126, 127, 131, 137, 139, 155
cytokines, viii, 63, 69, 70, 74, 75, 143, 144, 145, 146, 147, 148, 149, 150, 151, 152, 153, 154, 155, 157, 158, 159, 160, 161, 162, 163, 164, 165, 166, 168, 169, 170, 171, 172

D

depression, vii, ix, 5, 6, 7, 9, 10, 16, 40, 43, 44, 47, 48, 56, 104, 109, 114, 118, 120, 121, 122, 143, 144, 154, 159, 160, 162, 163, 164, 165, 166, 167, 168, 169, 170, 174, 177, 178, 179, 181, 184, 187, 188, 189, 191, 192, 193, 194, 196, 197, 198, 199, 200
disease processes, viii, 143, 144, 147, 154, 159, 162
divorce, ix, 187, 189, 193, 198
dizziness, 126

E

earthquakes, 43, 46
emotional development of children, 1
emotional distress, 106, 107, 126, 138, 170, 181, 189, 192, 216
erythrocytes, 69
exercise, 5, 43, 45, 46, 47, 50, 58, 69, 72, 76, 77, 78, 154, 155, 156, 158, 164, 166, 167, 169, 170, 172

F

family social support, vii, 1, 10
family stress, 8, 40
fatigue, 3, 126, 129, 130, 134, 136, 137, 143, 144, 154, 159, 160, 161, 162, 163, 164, 165, 166, 168, 170, 171, 175, 180
fear, vii, 1, 68, 104, 211, 212, 213, 215
feelings, viii, 4, 15, 35, 47, 103, 104, 105, 108, 109, 118, 120, 129, 130, 131, 132, 159, 173, 174, 188, 193, 194
females, 5, 16, 18, 20, 127, 128, 188, 191, 194, 195
femininity, viii, 173, 174

G

gender, 3, 4, 5, 6, 21, 47, 84, 88, 90, 92, 93, 140, 151, 169, 174, 194, 195
generalized estimating equations (GEE), 86, 89, 91, 92, 93, 94, 95
Global Severity Index (GSI), 129, 134, 135
glutamine, 71, 72, 73, 76, 77, 79
group therapy, viii, 164, 187, 190

H

headache, 126, 129, 130, 134, 136
health outcomes, viii, 83, 98, 143, 144, 159
heart rate, viii, 43, 44, 46, 47, 50, 58, 64, 65, 81, 82, 154, 155, 165, 169, 170, 174, 177
hypertension, 44, 45, 47, 48, 49, 50, 51, 52, 53, 55, 56, 57, 58, 59, 82, 169

I

immunosuppression, 71, 72, 73
infertility, viii, 173, 174, 175, 176, 177, 178, 179, 180, 181, 182, 183, 184, 185, 187, 188, 189, 190, 192, 193, 195, 196, 197, 198, 199, 200, 201
inflammatory bowel disease, 75, 78
intelligence, 11, 12, 13, 16, 19, 29, 33, 39, 40, 41
interventions, viii, ix, 37, 61, 144, 163, 165, 180, 181, 185, 187, 195, 198
irrationality, 195
ischemia, 43, 46, 47, 55, 77, 78
IVF cycle, 188, 190, 191, 196

K

Kruskall-Wallis Test, 134

L

language disorders, 13, 14, 30, 38
leukocytes, 63, 64, 65, 68, 69, 70, 72, 73, 74, 75, 77, 145, 146, 157, 158

M

males, 5, 16, 20, 58, 72, 162, 173, 174, 188, 191, 194, 195
mammography, ix, 203, 204, 211, 212, 215, 219
MANOVA, 116, 117, 118, 131, 132
masculinity, viii, 173, 174
maternal age, 103, 108, 112
maternal smoking, 81, 82, 83, 86, 95, 97, 98, 99
medication, ix, 6, 128, 130, 151, 159, 163, 187
mental stress, vii, viii, 43, 44, 45, 46, 47, 49, 50, 51, 52, 53, 55, 57, 58, 59, 69, 77, 125, 126, 127, 128, 129, 130, 131, 132, 134, 135, 136, 137, 138, 154, 155, 170, 171
military hospital, ix, 187
myocardial infarction, vii, 43, 44, 45, 46, 54, 55

N

neck, 126, 127, 129, 130, 134, 136
neutrophils, 62, 63, 64, 65, 68, 69, 70, 71, 72, 73, 77, 78, 79, 146

P

Parental Locus of Control Scale, 8
parental stress, vii, 1, 2, 8, 14, 16, 36, 37, 104
Parenting Stress Index, 6, 8, 16, 17, 21, 22, 24, 25, 27, 28, 29, 30, 37
parents, vii, viii, 1, 2, 3, 5, 6, 7, 8, 9, 10, 11, 12, 13, 14, 15, 16, 17, 18, 20, 21, 22, 23, 25, 26, 29, 30, 31, 32, 33, 34, 35, 36, 37, 40, 41, 52, 78, 83, 84, 103, 104, 105, 107, 108, 110, 111, 112, 113, 114, 115, 119, 120, 121
perceived stress, ix, 34, 57, 109, 164, 203, 204, 208, 209, 210, 211, 214, 216, 217
perceptions, ix, 2, 3, 8, 11, 15, 16, 21, 28, 29, 33, 39, 41, 203, 211, 216

personality, vii, 40, 43, 47, 48, 58, 119, 121, 167, 180
personality factors, vii, 43, 48, 180
physical capacity, 4, 5, 6, 164
physical fitness, 5
platelet function, 44
preterm infants, viii, 103, 104, 107, 108, 110, 111, 112, 114, 117, 118, 119, 120, 121

R

red cell haemodynamics, 63
relationship difficulties, ix, 187
relax-control condition, viii, 125, 126
ROS production, 70, 75

S

SCL-90, 129, 138, 139
self-esteem, viii, 10, 173, 174, 176, 196
serotonin, 152, 159
sexual activities, ix, 187
social support, 2, 8, 9, 10, 11, 14, 15, 17, 18, 21, 23, 26, 28, 31, 35, 36, 37, 38, 39, 40, 41, 42, 47, 103, 104, 108, 114, 122, 175, 193, 194, 195, 198, 199, 214

socioeconomic status, 3, 20, 23, 39, 42, 103, 108, 190
speech, 13, 14, 30, 33, 38, 155, 156, 157
stressors, 46, 49, 50, 56, 63, 65, 69, 70, 85, 126, 129, 135, 137, 138, 154, 155, 157, 162, 194
sudden life stressors, 43
surgery, ix, 2, 3, 6, 7, 12, 15, 31, 32, 38, 41, 122, 187, 216, 217
survival rate, 1, 190

T

tryptophan, 159

V

vasoconstriction, 44, 47

W

Wechsler Preschool and Primary Scale of Intelligence, 19, 30, 42
Whiplash Associated Disorder (WAD), v, viii, 125, 126, 127, 130, 131, 132, 133, 134, 135, 136, 137, 138

QP
82.2
.S8
S855

```
QP          Stress and health.
82.2
.S8
S855
2004
                                      46614
$79.00
```

DATE			

SOUTH UNIVERSITY
709 MALL BLVD.
SAVANNAH, GA 31406

BAKER & TAYLOR

SOUTH UNIVERSITY
709 MALL BLVD.
SAVANNAH, GA 31406